EAS® SPORTS NUTRITION REVIEW

The latest research on performance nutrition

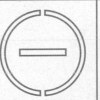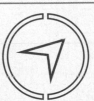

IMPORTANT NOTICE

Consult your physician or health care provider before commencing any new exercise, nutrition or supplementation program, particularly if you use prescription or over-the-counter medicines, or you are being treated by a health care provider for any chronic or medical condition. No representations are made about the result you may achieve from following the programs; as every individual is unique, there are no typical results you can expect from the following exercise, nutrition and supplementation recommendations.

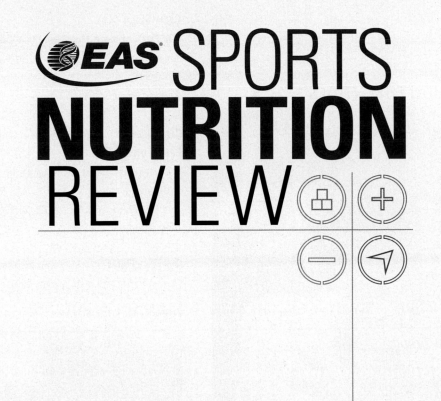

CONTENTS

PART ONE:
NUTRITION ESSENTIALS

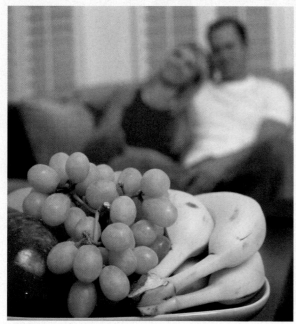

PART TWO:
WEIGHT LOSS AND WEIGHT
MANAGEMENT

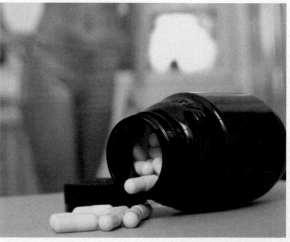

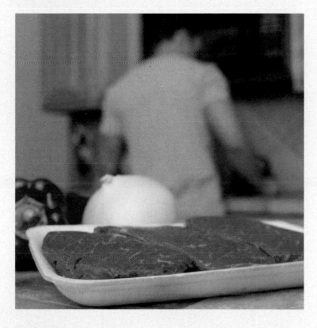

PREFACE

On behalf of the technical staff and experienced team at EAS, we are proud to present our first edition of the EAS *Sports Nutrition Review*. Since 1997, we've published a regular edition of the EAS *Sports Supplement Review*, which was devoted to the field of nutritional supplements, and provided the latest research on how to use nutritional supplements as part of your nutrition and training program. Although this book was valuable, we found it only targeted a small niche of our wide consumer audience. With our first edition of the *Sports Nutrition Review*, we hope to reach a much broader audience who is looking for accurate, up-to-date information on nutrition and exercise. The *Sports Nutrition Review* was developed to provide you with the most current and scientifically based information pertinent to nutrition and exercise as they are today.

The amount and depth of research on nutrition and exercise relative to sports performance has matured and expanded over the past 10 years. We have discovered that nutrition has a huge impact on sports and exercise performance and even the best training regimens can be thwarted by poor eating habits and bad nutrition. Without sound nutrition advice and implementation, it is virtually impossible for most people, especially for the athlete undergoing intense workouts, to achieve and excel at their goals. At the same time, any diet without an exercise plan in place is also not sufficient. The combination of diet, exercise, rest and hydration, with appropriate timing for all, is essential to achieve optimal health.

Even though research in sports nutrition has grown significantly over the past decade, the rise of obesity and associated health-related conditions among Americans has also grown at an alarming rate. Part of the problem is that with so much conflicting information out there, many individuals are unsure of a proper course of action to take. After all, you can spend years floundering and never improve your health and performance without sound nutrition and exercise knowledge. But, through knowledge, you can achieve your goals. Our mission with this book is to give you the tools you need to take charge of your health. Whether you are looking to shed extra weight, increase muscle mass or tone, improve athletic performance or a combination, the contents of the *Sports Nutrition Review* will help you achieve your goals.

Jim Heidenreich
Vice President—Marketing and Publisher
EAS

INTRODUCTION

The field of sports nutrition is constantly changing as new research is conducted, but in order to build upon this valuable knowledge, it helps to know the basics. Part One of the *Sports Nutrition Review* covers just that—nutrition basics. In Chapter 1, you'll have the chance to learn exactly what protein, carbohydrates and fat are, and how they work in your body. You build upon this knowledge in Chapter 2, where you'll learn about vitamins and minerals. Chapter 3 discusses a very elementary, but incredibly important topic: hydration. Chapter 4 analyzes the current USDA Food Guide Pyramid and provides a balanced nutrition alternative, while Chapter 5 gives you a chance to take everything you've just learned, put it together and create balanced, healthy meals when you're on the go, plus make meal-replacement drinks and ready-to-drink nutrition shakes into your healthy eating program.

In Part Two, we build upon the knowledge you have learned in Part One to create customized, balanced nutrition plans for fat loss and muscle growth. You'll also learn which nutritional supplements may help you take your fat loss and muscle growth to the next level. Part Three of the *Sports Nutrition Review* focuses on performance- and sport-specific nutrition and training. In Chapter 10, you'll learn how timing your intake of specific nutrients may improve your workouts. Chapter 11 explains how proper recovery is essential to better performance, improved health and injury prevention. Learn how to set goals you can achieve in Chapter 12, and find out which cardio and weight-training programs will enhance your balanced nutrition plan in Chapter 13 and Chapter 14.

The key to a lean, healthy physique involves careful planning, goal-setting, proper nutrition and consistent workouts, while nutritional supplements can help take your program to the next level. The *Sports Nutrition Review* addresses all of these important areas with the hope it will be your guide to building *your* best body ever.

ACKNOWLEDGEMENTS

The EAS *Sports Nutrition Review* could not have been created without our talented team of writers and experts. They are each experts in their respective fields, and their love for fitness and nutrition and the desire to teach others about it shows through in each and every chapter. In addition to talented writers, our team of editors worked tirelessly, day in and day out—many thanks to Cameran Erny, Ryan Mattingly and Amelia Rau Mattingly for their attention to detail, patience and good humor. And thank you to Chelsea Vurciaga, who volunteered to take on one of the most tedious jobs of all—researching, compiling and formatting all of the scientific references. In addition laying out this book in record time, our top-notch creative team of Silke Reuthlinger and Brian Harvat conceptualized the contemporary design scheme. Thank you to Todd Langley, Rick Souders, Stephen Shern and Jay Rusovich for providing the colorful photos that grace each page and to Matt Green, our production intern. Finally, thank you to Christine Steele. Not only did she start this project from scratch, but she has an incredible eye for noticing any out-of-place scientific fact, quoting the statistics (off the top of her head) from any scientific study, and finding whatever scientific references we needed at a moment's notice.

Gretchen Ferraro, M.A.

CONTRIBUTORS

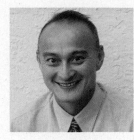

Jose Antonio, Ph.D., earned his doctorate at the University of Texas Southwestern Medical Center in Dallas. He is an original founder and the president of the International Society of Sports Nutrition (**www.sportsnutritionsociety.org**), a non-profit academic society dedicated to the dissemination of unbiased sports nutrition and supplementation information. He is a Fellow of the American College of Sports Medicine and a certified strength and conditioning specialist (C.S.C.S.). Currently, he teaches at Florida International University in Miami and is the editor-in-chief of STRONG Research magazine (**www.strong-research.com**).

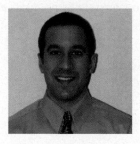

Ash Batheja, M.P.T., C.S.C.S., obtained a master's degree in physical therapy and has contributed his expertise to numerous areas of the training and nutritional landscape. In addition to working full time as a physical therapist, Ash has performed nutritional and supplementation research and has taught biomechanics at Creighton University. He has also authored dozens of articles and written textbook chapters, consulted for nutritional supplement manufacturers and has conducted presentations on supplementation at popular events across the country. Much of his involvement in a wide array of athletic interests stems from his lifelong pursuit of fitness, the dedication to which has allowed him to become a national champion power lifter.

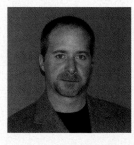

Brian Deeds, Senior Manager of Corporate Training and Organization Development at EAS, has over 10 years of experience in the field of training and training development, more than four of which have been with EAS. He is certified to offer a wide array of globally-recognized training systems. He is an internationally accomplished speaker and his training materials have been translated into several languages for use around the globe. Brian specializes in making difficult topics easy to understand and is able to emulate this unique style in his writing. These attributes have lent themselves well to the needs of his audience in the performance nutrition industry.

Kelly James-Enger escaped from the law in 1997, but don't worry—she's no fugitive. Since then, the former attorney's work has appeared in more than 45 national magazines including *Energy for Women, Muscle Media, Redbook, Self, Health* and *Continental*. She specializes in health, fitness and nutrition subjects and is a frequent speaker at events throughout the country. Kelly is also the author of *Ready, Aim, Specialize! Create Your own Writing Specialty and Make More Money* (The Writer Books, 2003) and the novels, *Did You Get the Vibe?* (Strapless, 2003) and *White Bikini Panties* (Strapless, 2004.) Visit **www.kellyjamesenger.com** for more information about her.

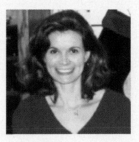

Gretchen Ferraro, M.A., is Editor-in-Chief of *Energy for Women* magazine, Executive Editor of *Muscle Media* magazine and Director of Publishing and Education at EAS, Inc. She was instrumental in the launch of *Energy for Women* magazine in 2001 and has helped edit a number of books, including Bill Phillips' bestseller *Body-for-LIFE* and the fourth issue of EAS' *Sports Supplement Review*. She received her master's degree in journalism from the University of Colorado-Boulder and she has written and edited for a number of magazines, including *Cooking Light, Glamour* and *Travel & Leisure Golf*.

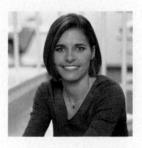

Matt Fitzgerald coaches runners and triathletes and is an All-American triathlete himself. He has authored *Triathlete Magazine's Complete Triathlon Book* and the forthcoming *Runner's World Guide to Cross-Training*. Matt has also written for *Muscle Media* magazine.

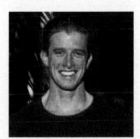

Victoria L. Freeman, Ph.D., has explored many aspects of health and fitness through her work as a freelance writer and editor in Denver, Colo. She has written for publications like *Energy for Women, Muscle Media, Delicious Living, REAL, Adolescence* and *Women's Edition* magazines. She is also a wellness coach and has authored a book chapter on exercise adherence for *Behavioral Medicine and Women* (Guilford Press, 1998). As a former competitive bodybuilder and power lifter, as well as completing graduate work in sports medicine, Victoria believes optimism, sound nutrition and a healthy lifestyle are our most powerful tools for creating health.

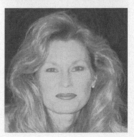

CONTRIBUTORS

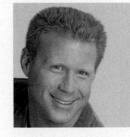

Brett Hall, R.D., is a nutrition and food science graduate from UC-Berkeley. A registered dietitian with 16 years of experience, he has worked as a sports nutrition specialist and consultant for various nutritional supplement companies. As a freelance writer, his goal is to cut through the complex scientific clutter surrounding nutrition, providing people with the proper tools to make healthier decisions. He is a regular contributor to *Muscle Media* and writes its monthly Feature Supplement and Sports Supplement Review columns.

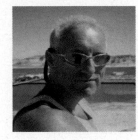

Charles Staley, B.Sc., M.S.S., moves with remarkable ease from coaching athletes in 22 different sports to helping the millions of people who bust their butts in the gym every day. With his behind-the-scenes knowledge of what makes the greatest athletes in the world reach Olympic conditioning, he is able to craft strength-training and fat-loss programs that adjust to you (something that most programs and coaches don't take into consideration). Whether you are a 108-pound, bikini-clad goddess looking to "tone" or a 300-pound lineman looking for that extra rep on your bench press, you've come to the right guy. Charles has written for *Muscle Media* and *Energy for Women* magazine.

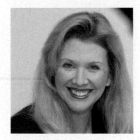

Christine Steele, Ph.D., is Director of Science and Quality at EAS, Inc. She heads the EAS Science Advisory Board for development of safe and efficacious nutritional products. Steele is the liaison between the diverse Science Advisory Board members and the EAS research and development team for coordinating and implementing their mutual goals into science-based, quality products. She has a Ph.D. in nutrition from Cornell University, as well as a master's degree in food science from Cornell University and a bachelor's of science degree from Purdue University. Steele holds memberships in numerous industry organizations, including the leading organizations in quality (ASQ), food science (IFT), clinical research (ACRP) and exercise science (ACSM, NSCA). She is certified as a strength and conditioning specialist (C.S.C.S.) through the National Strength & Conditioning Association and as a certified health & fitness instructor (HFI) through the American College of Sports Medicine.

Jeffery R. Stout, Ph.D., holds a B.S. in exercise science from Concordia University, a master's in exercise science and a Ph.D. in exercise physiology from the University of Nebraska. He is a Fellow of the American College of Sports Medicine (FACSM) and a certified strength and conditioning specialist (C.S.C.S.). Dr. Stout has peer-reviewed scientific publications in journals such as *Medicine and Science in Sports and Exercise* and *Journal of Applied Physiology* and has also made television appearances on CNN and The Discovery Channel. He has co-authored two books, *Supplements for Strength-Power Athletes* and *Supplements for Endurance Athletes* (Human Kinetics, 2002), as well as co-edited and contributed to the *Sports Supplement Encyclopedia* (Nutricia, 2002) and *Sports Supplements* (Lippincott Williams and Wilkins, 2001). He will be publishing his fifth book in 2004 entitled *Fit Kids-for-Life: A Parents Guide to Optimal Nutrition and Training for Young Athletes* (Basic Health Media).

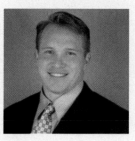

Hale Deniz-Venturi, M.S.,ATC/L,R.D.,L.D., has over 16 years experience in private practice, consulting and clinical work in various health care, sports nutrition, athletics, fitness, corporate health and clinical research settings acting as a registered dietitian, certified athletic trainer and exercise consultant. She has worked with numerous clients developing educational materials, group programs and translating technical research findings into practical applications for clients and the public. Hale is currently an instructor of clinical nutrition with emphasis on active lifestyle and sports nutrition at Rush University. She provides her expertise to assist with the American Dietetic Association's approved dietetic internship at Rush-Presbyterian-St. Luke's Medical Center in Chicago.

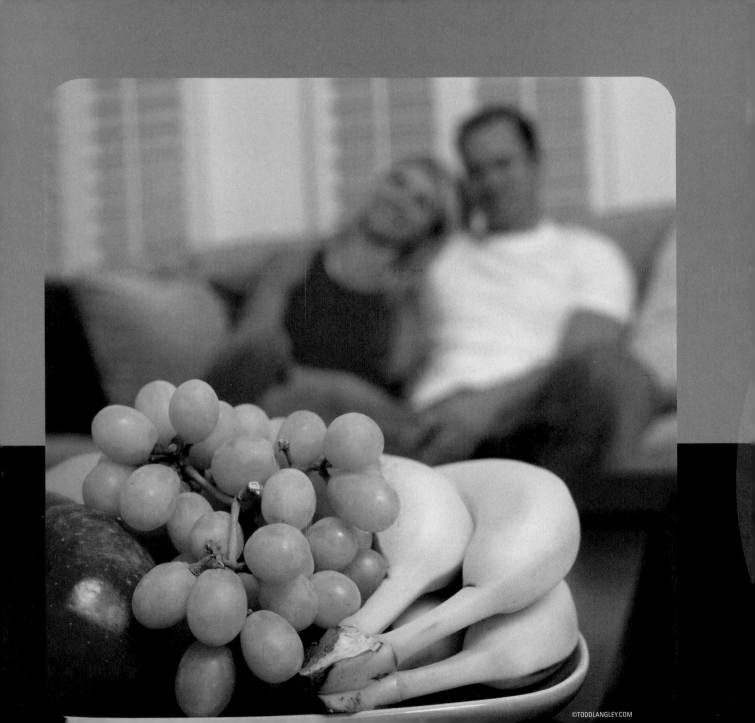

NUTRITION
BASICS

part one

1 UNDERSTANDING MACRONUTRIENTS
Carbohydrates, Protein and Fat
By Julie Upton, R.D.

CARBOHYDRATES—YOUR MUSCLES' PRIMARY ENERGY SOURCE

During exercise, your muscles need a continuous supply of energy from carbohydrates, proteins and fats that are in the muscle, liver and blood stream. The intensity and duration of the activity determine the predominance of which macronutrient is burned, but carbohydrates are the primary source of energy for muscles, as well as all of your body's main tissues.

Almost all dietary carbohydrates come from plant sources, with the exception of lactose, which is found in milk. Carbohydrates are made of carbon, hydrogen and oxygen through a process in plants that absorbs energy from the sun and converts it to carbohydrates that the plant uses for energy and stores within itself. When we eat these plants, we, in turn, are eating carbohydrates.

Carbohydrates are the only source of energy that the brain and central nervous system use. It is thought that the brain and central nervous system need about 130 grams (or 10 tablespoons) of glucose a day.[1] Our muscles also need a steady supply of carbohydrates, in the basic form of glucose, to contract. Carbohydrates also help spare muscle protein from being used as energy and to metabolize fat efficiently, some carbohydrate is needed. Carbohydrate-rich foods supply beneficial fiber to your diet that neither protein nor fat provide. The minimum amount of carbohydrates needed daily to prevent a deficiency is the Recommended Dietary Allowance of 130 grams of carbohydrates daily with an intake of 20 grams to 35 grams of fiber per day.[1]

Types of Carbohydrates

Carbohydrates are classified or named by their chemical structure. **Mono**saccharides are single unit carbohydrates; **di**saccharides are two monosaccharides linked together; and **poly**saccharides are carbohydrates with multiple single unit sugar molecules linked together to form one long-chain carbohydrate. Generally, most experts refer to carbohydrates as either simple, meaning one or two unit molecules, or complex, for the long-chain polymers.

Although there are some exceptions to the rule, simple carbohydrates are usually sugars or sweeteners and complex carbohydrates are starches or fibers. A healthful diet would obtain the majority of its carbohydrates from fruits and vegetables and whole-grain breads and cereals and lean dairy products.

Limiting added sugars and sweeteners is a nutrition recommendation set forth by several health organizations in an effort to curb obesity in the United States. The 2002 Dietary Reference Intakes suggested limiting simple carbohydrates to less than 25 percent of total calories.[1] The World Health Organization recommends no more than 10 percent of total calories from added sugars. Keep in mind that added sugars are not the same as sugars naturally found in foods. For active individuals eating some 2,500 calories, that would be 250 to 625 calories a day from added sugars. Active individuals should stick to up to 25 percent of total calories from added sugars, while sedentary individuals should limit these less nutritious calories to 10 percent of their daily intake.

Carbohydrate Utilization During Exercise

Carbohydrates are the major source of energy during exercise. At lower intensities, (<60 percent VO_2 max), fat oxidation can supply enough energy for exercise, but at higher intensities, carbohydrates are essential. Fatty acids can supply the majority of energy while exercising at a low intensity for several hours.[2]

When exercising at an intensity of over 60 percent of VO_2 max, carbohydrates supply the majority of energy for exercising muscles. As the intensity picks up, so does the reliance on carbohydrates to fuel muscles; for example, if you were doing an all-out 100-meter sprint, carbohydrates would supply 100 percent of the energy. As carbohydrates run low in the body, you have to slow down. Decades of research have indicated that high-carbohydrate diets are essential for optimal performance.[2,3]

Muscles have a limited supply of glycogen, the storage form of carbohydrates. A typical person will have 300 grams to 400 grams or 1,200 or 1,600 calories worth of carbohydrates stored in muscles; 300 to 400 calories stored in the liver and another 100 calories in the blood stream. That's a maximum of just over 2,000 calories worth of carbohydrates to be burned during exercise. Several studies have shown that eating a high-carbohydrate diet ensures that your body has adequate muscle and liver stores of carbohydrates to burn; conversely, studies have shown that when athletes are put on diets low in carbohydrates, muscle glycogen levels are lower and performance is impaired.[4]

Because your body only has a limited supply of stored carbohydrates, it's important to consume additional carbohydrates during endurance events if you want to be able to exercise at a higher intensity. The harder and longer you exercise, the more carbohydrates your muscles need to store. Without adequate carbohydrates in your diet, you may experience tiredness, staleness and lack of motivation to train. Carbohydrates are essential for mental acuity as well, so if you need to be sharp in your sport, don't skimp on carbohydrates. In addition, consuming carbohydrates during endurance activity helps reduce fatigue and even helps us perceive the exercise as being easier.[5] Chronic training with lack of carbohydrates has been linked to symptoms of overtraining (see chart) and may even compromise your immune system, increasing your chances of developing colds and other infections.[6]

Examples of Simple and Complex Carbohydrates and Common Food Sources:

Simple Carbohydrates and Food Sources

- Glucose: The single-unit carbohydrate that all other carbohydrates are broken down into for use by the body

- Sucrose: Beet and cane sugar, brown sugar, maple syrup, honey

- Fructose: Fruits, some vegetables, sweeteners such as high-fructose corn syrup, honey

- Lactose: Milk and dairy products

- Sucrose: Sugar, beets, fruit

Complex Carbohydrates and Food Sources

- Fibers and starches: Grains such as bread, pasta, beans, potatoes, corn and other vegetables

Carbohydrate Calculator

Whether you're running a marathon or 100 yards, lifting weights or playing basketball, carbohydrates are the primary provider of energy to muscles when working out.

Carbohydrates should supply about 40 percent of your total daily calories, although marathon runners or triathletes, who are exercising for hours most days a week, may even need up to 70 percent of their calories as carbohydrates.

The most accurate way to determine your carbohydrate needs is based on your body weight. Use the calculator at your left to determine the grams of carbohydrates you should be eating. When a range of carbohydrates is given, opt for the higher ends of carbohydrates if you are an endurance athlete or exercise twice a day or for over 90 minutes daily. If not, choose the lower end of the carbohydrate guidelines.

Carbohydrate Guidelines

These figures may be lower or higher depending on your fitness goals. Please see Chapter 6 and Chapter 8 for more information.

Daily:
3 to 4.5 grams carbohydrates per pound of body weight

Pre-Exercise:
.5 to 1.8 grams carbohydrates/pound, 1 to 4 hours prior to exercise

During Endurance or High-Intensity Exercise Lasting Over 90 Minutes:
30 to 60 grams carbohydrates per hour (120 to 240 carbohydrate calories)

After Strenuous Exercise:
.7 grams carbohydrates/pound body weight within 30 minutes

.7 grams carbohydrates/pound body weight again every 2 hours for 4 to 6 hours

Source: American College of Sports Medicine and American Dietetic Association. Joint Position Statement: Nutrition and Athletic Performance. *Med. Sci. Sports Exerc,* 32; 12:2130-2145, 2000.

Not All Carbohydrates Are Created Equal: Understanding the Glycemic Index and Glycemic Load

Glycemic Index (GI) is a term everyone is talking about these days, but it's greatly misunderstood. The Atkins, Zone, South Beach and many other popular diet books and programs advise against eating foods that rank high on the Glycemic Index. But what exactly is the Glycemic Index?

The Glycemic Index is a measurement to rank how fast carbohydrates are digested and absorbed, resulting in a rise in blood sugar levels. It's a way to compare foods gram for gram based on their effects on blood glucose levels. Carbohydrates that break down quickly have the highest glycemic indexes. Carbohydrates that break down slowly, releasing glucose gradually into the blood stream, have low glycemic indexes.

To measure the GI of a food, 50 grams of a carbohydrate in the food is fed to a subject and then blood glucose levels are measured for a specific period of time after consumption and compared to the blood glucose response of 50 grams of white bread or glucose.

A newer term being used now is glycemic load. The glycemic load provides a better indication of food choices because it is based on the total carbohydrate of a typical serving of the food, rather than a miniscule 50-gram (1.75 ounces) portion of food. The glycemic load equals the Glycemic Index of a food multiplied by the carbohydrate content. For people who have poor blood sugar control (i.e., diabetics), health professionals strive to lower the "glycemic load" of the diet.

What may come as a surprise is that white bread, instant rice, white potatoes, watermelon, carrots, raisins and some cereals are high in Glycemic Index while ice cream, beans and whole grains are low on the list. This is because fiber, fat, protein, acidity and other factors found in food may blunt the glycemic response. Since we often eat carbohydrate foods as part of a meal, the Glycemic Index does not apply to meals, only to the specific food tested.

Lowering the Glycemic Index and glycemic load has been shown to improve blood sugar levels and high blood cholesterol.[7] A diet rich in foods that elevate blood sugar levels are thought to be linked to obesity, high triglycerides in the blood, lower HDL "good" cholesterol, insulin resistance, Type 2 diabetes, heart disease and even colon and breast cancer.[7] However, because fiber, fat, protein and other factors affect Glycemic Index and glycemic load, it is not always practical or beneficial to use the index for planning meals; for example, ice cream and corn chips are lower on the Glycemic Index and glycemic load because of their fat content, but that doesn't necessarily make them healthier choices than lower-fat options.

Athletic Performance and the Glycemic Index

At this time there is insufficient evidence to suggest that active individuals consume foods that are either high or low in glycemic index to improve athletic performance.[3] As a general health rule, most scientists recommend eating foods that are lower on the GI prior to exercise and consume those that have higher GIs during and post-exercise to help replenish glycogen levels more quickly. More studies in the performance effects of eating a diet based on Glycemic Index or glycemic load need to be completed before any formal recommendations are given.

Use this chart to determine which foods are low, medium or high in glycemic load.

	Glycemic Index	Glycemic Load
BAKERY PRODUCTS		
High Glycemic Load		
Bagel (70g)	72	25
French bread (70g)	72	27
Donut (47g)	76	17
Croissant (57g)	67	17
Pancakes (80g)	102	22
Medium Glycemic Load:		
Apple muffin (60g)	44	13
Bran muffin (57g)	60	15
Cracked wheat bread (30g)	58	12
Wheat bread (30g)	52	10
Low Glycemic Load:		
Oat bran bread (30g):	44	8
Sourdough rye bread (30g):	53	6
CEREALS		
High Glycemic Load:		
Corn Flakes (30g)	92	24

Low Glycemic Index:
55 or less

Medium Glycemic Index:
56-69

High Glycemic Index:
70 or higher

Low Glycemic Load:
10 or less

Medium Glycemic Load:
11-19

High Glycemic Load:
20 or higher

	Glycemic Index	Glycemic Load
CEREALS continued		
Medium Glycemic Load:		
Cheerios (30g)	74	15
Bran Flakes (30g)	74	13
Shredded Wheat (30g)	83	17
Cream of Wheat (30g)	66	17
Just Right (30g)	62	14
Special K (30g)	69	14
Low Glycemic Load:		
All-Bran (30g)	30	9
GRAINS		
High Glycemic Load:		
Couscous (150g)	65	23
White rice (150g)	53	20
Spaghetti (180g)	47	23
Medium Glycemic Load:		
Bulgur (150g)	48	12
Long grain rice (150g)	41	16
BEVERAGES, (8 OUNCES)		
High Glycemic Load:		
Cranberry juice	68	24
Medium Glycemic Load:		
Cola	63	16
Orange juice	50	13
Apple juice	40	12
Gatorade	78	12
Hot chocolate	51	11
Low Glycemic Load:		
Soy milk	44	8
Tomato juice	38	4
Skim milk	32	4
Whole milk	27	3
FRUIT		
Medium Glycemic Load:		
Banana (120g)	51	13
Dried figs (60g)	61	16
Low Glycemic Load:		
Apple (120g)	40	6
Cherries (120g)	22	3
Grapefruit (120g)	25	3

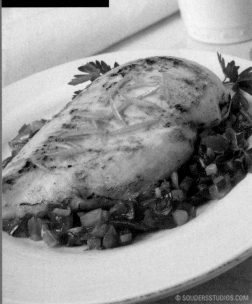

Fiber, fat, protein and acidity may blunt the glycemic response to a food.

© SOUDERSSTUDIOS.COM

NUTRITION ESSENTIALS

	Glycemic Index	Glycemic Load
FRUIT continued		
Grapes (120g)	46	8
Kiwi (120g)	53	6
Oranges (120g)	48	5
Pear (120g)	33	4
VEGETABLES		
High Glycemic Load:		
Baked potato (150g)	85	26
Medium Glycemic Load:		
Sweet potato (150g)	61	17
Mashed potatoes (150g)	74	15
Sweet corn (80g)	60	11
Low Glycemic Load:		
Baked beans (150g)	48	7
Green peas (80g)	48	3
Carrots (80g)	47	3
DESSERTS/SNACKS		
High Glycemic Index:		
Jelly beans (30g)	78	22
Mars bar (60g)	68	27
Nutrition bar (65g)	56	24
Medium Glycemic Index:		
Doritos (50g)	42	11
Low Glycemic Index:		
IronMan PR bar (65g)	39	10
Ice cream (50g)	61	8
Low-fat, reduced-sugar ice cream (50g)	37	5
Pudding (100g)	47	7
Reduced-fat yogurt (200g)	26	3
Peanut M&Ms (30g)	33	6

Adapted from: Foster-Powell, K, Holt, S, and Brand-Miller, C., "International table of glycemic index and glycemic load values." *Am J Clin Nutr* 2002;76:5-56.

tip

Key Glycemic Points:
- The Glycemic Index measures how fast a 50-gram dose of carbohydrates is digested and absorbed.
  - Carbs that break down quickly are high glycemic.
  - Carbs that break down slowly are low glycemic.
- The Glycemic Load is based on how fast a typical serving of carbohydrates is digested and absorbed.

Carb-Loading: What It Is and How It Works

Contrary to popular belief, carb-loading doesn't mean pigging out on pasta the night before a marathon, triathlon or other endurance event. The scientific term for carbohydrate loading is actually glycogen supercompensation. It's a technique used to stimulate the muscles to store more carbohydrates by manipulating training and diet composition for a week prior to an endurance event. Studies have shown that endurance athletes who follow the protocol store additional carbohydrates in the form of glycogen.[8] Because glycogen stores hold water, athletes may feel heavy and bloated when carb-loading, but the advantages of additional carbohydrates during the later phases of an endurance event outweigh the feeling of heaviness; however, for shorter events, carb-loading is not recommended.

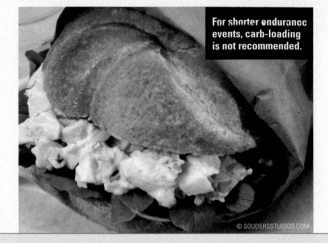

For shorter endurance events, carb-loading is not recommended.

Carbohydrate Counter

Use this chart to help plan your meals and snacks around carbohydrate-rich choices.

BREADS, CEREALS AND GRAINS

One serving of these foods provides about 15 grams of carbohydrates:

Bread
1 ounce (1 slice) whole-wheat bread
½ English muffin

Cereals
1 ounce (about 1/2 cup) cereal
1/4 cup granola
1 ½ cups puffed cereal
½ cup cooked oatmeal or other cooked cereal
½ cup cooked grits
2 ½ tablespoons Grape-Nuts cereal

Grains and Other Carbohydrates
½ cup cooked pasta
½ cup cooked rice, bulgur or other grain
1 small waffle
2 small pancakes
2 saltines
1 small (6-inch) flour tortilla
¾-ounce pretzels

STARCHY VEGETABLES

15 grams of carbohydrates per serving:
½ cup baked beans
½ cup black, garbanzo, lima, pinto beans
½ cup peas, corn, squash
½ cup mashed potatoes
½ medium baked potato
¾ cup mashed squash
½ medium sweet potato
1 cup cooked beets

FRUITS AND FRUIT JUICES

15 grams of carbohydrates per serving:
1 small apple
½ cup applesauce, unsweetened
3 dried apple rings
4 ounces apple, cranberry, grape, grapefruit, orange or pineapple juice
12 ounces vegetable juice
4 medium apricots
1 medium banana
¾ cup blackberries, blueberries, cantaloupe, pineapple
1 medium orange, peach

Here is the specific carb-loading technique prior to an endurance event.

Days Before Event	Exercise	Diet
6	90 minutes exercise	5g carb/kg body weight
5	40 minutes exercise	5g carb/kg body weight
4	40 minutes exercise	5g carb/kg body weight
3	20 minutes exercise	10g carb/kg body weight
2	20 minutes exercise	10g carb/kg body weight
1	Rest	10g carb/kg body weight
Event		

Source: *Sports Nutrition: A Guide for the Professional Working with Active People* 3rd edition, Rosenbloom C. (American Dietetic Association, 1999).

½ large grapefruit
2 dried figs
½ cup fruit salad
½ cup (15) grapes
1 ½ cups watermelon
1 cup strawberries or raspberries
1 ½ tablespoons raisins

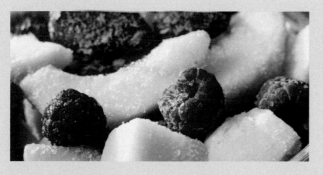

SWEETS

15 grams of carbohydrates per serving:
1 tablespoon jam/jelly
1 tablespoon brown sugar
1 tablespoon white sugar
1 tablespoon honey
1 tablespoon regular syrup

2 tablespoons light syrup
1 ½ Fig bar
½ cup soda, fruit punch or fruit "ades"

MILK, DAIRY PRODUCTS AND DAIRY ALTERNATIVES

12 to 40 grams of carbohydrates per serving:
1 cup skim, 1 percent, 2 percent or whole milk (12 grams)
1 cup chocolate milk (26 grams)
1 cup non-fat plain yogurt (16 grams)
1 cup vanilla yogurt (36 grams)
1 cup fruit flavored yogurt (40 to 60 grams)
1 cup rice milk (25 grams)
1 cup soy milk

VEGETABLES

5 grams of carbohydrates per serving:
½ artichoke
½ cup asparagus
½ cup broccoli, cabbage, squash, green beans, mushrooms
1 tomato

Source: Nutrients in Food. Hands ES. Lippincott Williams and Wilkins. Philadelphia, PA 2000 and USDA Nutrient Database; www.nal.usda.gov/fnic/foodcomp/

POWER UP WITH PROTEIN—THE BUILDING BLOCK OF MUSCLES

Since ancient times, protein was thought to be the nutrient responsible for strength and stamina. Writings about the first Olympic games in 776 B.C. tell of various animal meats such as oxen, goat and deer that the athletes ate before their competitions. Even reports from the 1936 Olympic games in Berlin commented on how the German athletes would eat over 2 pounds of meat per day. A pre-event meal often consisted of one or more steaks and several eggs.[9]

Slowly, research started to show the importance of carbohydrates and fat for energy production and optimal performance. Although carbohydrates are now known to be the muscles' primary fuel and fat provides the most concentrated storage form of energy for the body, protein is essential for anyone concerned about performance. Depending upon how muscular you are, the majority of your body weight is derived from protein.[10]

What Is Protein?

Protein is a macronutrient like carbohydrates and fat. All macronutrients contain carbon, oxygen and hydrogen molecules. Protein differs from carbohydrates and fat in that it also contains nitrogen, sulfur and some minerals. When 100 or more amino acids link together, a protein is formed. Proteins are made following specific genetic codes, so the amino acids are linked together in ways that turn on or off genes and code for specific proteins. There are over 10,000 different proteins that help make you who you are.

The building blocks of protein are 20 different amino acids. Of the 20 amino acids, nine are considered essential because the body cannot produce them. Because the body needs a daily supply of these amino acids, protein is an essential nutrient that needs to be consumed daily.

Nine **Essential** Amino Acids	**Nonessential** Amino Acids
Histidine	Alanine
Isoleucine (branched chain amino acid)	Arginine
Leucine (branched chain amino acid)	Asparagine
Lysine (branched chain amino acid)	Aspartic acid
Methionine	Cystine
Phenylalanine	Glutamic acid
Threonine	Glutamine
Tryptophan	Glycine
Valine	Proline
	Serine
	Tyrosine

Adapted from: *Sports Nutrition: A Guide for the Professional Working with Active People.* 3rd edition Rosenbloom, C (The American Dietetic Association, 1999)

Roles of Protein in the Body

Everyone knows that protein is important for building muscle and repairing muscle fibers after exercise, but proteins in the body have thousands of other essential roles, including:

- Producing antibodies for the immune system
- Manufacturing hormones and enzymes that are involved in most reactions in your body
- Aiding in the digestion and absorption of food
- Being a source of fuel when muscle glycogen levels are low
- Maximizing the transport of oxygen to tissues
- Providing structure for muscles, tendons, ligaments, organs, bones, hair, skin and all other tissues

You need protein on a daily basis to help build and repair muscles.

© SOUDERSSTUDIOS.COM

Protein Digestion and Absorption

You need to eat protein-containing foods daily to obtain your daily requirements for essential amino acids. About 90 percent of the protein you eat is broken down into amino acids and becomes part of the amino acid "pool" that the body draws upon when it needs to build or repair muscles or other tissues or to do any of the other roles that the amino acids play. (The body excretes the other 10 percent.) Unlike carbohydrates and fat, which the body can store as glycogen or triglycerides respectively for use later, amino acids have no form of storage in the body, so it's important to have some protein every day.

When you eat foods containing protein, the protein molecule is broken down in the mouth and small intestine into its amino acids. Once broken into amino acids, three things can happen. The amino acids can be:

- Converted into glucose
- Converted into triglycerides and stored as body fat
- Released into the blood stream as the plasma protein or free amino acids to be used as energy

When you eat enough protein to cover your body's amino acids needs, your body is considered to be in protein equilibrium; however, if you don't eat enough protein, protein (usually from the muscles) is broken down to fulfill the amino acids "pool." If you consume more protein than your body needs, the excess amino acids are broken down further and the nitrogen, ammonia, uric acid and creatine are secreted in urine, and part of the amino acid remaining can either be stored as body fat or muscle.

Daily Protein Needs

The National Academy of Sciences (NAS) sets the protein requirements for children and adults. They are based on the needs of average Americans and not active individuals. The protein recommendations are based on body weight or the average weight of a male and female adult. The NAS also recommends that protein intake should provide 10 percent to 35 percent of total calories. This wide range represents a shift in thinking that there is no "one-size-fits-all" guideline for nutrient recommendations; for example, individuals who consume fewer calories need to have a higher percentage of those calories from protein while an athlete eating 3,000 calories a day or more can eat a lower percentage of calories from protein to meet his or her protein needs. There are currently not official NAS Recommended Dietary Allowances (RDAs) developed for athletic individuals. The NAS recommendations are considered too low for most active individuals.[11]

National Academy of Sciences Protein Recommendations:
.4 grams protein/pound body weight

National Academy of Sciences Recommended Dietary Allowance:
46 grams protein/day for women
56 grams protein/day for men

Protein Requirements for Active Individuals

The dietary recommendations for protein for physically active individuals have been hotly debated for years. The protein requirements appear to be affected by a variety of factors, including age, sex, exercise type, intensity and duration, training history, total calorie intake and timing of meals.

The protein requirements for athletes are based on the requirements for specific essential amino acids; for example, the branched chain amino acid leucine is used as fuel during exercise. One study found that during two hours of exercising at 50 percent VO_2max nearly 90 percent of the total daily requirement of leucine was burned as fuel.[12]

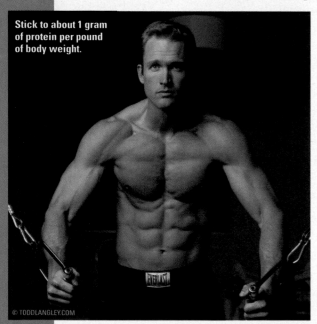

Stick to about 1 gram of protein per pound of body weight.

© TODDLANGLEY.COM

Both intensity and duration will increase protein requirements. Resistance exercise and endurance exercise both affect protein utilization. When beginning a training program, the body uses a lot of additional protein until the body adapts to the exercise program, usually happening in two or three weeks.

If you're trying to lose weight, protein needs per pound of body weight are also increased. This happens because as you lose weight, muscle protein is broken down as an energy source. Research has shown that consuming 1.6 grams of protein per pound of body weight while dieting enabled subjects to maintain more muscle mass compared to those who followed a traditional diet with .8 grams per pound of body weight. In order to make the most of calories, high-quality protein sources are important when dieting to help maintain muscle mass to keep metabolic rate high.

Despite increased protein requirements for active athletes, there is no need to believe that more is better. The maximum protein the body can utilize daily is about 1 gram of protein per pound of body weight or 2.2 grams of protein per kilogram of body weight. Too much protein can lead to weight gain (as fat), interfere with other nutrients and increase the load on the kidneys to excrete additional nitrogen.

Protein Requirements for Active Individuals

(For ease of calculation, use 1 gram/pound.)

Moderate Strength Training	Primarily Aerobic Exercise
1.2 to 1.4 grams/pounds per day	.5 to .64 gram/pound
Competitive Athletes, Adults	
1.2 to 1.8 grams/pounds per day	.5 to .82 gram/pound
Competitive Athletes, Children	
1.8 to 2.0 grams/pounds per day	.82 to .91 gram/pound
Heavy Strength Training	
1.6 to 1.8 grams/pounds per day	.73 to .82 gram/pound
Athletes Restricting Calories	
1.4 to 2.0 grams/pounds per day	.64 to .91 gram/pound

Adapted from: *Sports Nutrition: A Guide for the Professional working with Active People.* 3rd edition. Rosenbloom, C. (American Dietetic Association, 1999).

Protein Timing and Type

When to eat protein is also important for active individuals. There is some evidence that pre- and post-exercise meals containing some essential amino acids result in greater gains in muscle mass compared to gains from training alone. For endurance athletes, a post-exercise meal containing essential amino acids is important for added strength gains. At this time, the best guideline is to eat small amounts of protein at each meal and have protein with carbohydrates immediately after a strenuous exercise session to help the muscles facilitate glycogen storage upstores as quickly as possible. Post-exercise protein recommendations suggest eating a ratio of protein to carbohydrate of 1:3. What that means is that for every 3 grams of carbohydrates you have a gram of protein.[13] There are several sports bars and drinks designed to provide this combination of nutrients, or it can easily be done with whole foods such as a turkey sandwich or fruit smoothie with protein powder.

Second, protein type may also be important due to variable speeds of absorption and availability, differences in the types of amino acids and the hormonal responses that occur as a result from the protein. Researchers are looking into how certain amino acids stimulate anabolic hormones such as insulin and subsequent muscle growth; for example, studies have shown that high-quality animal protein containing all the essential amino acids produces greater hormonal responses in athletes compared to consuming incomplete vegetable-based protein.[14,15]

Taken together, these data suggest that the time course and magnitude of amino acid delivery to muscle are affected by protein type. At this time, the best recommendation

How Much Protein is in a Pound of Muscle?

Your muscle is primarily water, and contains up to 20 percent protein by weight.

Here's how a pound of muscle breaks down into components:

Water:	70 to 75 percent
Protein:	15 to 20 percent
Fat, glycogen, minerals:	5 to 7 percent

is to eat a wide variety of protein sources (including various animal and vegetarian sources daily) to ensure that you have a good mix of amino acids delivered to your body.

Distinguishing Between High- and Low-Quality Protein

Protein is classified as complete or incomplete, depending upon its amino acid profile. If the protein contains all the amino acids needed to construct new proteins, it's considered a complete protein. Animal sources of protein such as meat, poultry, fish and dairy products are complete proteins. Other protein sources may lack one or more of the essential amino acids and are therefore called incomplete proteins. Incomplete proteins come from plant-based foods such as fruits, vegetables, grains and nuts. One exception is soy protein. Soy protein is considered a complete protein because it contains all of the essential amino acids.

In addition, proteins are also compared to each other based on several different types of analyses to determine how efficiently they provide the body with the essential amino acids. These analyses provide measures for protein digestibility and are called "protein efficiency ratio," "protein digestibility-corrected amino acid scores (PDCAAS)" or "biological value." All measure the ability to supply complete proteins that are the best absorbed and utilized by the body. Use the chart below to see how the protein quality of other foods stacks up. Generally, animal-based protein sources rank high on protein scores, whereas vegetable-based protein sources rate lower, with the exception of soy protein.

Two or more incomplete, vegetable-based proteins can be eaten so the body has all of the essential amino acids and form a complete protein. Examples of combined, complete plant proteins are rice and beans, milk and wheat cereal, and corn and beans. There's no need to combine specific foods at meals to create complete proteins, as once thought. If you eat adequate calories and a variety of plant-based foods, your body will create enough complete proteins out of the amino acid pool.

Food Sources of Protein	Grams of Protein
Fish, poultry or lean meat, cooked (3 ounces)	20 to 30 grams
Tofu, firm (½ cup)	20 grams
Cottage cheese, low-fat (½ cup)	15 grams
Yogurt, low-fat (6 to 8 ounces)	10 to 12 grams
Lentils, cooked (½ cup)	9 grams
Kashi GoLean cereal (¾ cup)	8 grams
Milk, 1 percent or skim (8 ounces)	8 grams
Peanut butter (2 tablespoons)	8 grams
Cheese (1 ounce)	7 grams
Peanuts (1 ounce or 28 nuts)	7 grams
Egg (1)	6 grams
Baked potato (1)	5 grams
Pasta, cooked (1 cup)	5 grams
Hummus (¼ cup)	3 grams
Vegetables, cooked (½ cup)	2 grams

Source: *Bowes & Church's Food Values of Portions Commonly Used*, 17th edition, 1998.

Vegetarian Athletes' Special Needs

There are several different types of vegetarians; for example, lacto-ova vegetarians eat dairy and eggs, while vegans abstain from all animal-derived foods. Vegetarian diets can be healthy and provide all the nutrients needed for optimal performance, but strict vegetarians need to make good food choices to ensure they meet their protein requirements. Use these tips to obtain daily protein requirements:

- Choose soy-based meat and dairy alternatives for complete protein.
- Include plenty of legumes, seeds and nuts, which are more complete than protein in grains and vegetables.
- Consume adequate calories. If your body burns more calories than you consume, your protein needs increase to account for increased muscle mass degradation.
- Choose fortified breakfast cereals that are rich in protein.

FACTS ABOUT FAT

What Is Dietary Fat?

The fats in food are referred to as lipids, from the Greek word "lipos" which means fat. Lipids are all made up of carbon, hydrogen and oxygen, similar to carbohydrates and protein. They are either oils (liquid at room temperature), fats (solids at room temperature) or waxes and other related compounds. The lipids we will focus on are the primary lipids we eat and how they affect athletic performance.

The fat in food is an essential nutrient, just like carbohydrates, protein, vitamin C, E or any other essential nutrients. Fat is the most concentrated energy source of any of the macronutrients. It's also necessary to digest and absorb vitamins A, D, E and K and hundreds of beneficial carotenoids, such as lycopene and lutein. Fats also provide the body with essential fatty acids, linoleic and linolenic acids, that help to maintain the immune system, strong nails, shiny hair and clear skin. Fatty acids produce hormones that affect everything from hunger and sex drive to your moods.

All Fats Are Not Created Equal

There are "good" and "bad" fats that either help protect you from diseases or increase your risk for chronic conditions. The so-called healthy fats are monounsaturated or polyunsaturated fats and the bad fats are saturated fats or trans fats. When monos or polys are substituted for saturated fat or trans fats in the diet, they lower total blood cholesterol and triglycerides and raise healthy, HDL-cholesterol levels in the blood. They also improve insulin sensitivity and blood pressure. Saturated fat and trans fats may promote heart disease, diabetes, certain cancers and obesity because they raise LDL cholesterol levels, aggravate inflammation in the arteries, elevate triglycerides and trans fats lower healthy HDL cholesterol levels.[16]

Fat Metabolism

Fat is broken down into short, medium or long-chain fatty acids and glycerol and then is further metabolized into triglycerides, which are the storage form of lipids in the body. Triglycerides are stored in the liver, muscles or fat tissue for use as energy at a later time. The body can store unlimited amounts of fat (as body fat). For most normal-weight individu-

Sources of Fat in the Diet

Of the 76 grams of fat Americans eat on average daily, here are the foods that pack the most fat into the typical American diet:[21]

Food	Percent of total fat
Meat, fish and poultry	30
Grains and grain-based foods	8
Dairy products	13
Fats and oils	10
Pastries and bakery items	7
Eggs	3
Nuts	3

Source: Chanmugam, P, Guthrie JF et al., "Did fat intake in the United States really decline between 1989 to 1991 and 1994 to 1996?" *JADA* 2003;103(7):867-72.

als, fat stores contain at least 100 times more available energy compared to stored carbohydrates.[17]

All this stored triglyceride can be burned for fuel during exercise; however, the amount of fat versus carbohydrate burned during exercise depends upon the duration and intensity of your workouts. At low intensities, fat oxidation provides the bulk of energy to the muscle but as intensity increases, the percentage of carbohydrates oxidized for fuel increases. Once you reach 70 percent to 80 percent of your VO_2 max, fat oxidation is limited and carbohydrate provides 70 to 80 percent of the energy.[18] Compared to burning one glucose molecule for energy, a fatty acid creates nearly four times as much energy; however, fat oxidation requires more oxygen than carbohydrate oxidation, so when you start breathing hard, your ability to burn fat as fuel diminishes.

Aerobic training makes the body more efficient at burning fat as fuel by increasing the enzymes that are necessary to turn fatty acids into energy. This helps spare carbohydrates, thereby enhancing endurance. A marathon runner, for instance, will have the ability to burn more fat as fuel at the same percentage of VO_2 max compared to an untrained individual.[18,19]

Fat Recommendations for Active Individuals

Studies have looked at the performance-enhancing benefits of high-fat diets or diets rich in specific fatty acids, but there appears to be little evidence that higher-fat diets or specialty fats are performance-enhancers.[14] At this time, there are no special recommendations for limiting fat or loading up on fat for optimal performance.[20] Athletes with calorie needs over 3,000 calories a day may find that consuming more fat-rich foods enables them to meet their calorie needs more easily. It requires constant feedings to meet the high-energy needs with low-fat, low-calorie foods.

The Institute of Medicine recommends that all adults consume 20 percent to 35 percent of total calories in fats, with an emphasis on healthier unsaturated fats, to ensure that you're getting enough fat in your diet. That translates into 55 to 97 grams of fat daily for someone eating 2,500 calories a day. Studies show that fat intake among athletes varies greatly, from 15 percent of calories to over 40 percent of calories.[17] Sticking to healthful fats will not only be better for disease prevention, but these types of fats may be more readily burned as fuel

FAT CHART

Fats	How much
Monounsaturated fats: Olive, canola, peanut oils; nuts and avocados.	10 percent to 15 percent of calories.
Polyunsaturated fats: Include omega-6 and omega-3 polyunsaturated fats **Omega-6 fats:** Corn, safflower, sesame, soy and sunflower oils (and in margarines, salad dressings and mayonnaise made with these oils) nuts and seeds. **Omega-3 fats:** Cold-water fish like herring, mackerel, salmon, sardines and tuna; flax seed, canola oil and walnuts.	Up to 10 percent of calories.
Saturated fats Meat, poultry, butter, cheese, cream and whole milk; coconut, palm and palm kernel oils; processed foods such as cookies, crackers, chips and other baked goods.	Up to 10 percent of calories.
Trans fats: Stick margarines, shortening, packaged baked goods such as cookies, pastries and crackers, candy, snack foods, French fries and other fried foods. A very small amount also occurs naturally in meat, poultry and dairy products.	As little as possible.

compared to unhealthy fats.

Because dietary fat contains nine calories per gram (protein and carbohydrates contain four calories per gram), fat is considered the most calorically dense nutrient. When trying to lose weight or maintain weight loss, eating a diet that eliminates unhealthy sources of fat will also cut out a lot of calories. Dietary fat is also easily converted into body fat if you don't need the energy of fat, so too much dietary fat can make it easier for you to pack on pounds.

TRANS FATS: How to Avoid Them

You might know that fried fast food, margarine or doughnuts contain unhealthy trans fats, but so do many wholesome-sounding foods like whole-wheat crackers, frozen waffles and some cereals. The Food and Drug Administration (FDA) recently ruled that by January 1, 2006, all food labels with fat will be required to list the amount of trans fat per serving. According to the FDA, three years after January 1, 2006, trans fat labeling may prevent 600 to 1,200 cases of coronary heart disease and 250 to 500 deaths each year. While more companies are starting to include the grams of trans fat per servings now, many companies don't include trans fats on their labels. Here's how you can avoid eating too many of these undesirable fats:

Avoid foods made with hydrogenated or partially hydrogenated oils, a major source of trans fats and choose soft or liquid margarine instead of hard or stick margarines. Better yet: use olive or canola oil instead of margarine.

Source: Votruba, SB, Atkinson, RL et al., " Prior exercise increases subsequent utilization of dietary fat." *Med. Sci. Sports Exerc.,* Vol. 34, No. 11, pp. 1757-1765, 2002.

REFERENCES CITED:

[1] Trumbo, P et al. Dietary reference intakes for energy, carbohydrate, fiber, fat, fatty acids, cholesterol, protein and amino acids. *J Am Diet Assoc* 102.11 (2002): 1621-30.

[2] Rosenbloom, C. *Sports Nutrition: A Guide for the Professional working with Active People (Third Edition).* (The American Dietetic Association, 1992).

[3] Joint Position Statement: nutrition and athletic performance. American College of Sports Medicine, American Dietetic Association. *Med Sci Sports Exerc* 32.12 (2000): 2130-2145.

[4] Costill, DL, Flynn, MJ et al. Effect of repeated days of intensified training on muscle glycogen and swimming performance. *Med Sci Sports Exerc* 20 (1988): 249-54.

[5] Utter, AC, Kang, RJ et al. Effect of carbohydrate ingestion on ratings of perceived exertion during a marathon. *Med Sci Sports Exerc* 34 (2002): 1779-84.

[6] McArdle, WD, Katch, FI and Katch, VL. *Sports and Exercise Nutrition* (Lippincott Williams & Wilkins, 1999).

[7] Jenkins, JA, Kendall, CW, Augustin, LS et al. Glycemic index: overview of implications in health and disease. *Am J Clin Nutr* 76.1 (2002): 266S-73S.

[8] Sherman, WM, Costill, DL, Fink, WJ and Miller, JM. The effect of exercise and diet manipulation on muscle glycogen and its subsequent use during performance. *Int J Sport Med* 2 (1988): 114-18.

[9] McArdle, WD et al. *Sports and Exercise Nutrition* (Lippincott Williams & Wilkins, 1999).

[10] Crim, MC and Hamish, MN. *Proteins and amino acids. Modern Nutrition in Health and Disease. (Eighth edition).* (Lea & Febiger; Waverly Co, 1994).

[11] Lemon, PW. Protein requirements of athletes. *Sports Med* 12 (1991): 313-25

[12] Young, VR, Bier, DM et al. A theoretical basis for increasing current estimates of the amino acid requirements in adult men with experimental support. *Am J Clin Nutr* 50 (1989): 80-92.

[13] Rosenbloom C. *Sports Nutrition: A Guide for the Professional working with Active People (Third Edition).* (The American Dietetic Association, 1992).

[14] Lemon, PW. Beyond the zone: protein needs of active individuals. *J Am Coll Nutr* 19.5 suppl. (2000): 513S-521S.

[15] Lemon, PW, Berardi, JM and Noreen, EE. The role of protein and amino acid supplements in the athlete's diet: does type or timing of ingestion matter? *Curr Sports Med Rep* 1.4 (2002): 214-21.

[16] Duyff, RL. *American Dietetic Association Complete Food and Nutrition Guide.* (Second Edition). (John Wiley & Sons, Inc, 2002).

[17] Rosenbloom, C. *Sports Nutrition: A Guide for the Professional working with Active People.* (Third Edition). (The American Dietetic Association, 1999).

[18] Ranallo, RF and Rhodes, EC. Lipid metabolism during exercise. *Sports Med* 26 (1990): 29-42.

[19] Votruba, SB, Atkinson, RL et al. Prior exercise increases subsequent utilization of dietary fat. *Med Sci Sports Exerc* 34.11 (2002): 1757-1765.

[20] American College of Sports Medicine and American Dietetic Association. Joint Position Statement. Nutrition and Athletic Performance. *Med Sci Sports Exerc* 32.12 (2000): 2130-2145.

[21] Chanmugam, P, Guthrie, JF et al. Did fat intake in the United States really decline between 1989-1991 and 1994-1996? *JADA* 103.7 (2003): 867-72.

2 VITAMINS AND MINERALS

What They Are, What They Do and Why We Need Them

By Brian L. Deeds, Sr. Mgr. of Training and Corporate Development, EAS

Most people are aware that vitamins and minerals are essential to good health but knowing exactly *what* they are and *how* they work are a completely different story. Sure, you can read books, magazines, medical references and countless studies, but when you're finally through with your research it's likely that you'll find yourself right back where you started—overwhelmed and confused. This chapter was written to take some of the mystery out of the broad and complex topic of vitamins and minerals.

This chapter contains two distinct sections: a layman's explanation followed by an overview of vitamin and mineral functionality. There will be periodic summaries of concepts to help make the information "digestible." If you know everything there is to know about this subject, you're welcome to skip ahead, but you might be missing out on some interesting concepts. If you're just a beginner on the topic of vitamins and minerals, you'll want to read the entire chapter from beginning to end to build a foundation of knowledge.

PART I: WHAT IT IS ALL ABOUT—A LAYMAN'S EXPLANATION

The "Big" Question

The foremost question on everyone's mind is probably: "Do I *really* need additional vitamins and minerals, or am I getting enough from eating foods?" Well, the basic answer is "maybe." You see, there are many variables involved in meeting your daily vitamin and mineral requirements. It is nearly impossible to give a solid answer that covers everyone's needs. What we'll do is take a look at some of these variables so you can decide if increasing your vitamin and mineral intake is warranted.

It's Dinner Time … Do You Know Where Your Vitamins Are?

Theoretically, you can meet your daily requirements of vitamins and minerals from eating a wide variety of whole foods. That means consuming plenty of fruits, vegetables, grains and meats every day. In other words, different types of foods will offer different types of vitamins and minerals; for example, lean ground beef offers plenty of iron, milk provides calcium, nuts and seeds provide vitamin E.[1] If you're eating a widely varied diet that includes meats, fruits, vegetables, dairy, nuts and seeds you may have adequate vitamin and mineral intake.

Did you know that excessive cooking under high temperatures may reduce the vitamin content of perfectly good vegetables into a mushy mess? Do the vegetables you eat each and every day include the red ones, orange ones, yellow ones, and the leafy greens and fibrous types such as broccoli? If you can honestly say that you don't overcook your vegetables, that you eat plenty of various colors and varieties of raw vegetables every day, congratulations! However, if your eating habits are like most of the U.S. population, then a fast-paced lifestyle, access to junk food and eating processed foods have gotten the better of you. Let's face it: finding and consuming quality foods is challenging even for those who follow a proper nutritional regimen. How can you be sure, even if you are a die-hard health nut, that you're eating what you *think* you're eating? Maybe the meaning can be clarified by asking this question: "How do you know that the fruits and vegetables you're eating contain adequate levels of vitamins and minerals?"

The Decay of Modern Vitamins

There is speculation that our soils are depleted of key nutrients as a result of over-farming. This means that many fruits and vegetables may not have had the opportunity to absorb sufficient levels of vitamins and minerals from the soil. Even fertilizing between harvests may not be enough to replenish the fields for the next series of crops.

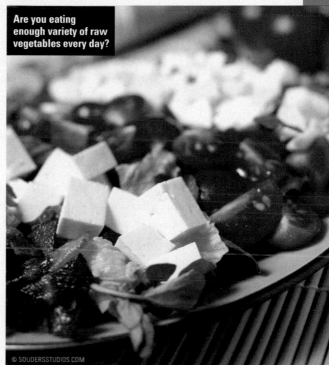

Are you eating enough variety of raw vegetables every day?

© SOUDERSSTUDIOS.COM

Apparently, the RDA (Recommended Dietary Intake) takes these factors into consideration. Their recommendations are based on foods that can be found directly on the shelves in grocery stores. Where specifically were the fruits and vegetables grown? One farm's produce may offer levels of nutrients that another may not. What kinds of pesticides were used for a particular batch of crops? Was one batch picked "greener" than another? Again the question is presented: "How can you be sure that you're eating what you *think* you're eating?"

Party On

Now let's throw another variable into the equation—smoking. Yes, smoking cigarettes is detrimental to your health: That's a given. You've been lectured enough on that already. The point to be made is how smoking destroys vitamins in your body. Even if you don't smoke you're not quite off the hook. The secondhand smoke you breathe may have a similar effect on *your* vitamin stores. Specifically, smoke from cigarettes diminish your calcium stores, plus your stores of vitamins C and B.[2,3,4,5,6,7,8]

If you're out in a bar around all that smoke, you might as well enjoy a martini or two. Since you're already on your way to destroying your vitamin stores, have some alcohol to finish the job. Alcohol triggers the release of water stores from your body, causing the frequent restroom breaks.[9] Just know that you could be eliminating some of your vitamin and mineral stores right down the drain every time you have to excuse yourself.[10,11] By the way, the elimination of key vitamins and alteration of body nutrient stores due to consuming alcohol is thought to be a contributing factor to disorders of long-term, excessive alcohol consumption.

Thanks a Latte

You're not out of hot water just yet (so to speak). If you're like millions of other Americans, you're a sucker for a hot cup of coffee. Although there's nothing better than a nice frothy cappuccino or a strong cup of coffee, there is a downside to drinking it, relative to vitamins and minerals: Caffeine may cause your body to excrete excess calcium.[12]

Happy, Happy, Joy, Joy!

Certainly you're a well-adjusted individual who is generally easygoing and happy-go-lucky. Nothing ever gets you down at work, right? You smile happily when someone cuts you off in traffic. For people like you, the loss of B vitamins due to stress just isn't an issue. For the rest of us, stress plays a role in reducing vitamin stores.

RECAP

Let's stop for a minute and summarize some of the key points. Although you could theoretically meet your entire vitamin and mineral needs through nutritional whole foods, there are a few variables to consider. Some of these variables are summarized as follows:

- There is a theory that farming soils are depleted of nutrients because of over-farming, contributing to fruits and vegetables having less than optimal levels of nutrients.
- You need to eat a wide variety of fruits and vegetables daily.
- Extreme cooking of vegetables under high temperatures can significantly reduce their vitamin content.
- Smoking may contribute toward losses in calcium, vitamin C and B vitamins.
- Alcohol consumption may contribute toward losses in C and B vitamins.
- Coffee may contribute toward losses in calcium, vitamin C and B vitamins.

If any of these factors are of personal concern, there is a possibility that consuming additional vitamins and minerals may benefit you.

RISKY BUSINESS

There are some groups of people who may be categorically at risk for vitamin and/or mineral deficiencies. Some examples of these groups are women, female athletes, endurance athletes and people who engage in high intensity training such as bodybuilders, wrestlers, those who are on calorie-restricted diets, ultra-high endurance athletes and vegetarians.

Women and Deficiency Risk

Women as a group are at risk for iron deficiencies. Consider that only 25 percent of American women meet their Recommended Dietary Allowance (RDA) for iron, 12 percent of the female population, ages 19 to 50, is iron deficient and about 3 percent have been diagnosed with anemia.[13,14,15] An iron deficiency results in suppressed red blood cell production, which in turn, equates to a lack of oxygen in the body (anemia).[16,17] Simply put, anemia causes low energy levels due to poor oxygen circulation.

The Female Athlete Triad

Female athletes may be at risk for a condition called the "female athlete triad."[18,19,20] This condition is comprised of amenorrhea (irregular menstrual cycles), disordered eating and osteoporosis (bone fragility). The major cause of this condition may be the disordered eating part of the triad.[21] Why? Female athletes may be more likely than males to follow a calorie-restricted diet as a means to control body fat; unfortunately, fewer calories mean that fewer essential nutrients (including vitamins and minerals) are being ingested. This may ultimately lead to deficiencies;[22,23] for example, some female athletes avoid drinking milk in order to reduce their fat intake. A complete elimination of dairy from the diet may lead to lower dietary calcium intakes and a potential deficiency over time. A long-term deficiency of calcium may lead to osteoporosis.[24,25]

Nutrient Intake in Vegetarians

Unless they are very careful to balance their diet, vegetarians and vegans could be especially at risk for protein, zinc, vitamin B_{12}, vitamin D, iron and calcium deficiencies.[26,27] Vegans may be at the most risk as they abstain from consuming foods derived from any animal source, meaning that even cheese may be completely eliminated from the diet. This minimizes their food selections and ultimately may limit their intake of optimal amounts of vitamins and minerals.[28,29] Additionally, excess fiber intake may hinder the absorption of some vitamins and minerals and may further impact those who consume foods derived from fruit and vegetable sources only.

High Endurance, Low Intake

Athletes who engage in very intense training activities may have greater requirements for vitamins and minerals. Specifically they may lose some minerals through sweat.[30,31] These minerals include the electrolytes sodium, potassium and chloride. Also, athletes and fitness enthusiasts who regularly engage in calorie-restricted diets may put themselves into a state of nutritional deficiency; for example, many wrestlers and boxers go on calorie-restricted diets to "make weight" for a competition. During this period of fasting, their nutritional requirements may be far from being met. Likewise, bodybuilders, fitness competitors and dancers who engage in periodic sessions of fasting and/or calorie restrictions may be putting themselves at risk for at least short-term nutrient deficiencies.

RECAP

Although some nutritionists frown upon vitamin and mineral supplementation, there is *some* agreement that certain groups of the population may benefit. These groups include the following examples:

- Female athletes categorically are at risk due to their tendency to minimize their caloric intake. A known condition of female athletes is called the "female athlete triad."
- Women in general are at risk for iron deficiencies.
- Strict vegans and vegetarians are at risk. Some key nutrients can only be obtained from consuming foods from animal sources or consuming fortified foods.
- High-fiber diets may suppress the optimal absorption of micronutrients.
- Athletes who regularly engage in calorie-restricted diets while maintaining an active lifestyle may be at risk for nutrient deficiencies.

The "Establishment"

If you're semi health-conscious you may look at a nutritional label from time to time and notice sections regarding Recommended Dietary Allowance (RDA) and Daily Values (DV). These refer to suggested daily intake levels for nutrients. You may even take into consideration the actual percentages of vitamins (and minerals) that are contained in a particular product. But if you're like the average consumer, you may just glance at the product label, see that it lists some vitamins and feel good that you're getting at least *some* of your daily requirements of essential nutrients.

The percentages listed on labels are the amount of vitamins and minerals contained in the product relative to the amount that a panel of scientists and nutritionists feel you need on a daily basis; for instance, if you see that a product label that states that a serving contains 10 percent of the daily value (DV) for vitamin C, then that is 10 percent of the total amount that has been established for a typical daily intake of 2,000 calories per day. You should be able to look at various product labels to determine how many vitamins and minerals you are consuming each day, although keep in mind that if you're an active individual or an athlete, you may require more or fewer calories per day than the recommended 2,000, meaning your vitamin and mineral needs may change as well.

The original guidelines for consumption of vitamins and minerals (RDA) were established in order to keep the average person healthy while warding off some common diseases—nothing more, nothing less.

The Birth of Confusion and Controversy

The Food and Nutrition Board (FNB) of the National Academy of Sciences was established in 1940 and issued the first set of RDAs in 1941 for calories and nine essential nutrients, including protein, iron, calcium, vitamin A, vitamin D, thiamin, riboflavin, niacin and vitamin C. Since then, the FNB has expanded their recommendations on nutrient intake guidelines as science progressed. The guidelines established the definition of recommended dietary allowances as follows: "The levels of intake of essential nutrients that, on the basis of scientific knowledge, are judged by the Food and Nutrition Board to be adequate to meet the known nutrient needs of practically all healthy persons." The "practically all healthy persons" portion of that definition is one of the key foundations for

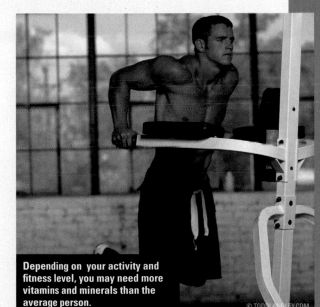

Depending on your activity and fitness level, you may need more vitamins and minerals than the average person.

controversy, specifically between scientists/dieticians and the athletic community. On one hand, you've got the scientific community stating that their established guidelines for vitamins and minerals are plenty for most people, including people with very active lifestyles. On the other hand, you've got supplement companies and athletes standing firm in their defense of ingesting higher levels of these nutrients.

There are few studies that validate the benefit of consuming elevated levels of vitamins and minerals (over the established recommendations). There are far more studies that conclude the exact opposite; however, studies can be deceiving. The practice of studying vitamins and mineral requirements for physically active individuals is relatively uncharted territory. Specifically, ongoing studies that establish vitamin and mineral requirements of extreme athletes (runners, bodybuilders, cyclists and wrestlers, for example) are not easy to find or they are non-existent altogether. This leads to a big grey area in clarifying the nutrient needs for performance athletes.

A Closer Look

Let's go back to exploring the RDA for a moment to gain a better understanding of what's behind this difference in thinking. The RDA is a set of recommendations established by the Food and Nutrition Board of the National Research Council for the intake of substances that the body needs to function normally. These amounts are estimates that are updated regularly (usually about every five years) to reflect the latest research findings. Since the goal is to establish nutrient intake for "normal" functions and not "optimal" performance, exercise enthusiasts may be skeptical of these generalizations.

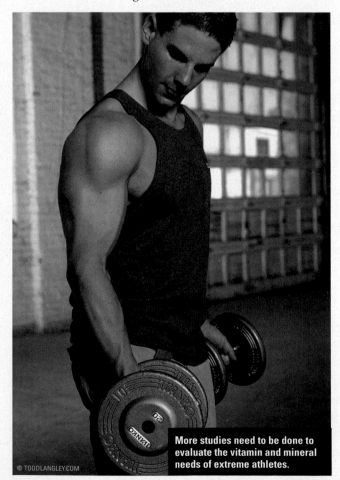

© TODDLANGLEY.COM

More studies need to be done to evaluate the vitamin and mineral needs of extreme athletes.

This brings us to the DV (Daily Value), which is based on parameters established by the Federal Department of Agriculture (FDA). These parameters include daily reference values (DRVs)—recommended intake of protein, carbohydrates, fat and fiber—and referenced daily intakes (RDIs), which are based on the RDA. The DV percentage is a blanket value that encompasses the average nutritional needs of most healthy individuals within all of these various RDAs. It is this blanket DV value that is used on food labels, and it provides a way for you to gauge the amount of a vitamin or mineral present in a serving of food.

However, the term "healthy" for the RDA and "healthy" for a fitness enthusiast may mean two completely different things. Also, "average" is a word that may need clarifying. How can you tell whether or not you're an average American? If you feel completely out of place in a fast food restaurant, you may *not* be average. If your favorite activity isn't sitting on the couch eating potato chips, you may *not* be average. If you'd rather go for a hike instead of play a video game, you may *not* be average.

So, where does this leave you? It may still seem ambiguous as to what the recommendation really is. "Should I up my intake of vitamins and minerals or not?" Well, the point of this chapter isn't to give you a definitive "yes" or an absolute "no." Rather, the goal is to give you an overview of facts that may help you to make an informed decision based on your diet and assess potential gaps in your vitamin and mineral intakes. Maybe this questionnaire will help you to start formulating a decision.

	QUESTION	Yes	No
1.	Are you a vegetarian or strict vegan?		
2.	Do you regularly engage in strenuous activities?		
3.	Are you guilty of not eating several servings of green vegetables each day?		
4.	Are you guilty of not eating several servings of red, yellow and orange vegetables each day?		
5.	Do you eat canned vegetables?		
6.	Do you boil or fry your vegetables?		
7.	Do you ever engage in calorie-restricted diets?		
8.	Do you have a high-stress job?		
9.	Are you regularly stressed due to personal situations?		
10.	Do you smoke?		
11.	Do you drink regularly?		
12.	Are you a "partier" (regular, excessive drinking)?		
13.	Do you drink caffeinated beverages such as coffee, tea or colas?		
14.	Do you regularly eat fast food?		
15.	Do you regularly get sick (barring real medical issues), such as frequent colds?		
16.	Do you eat "store-bought" vegetables and not the vine-ripened organic ones?		

Now add up your "yes" and "no" answers. If you answered "yes" more than you answered "no", you could be a candidate for needing additional vitamin and mineral intake. Check the "yes" or "no" boxes as they apply:

Size Matters

With a lengthy background to vitamins and minerals behind us, we can finally address the burning question; "What exactly *are* vitamins and minerals?" To explain what vitamins and minerals are is a daunting task to be sure. The deeper you delve into this subject, the more complicated it can get. Maybe that's the reason why many people just pop a few multivitamin pills and forget about it. Taking vitamins and minerals for granted is fine for the average consumer but if you're reading this book, you're far from average. You want to know how vitamins and minerals fit into the equation of your quest to meet and exceed your fitness goals.

Generally speaking, vitamins and minerals are obtained from the foods we eat. These vitamins and minerals are nutrients that are considered essential, meaning our bodies can't synthesize them and therefore, we must consume foods containing them. Nutrients are categorized into two general classifications: "micronutrients" and "macronutrients." Vitamins and minerals are considered to be micronutrients. A micronutrient is one that is needed in small (micro) amounts; they are typically measured in microgram or milligram quantities. This is in contrast to the other classification of foods—the macronutrients—and include protein, fats, carbohydrates and water. Our bodies absorb the vitamins and minerals from the macronutrients that we eat.

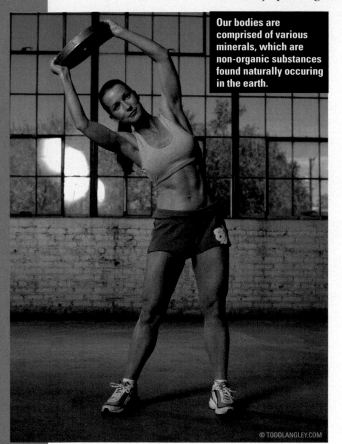

Our bodies are comprised of various minerals, which are non-organic substances found naturally occuring in the earth.

© TODDLANGLEY.COM

Minerals: Inexpensive yet Invaluable

Minerals are considered to be "non-organic" because they are found naturally occurring in the earth. In other words, they aren't produced by any living organism— they're just there; therefore, minerals are some of the lowest common denominators of life. They cannot be broken down, metabolized or processed into another form. Some of these basic elements include calcium, potassium, magnesium, zinc, copper, iron, sodium and selenium. These minerals (and many more) are the very foundation of our body's structure and existence. Aside from all of the water (around 70 percent) our bodies are largely comprised of various minerals. You know the phrase, "ashes to ashes and dust to dust?" Eventually, we are all reduced back into dirt. The real value of these minerals, relative to their functions in the body, is very hard to estimate. How do you put a value on calcium's role in building bone mass? Ask someone with osteoporosis; they'll tell you. What is the value of iron to a woman who is anemic? What value would you place on chromium, since it helps insulin to effectively deliver proteins, carbohydrates and other nutrients to tissues? The point is that although the commercial value of the elements in your body is pretty cheap, the functional value they offer is immeasurable.

Vitamins: A Living Phenomenon

Vitamins are considered to be organic because they are produced from living organisms. Some vitamins can be produced within the human body; for example, vitamin D can be synthesized in the skin when it is exposed to sunlight.[32] Vitamin K is produced within the digestive tract by microorganisms.[33,34] The rest of the vitamins can only be obtained from eating a variety of foods, some of which are from animal sources. Vitamin B_{12} for instance, can *only* be found naturally in animal sources such as beef, liver, eggs and cheese. If you do not eat animal foods, you would need to meet your vitamin B_{12} needs by eating fortified foods.

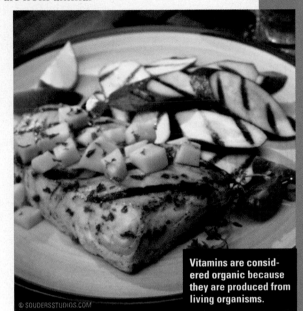

© SOUDERSSTUDIOS.COM

Vitamins are considered organic because they are produced from living organisms.

Certain vitamins act as catalysts for processes in the body. They help to optimize countless biological functions, ensuring that your body is working to its full potential; however, vitamins do not provide energy in themselves; instead they assist in producing energy. For example, B vitamins play a very important part in releasing energy from foods, assisting in the production of ATP, the metabolism of carbohydrates, red blood cell formation, and assisting in maintaining the lining of nerve cells.

Vitamins are classified into two, general categories: fat and water soluble. The terms "fat soluble" and "water soluble" simply refer to how vitamins are transported and stored in the body. The fat-soluble vitamins A, D, E and K are transported with fats throughout the body and are stored in fatty tissues and the liver. Since they are stored in fatty tissues, fat-soluble vitamins stay in the body for an extended period of time. Water-soluble vitamins (vitamin C and B vitamins) move a little freer as they are transported along with water. They are eliminated from the body fairly quickly, which is why your urine may take on a "highlighter-yellow" color an hour or so after taking a multivitamin.

No Escape

Many vitamins and certain minerals can play a role in antioxidant protection against the damaging effects of free radicals.[35] The terms "free radical" and "antioxidant" are overused and often misunderstood. A lot of products tout ingredients with "powerful antioxidant" effects as a major selling point. "Combat free radicals" is another overly used slogan. Through all of the marketing hype, the average consumer may recognize the importance of ingesting antioxidants as a means to fight free radical damage. It is generally understood that free radicals are linked to ailments such as arthritis, heart disease and immune system dysfunction;[36,37,38] however, ask five different people what free radicals are and you'll get five different answers.

Free radicals are molecules that lack a stable electronic charge. They are currently thought to play a significant role in the formation of many diseases, including atherosclerosis and neurodegeneration. Our bodies have elaborate defense systems to fight these free radicals, and this defense system includes antioxidants such as vitamins E and C, carotenoids and enzymes such as superoxide dismutase, catalase, glutathione peroxidase and glutathione reductase.[39,40,41]

Since free radicals lack that stable electric charge, they may "steal" an electron from unsuspecting nearby compounds in a healthy cell in your body. The healthy cell could be from muscle, fat, tendon, bone or almost any other example you can think of. Once the free radical "steals" the electron from a compound inside the healthy cell, the healthy cell now contains a compound that is unstable and essentially becomes a free radical. It "steals" an electron from the neighboring cell, which in turn, becomes unstable. This process can easily get out of hand and spread through healthy tissues like wild fire.

If left unchecked, free radicals can weaken the integrity of the cell to which they have attached. Visualize the free radical as "shorting out" the cell and draining its energy, kind of like a car battery with an exposed wire. If you have exposed wires on your battery cables that are touching metal, chances are your battery will be dead the next time you try to start your car. When that happens, healthy cells can be drained of their energy, weakened or destroyed altogether.

Unfortunately, there's no way to avoid free radicals. They're everywhere. A major misconception is that they only come from pollution—not true. Although pollutants such as exhaust fumes and smoke may increase free radicals, so do a lot of other things. Moving away to the pristine wilderness won't get you away from them. You'll ingest free radicals no matter what you do, no matter where you go. There is no escape. Take a drink of coffee—you're getting them. Have a sandwich, they're probably there. Even strenuous exercise can increase the effects of free radicals in the body. The answer to combating free radicals is in the refuge of antioxidants.

Antioxidants are a class of compounds that have the ability to "share" that missing electron with a free radical. The end result is a free radical that attaches to an antioxidant instead of a healthy cell. When this occurs, the free radical becomes stable and is rendered harmless. It may then be excreted from the body. There are a lot of substances that offer antioxidant effects, many of which are vitamins and minerals. Examples of common vitamin and mineral antioxidants include vitamin C, vitamin E and the mineral selenium.[42]

We are fortunate that some vitamins are water soluble and some vitamins are fat-soluble. This helps us to get antioxidant support in all areas of our bodies; both the liquid and the fatty regions.

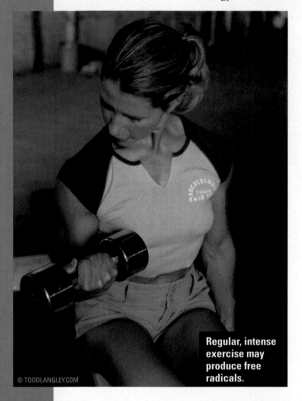

Regular, intense exercise may produce free radicals.

© TODDLANGLEY.COM

Too Much of a Good Thing?

One of the big concerns—and hypes—has to do with the toxicity of vitamins and minerals. Some sources might suggest that consuming in excess of 200 percent of the RDA could lead to a toxic buildup of certain micronutrients. But is this true? Well, there is a potential for a buildup of certain vitamins and minerals from consuming elevated doses of these nutrients. The fat-soluble vitamins, for instance, are often at the receiving end of this finger-pointing. Since fat-soluble vitamins are stored in fatty tissues, they may stay in the body for an extended period of time. Theoretically, you could build excessive stores of fat-soluble vitamins if your rate of intake exceeds your use and excretion. In other words, an overlapping effect could occur if you ingest vitamins at a rate faster than your body can eliminate them.

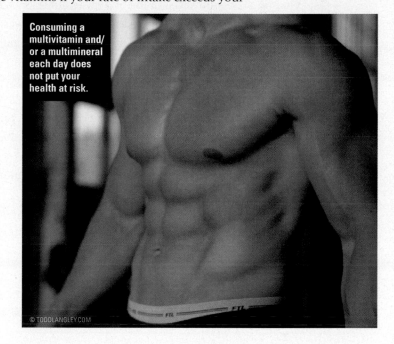

Consuming a multivitamin and/or a multimineral each day does not put your health at risk.

© TODDLANGLEY.COM

Although the word "toxic" may bring up visions of industrial waste and strange mutations, those fears generally don't apply to vitamins and minerals. The word generally was used because you definitely want to limit your intake of certain micronutrients; heavy metals such as mercury and hazardous elements such as arsenic are two good examples. Those minerals would definitely cause some reactions. Relative to normal consumption of micronutrients such as with multivitamin/mineral products and vitamin/mineral-fortified foods, the word "toxicity" isn't necessarily synonymous with "life threatening."

For the sake of our topic of vitamins and minerals, maybe we should rephrase the word "toxic" to "noted observable effect" due to overload or chronic high doses. A noted observable effect from vitamins and minerals could be as insignificant as a minor headache or as uncomfortable as diarrhea. For instance, some people may experience an upset stomach or suffer diarrhea when they consume high doses of vitamin E from supplements. A large dose of niacin may cause a flushing effect. High doses of beta carotene may cause the skin to take on an orange hue. All of these effects are not permanent and are eliminated when the particular vitamin and/or minerals doses are reduced.

Now, these points weren't made to minimize the potential hazards of vitamin and minerals. You shouldn't walk away from this chapter scoffing at the established vitamin and mineral recommendations. These recommendations were established for your safety; however, it isn't likely that consuming a multivitamin/mineral product each day will put you at risk for micronutrient toxicity.

RECAP

Where does this leave us? Let's take a moment to summarize:

- Vitamins and minerals are considered to be "micronutrients."
- Minerals are non-organic compounds found naturally occurring in the earth.
- Most vitamins are naturally occurring organic compounds and can be found in plants; some are derived from animal sources.
- Vitamin D is synthesized in the body when the skin is exposed to direct sunlight.
- Vitamin K is produced by microorganisms in the digestive tract.
- Vitamins can be classified as fat-soluble or water-soluble.
- Fat-soluble vitamins are A,D,E,K.
- Water-soluble vitamins are vitamin C and B vitamins.
- Fat-soluble vitamins are stored in the body for an extended period of time.
- Water-soluble vitamins are flushed out of the body continuously throughout the day.
- Vitamins themselves do not provide energy. Rather, they assist the body in optimizing countless functions.
- Certain fat-soluble vitamins, such as preformed vitamin A and vitamin D, may have the most risk for toxicity.
- Sensible use of vitamin- and mineral-fortified foods won't put people at risk.
- In most cases, you would have to work hard at reaching the safe upper limits of vitamin and mineral consumption.

PART II: VITAMINS, MINERALS AND SPORTS PERFORMANCE

The purpose of this section is not to promote increasing your intake of a particular vitamin or mineral; it is to further define the profound importance of these micronutrients. Consider that a deficiency in any one vitamin or mineral means that some process, somewhere in your body, may not be functioning optimally. This could ultimately hinder your performance, recovery, energy levels and ability to grow new muscle tissue.

Although vitamins and minerals may have overlapping effects in the body, they will be categorized here as they relate to insulin support, bone formation, blood formation, energy metabolism and muscular function. A complete list of vitamins and minerals, along with their functions, doses, sources and upper limits can be found at the end of this section.

Insulin: It Does a Body Good

The word insulin is often associated with diabetes; however, insulin is not just a concern for diabetics. It's a concern for all of us. Insulin is a hormone with a primary function of nutrient delivery and storage. Insulin is released from the pancreas when foods are ingested, escorting glucose (blood sugar) and nutrients to the body's tissues and organs.[43] Due to its nutrient-storing abilities, insulin is considered to be anabolic (muscle-building) in nature.[44]

Because insulin plays such a key role in delivering nutrients throughout the body, performance athletes are highly interested in optimizing its effects. In essence, the more efficiently insulin can deliver nutrients to tissues, the faster recovery and new growth can occur; however, insulin is simply a messenger. It just delivers nutrients to where they are needed, meaning that insulin will deliver nutrients to fat cells as well as muscle cells. For this reason, fitness enthusiasts want to maximize the effects of insulin in the muscle cells and not in the fat cells.

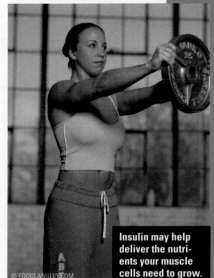

© TODDLANGLEY.COM

Insulin may help deliver the nutrients your muscle cells need to grow.

If insulin is able to do its job with maximum efficiency, more nutrients are able to be delivered and packed into muscle cells. This may equate to better "pumps," volumization, nutrient stores for energy and an increased potential for faster recovery and new muscle growth. Although chromium plays a role in insulin action, consuming excess levels won't necessarily "super-charge" the effects of insulin in healthy athletes; however, people with a chromium deficiency may experience improved insulin activity by upping their intake of chromium.

A Bone to Pick with You

Bones are not just solid, dead structures as some would believe. On the contrary, bones are comprised of intricate, multi-layered tissues fed through nerves and blood vessels. Bones are composed of the ridged, calcified tissue that makes up the skeletal structure. The importance of "feeding" your bones with vitamins and minerals may best be illustrated by the following list of attributes:

- **Mineral Storage:** Bones store calcium, phosphorous and other minerals used by the body.
- **Protection:** Bones protect the body and internal organs from injury. For instance, the spine and skull protect the central nervous system.
- **Movement:** Bones provide a structure for muscular attachment. When a muscle contracts, the bones act as levers.
- **Blood Cell Formation:** Red blood cells and some white blood cells are formed in the marrow of bones. Red blood cells carry oxygen throughout the body and white blood cells fight infections.
- **Structure and Support:** The skeletal system provides a framework of support for the body. For instance, the bones of the leg and back support your body's entire weight.

With such an array of vital functions, it should be apparent that bones need to be fed with a constant supply of key vitamins and minerals. Some of the most important micronutrients for bone health include calcium, phosphorous and vitamins A, D and K.[45,46,47,48,49,50,51]

Calcium is well-known for its role in bone health; however, the body prioritizes the balance of calcium in the blood stream over bone tissue. This means that when a deficiency of calcium exists in the body, calcium is stripped from bone tissue in order to regain normal blood-calcium levels. If calcium is not replaced through the diet, the bones will be subject to osteoporosis. By the way, osteoporosis translates into "bone holes." Too many of these "holes" will equate to a weakened skeletal structure that cannot support an active lifestyle.

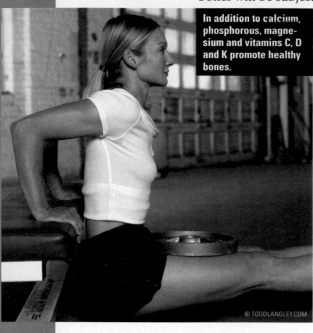

In addition to calcium, phosphorous, magnesium and vitamins C, D and K promote healthy bones.

© TODDLANGLEY.COM

Phosphorous is highly a concentrated mineral in bone matter. Not only is it used to create strong bones and teeth, it is released to be used in many processes in the body, including the formation of ATP in muscle cells. Fortunately, phosphorous deficiencies are rare in the U.S. because it is readily found in many foods and beverages such as in soft drinks. Although phosphorous content may be a redeeming factor of soft drinks, that's not necessarily a reason to go out and start guzzling more of them.

Magnesium and vitamins C, D and K all play a vital role in promoting healthy bones. Collectively these nutrients assist in binding calcium and phosphorous into bone, support the production of osteocalcin (produced by the bone forming cells, osteoblasts) and the connective tissue that attaches to bone called collagen.

Some Bloody Good Stuff

Blood is certainly the elixir of life. It circulates through your veins and arteries to deliver oxygen and nutrients. It transfers waste products to organs that can eliminate them, transports white blood cells and antibodies to fight infections and circulates heat throughout the body. It goes without saying that consuming vitamins and minerals that support a healthy blood supply are of utmost importance. Simply put, healthier blood equals better oxygen delivery, which equals the ability to perform exercise with greater intensity.

Iron is most often recognized as a blood-supporting nutrient. It is necessary for the formation of hemoglobin in red blood cells that carry and deliver oxygen throughout the body. Hemoglobin also carries carbon dioxide (a waste product) from tissues to the lungs where it can be eliminated into the air by exhaling. But iron can't create hemoglobin on its own; it needs copper to transform dietary iron into a form that the body can use.

Folate and vitamin B_{12} may be overlooked as blood-supporting nutrients. Folate and B_{12} are used in the process of cell division, particularly in red blood cells. A deficiency of folate or B_{12} may lead to abnormally large blood cells that do not function properly. Specifically, these large cells cannot carry oxygen or remove carbon dioxide effectively. Basically this means that a folate or B_{12} deficiency could leave you gasping for air during intense exercise.

Set Them Free: Releasing Energy from Foods

The breakdown and release of nutrients from foods could not occur without the help of some key vitamins: the B vitamins and biotin (vitamin H) to be specific. The exact processes through which these vitamins help to release energy from foods are far too complicated for this article. Go to a scientific journal to learn more about them if you would like. The most important thing to know is that these vitamins assist in protein, fat and carbohydrate metabolism. Some of these processes occur during exercise itself, such as in the release of blood sugar for energy from glycogen stores (sugar in the muscles).

Individuals who exercise may have higher energy and protein requirements and may equate to a need for increased intakes of B vitamins. The logic goes like this: Since B vitamins are required for the metabolism of protein and carbohydrates, an elevated intake of those nutrients may require an elevated level of B vitamins to metabolize them; however, to definitively say "yes" you *need* additional B vitamins just because you exercise or eat a lot of food is not feasible. As described earlier in the chapter, there are a lot of factors to consider when determining if vitamin and mineral supplementation is right for your particular needs and/or lifestyle.

Vitamins, Minerals and Muscular Function

There are a multitude of vitamins and minerals that effect muscular function, both directly and indirectly. For the sake of this article, we should try to stick with some of the micronutrients that have a more direct effect. These nutrients include sodium, potassium, phosphorous, calcium and B vitamins.

Sodium and potassium are two minerals that are sometimes called "electrolytes" because of their role in the body as conductors. These micronutrients allow electrical impulses to pass throughout the body and control vital functions such as muscular activity. These minerals are

Common Terms

Daily Values (DV)—Recommended nutrient intake levels used in food labeling based on referenced daily intakes (RDIs) and daily reference values (DRVs) for a standard 2,000-calorie diet.

Dietary Reference Intakes (DRI)—A set of four reference values, including EAR, RDA, AI and UL. The DRIs are levels of nutrient intake intended for use as reference values for planning and assessing diets for healthy people.

- Estimated Average Requirements (EAR)—Nutrient intake levels recommended to meet the needs of half the population of healthy people.
- Adequate Intakes (AI)—Tentative recommended nutrient intake levels based on less conclusive scientific information but are the best guess based on available scientific knowledge to date.
- Tolerable Upper Intake Levels (UL)—Upper limits of recommended nutrient intake values for health and without adverse incident in the majority of the population.
- Recommended Dietary Allowances (RDA)—Recommended nutrient intake levels to meet the needs of practically (over 98 percent) all healthy people while decreasing the risk for certain chronic diseases. The RDAs are based on age and gender, with recommendations for pregnancy and lactating women.

also important for maintaining proper fluid balances in the body, including the volumization of muscle cells. Those who sweat profusely during intense exercise may need to replace their electrolyte stores regularly.

Phosphorous and calcium play critical roles in muscular contractions. Phosphorous is a key component of ATP molecules (adenosine tri-phosphate) which are the "energy machines" inside of muscle cells. ATP is most beneficial for short duration, high intensity activities such as weight lifting. Three phosphate minerals are attached to each adenosine molecule. When one of the phosphates breaks loose, energy is released and muscular contractions can occur.

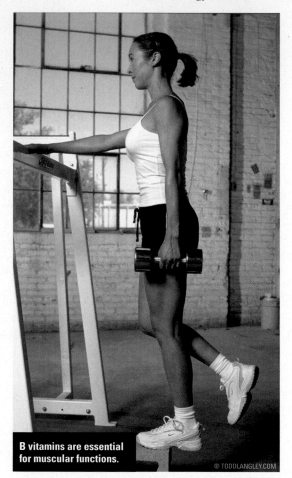

B vitamins are essential for muscular functions.

© TODDLANGLEY.COM

The only problem is that you are left with ADP (adenosine di-phospate). This is an adenosine with two phosphates instead of the preferred three. In order to increase your power output, you want the adenosine to have an instant supply of free phosphates to turn ADP back into ATP. Phosphorous supplies the body with the phosphates necessary to complete this process. Simply stated: no phosphates, no ATP. No ATP, no muscular contractions. Calcium is also involved with this process, although the specifics are complicated to describe. Just know that the presence of calcium in muscle allows the individual muscle fibers to pull against each other to create the actual contractions.

B vitamins may be overlooked as essential nutrients for muscular functions; however, without them, your body wouldn't be able to create energy from the foods you eat. Specifically, B vitamins assist in releasing and metabolizing carbohydrates, proteins and fats from foods. Although that summarizes their function as a whole, the individual B vitamins offer specialized activities in the body. For instance, some B vitamins assist in the production of ATP and others help in turning muscle sugar (glycogen) into blood sugar (glucose) for immediate energy.

Since B vitamins are water soluble, they are flushed out of the body on a continual basis. For fitness enthusiasts, this makes replacing B-vitamin stores in the body an important issue.

The importance of vitamins and minerals for your overall health and fitness performance should be glaringly apparent. Micronutrients assist in processes throughout the body and directly impact your ability to exercise, recover and form new muscle tissue and a strong skeletal system. Does this necessarily mean that you need to run out and start hyper-dosing on vitamins and minerals? No, this just means that you need to pay close attention to what you are eating. A deficiency in any one vitamin or mineral may mean that some biological process somewhere in the body may not be working at optimal levels. This could ultimately hinder your performance. You know the phrase, "You are what you eat."

For more information on recommended amounts of vitamins and minerals, and their functions in your body, please turn to the Appendix.

Chapter Summary

Dieticians and nutritionists are to some degree opposed to vitamin and mineral supplementation. On the other hand, fitness enthusiasts believe that "more is better." The purpose of this chapter wasn't to sway your thinking in either direction; only to give you a reasonable perspective on the subject matter so you could come to your own conclusions. Since there are so many variables involved with consuming and maintaining adequate levels of micronutrients, it may make sense for some people to use additional vitamins and minerals as an "insurance policy" against deficiencies.

Consider that those concerned with their fitness want to ensure that their bodies are functioning at optimal levels at all times. Any single biological process that is not working to its full potential may ultimately lead to hindered performance. This potential is unacceptable for those wanting to better their athletic performance. Under certain conditions, even the "average Joe" may need a little help achieving their RDA. These "conditions" include poor dietary habits, excessive stress, smoking, drinking and living in areas with elevated levels of pollution.

If you've determined that supplementing with additional vitamins and minerals is right for your particular needs then your next questions are probably, "What's the

RECOMMENDED READING

Manore, M and Thompson, J eds. *Sports Nutrition for Health Performance* (Human Kinetics, 2000)

Phlllips, B. *Sports Supplement Review* (Third Edition) (Mile High Publishing, 1997)

Fogelholm, M and Burke, L, Deakin, V eds. Vitamin, mineral and antioxidant needs of athletes. In *Clinical Sports Nutrition* (Second Edition) (McGraw Hill Publishing, 2000)

Volpe, S and Rosenbloom, CA ed.Vitamins and minerals for active people. In *Sports Nutrition: A Guide for the Professional Working with Active People* (Third Edition) (American Dietetic Association, 2000)

best vitamin/mineral supplement and where can I get it?" Although those are valid questions, they won't be completely answered here. This isn't a review of vitamin and mineral products. There are a lot of vitamin and mineral products available, some of them are good, some of them are not worth the money. Just do your homework, ask some questions at your local retailer and go with what makes sense for you.

An easy way to guard against nutritional deficiencies is to consume one or two vitamin/mineral-fortified meal replacement products each day. For more information on meal-replacement products, please go to Chapter 4. Many of these products, such as EAS Myoplex®, include up to 50 percent or more of the RDA of vitamins and minerals. If you don't like meal-replacement products or if you are an extremely busy individual, then vitamin/mineral tablets or capsules may make sense, but try not to take them on an empty stomach. Food helps to hold the product in your stomach and small intestine for an extended period of time, increasing the likelihood that it will be more completely broken down and absorbed.

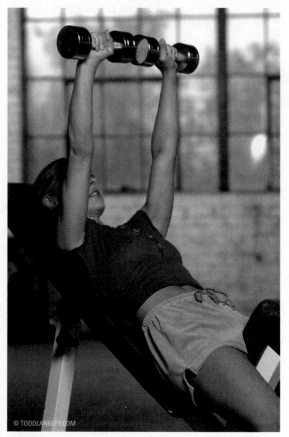

© TODDLANGLEY.COM

The final point has to do with vitamin and mineral "toxicity." Many nutritionists sternly warn against exceeding 200 percent of your recommended daily allowance; however, as the vitamin and mineral chart demonstrates, it would take substantially more than 200 percent of your RDA to even start reaching levels that would result in any noted observable effects (barring real medical issues, of course). If you want to take a vitamin/mineral supplement but don't think you need the full dose as recommended on the bottle try this: consume quality whole foods and maybe have one vitamin/mineral capsule per day. This may help you to guard against nutritional deficiencies while stretching your supplement dollar.

Always remember that no pill, capsule, tablet or supplement can take the place of a sensible nutrition plan and hard training. Nutritional products should only be used to enhance an already sound regimen. In this manner they may help to optimize your nutritional plan and performance by guarding against nutritional deficiencies.

REFERENCES CITED:

[1] US Department of Agriculture, Agricultural Research Service USDA National Nutrient Database for Standard Reference, Release 16. Nutrient Data Laboratory Home Page, http://www.nal.usda.gov/fnic/foodcomp (2003)

[2] Need, AG, Kemp, A et al. Relationships between intestinal calcium absorption, serum vitamin D metabolites and smoking in postmenopausal women. *Osteoporos Intl* 13.1 (2002): 83-88.

[3] Brot, C, Jorgensen, NR, Sorensen, OH. The influence of smoking on vitamin D status and calcium metabolism. *Eur J Clin Nutr* 53.12 (1999): 920-926.

[4] Schectman, G, Byrd, JC and Gruchow, HW. The influence of smoking on vitamin C status in adults. *Am J Public Health* 79.2 (1989): 158-62.

[5] Liu, CS and Chen, HW et al. Alterations of small-molecular-weight antioxidants in the blood of smokers. *Chem Biol Interact* 116.1-2 (1998): 143-154.

[6] Faruque, MO, Khan, MR et al. Relationship between smoking and antioxidant nutrient status. *Br J Nutr* 73.4 (1995): 625-632.

[7] Vermaak, WJ and Ubbink, JB et al. Vitamin B-6 nutrition status and cigarette smoking. *Am J Clin Nutr* 51.6 (1990): 1058-1061.

[8] Tungtrongchitr, R, Pongpaew, P et al. Relationship of tobacco smoking with serum vitamin B12, folic and haematological indices in healthy adults. *Public Health Nutr* 6.7 (2003): 675-681.

[9] Eggleton, MG. The diuretic action of alcohol in man. *J Physiol (Lond)* 101 (1942): 172-191.

[10] Jacques, PF, Sulsky, S et al. Moderate alcohol intake and nutritional status in nonalcoholic elderly subjects. *Am J Clin Nutr* 50.4 (1989): 875-883.

[11] Bregheim, I, Parlesak, A et al. Nutritional deficiencies in German middle-class male alcohol consumers: relationship to dietary intake and severity of liver disease. *Eur J Clin Nutr* 57.3 (2003): 431-438.

[12] Hasling, C, Sondergaard, K et al. Calcium metabolism in postmenopausal osteoporotic women is determined by dietary calcium and coffee intake. *J Nutr* 122.5: 1119-1126.

[13] Department of Health and Human Services Dietary Intake of Macronutrients, Micronutrients, and Other Dietary Constituents: United States, 1988-1994. Vital and Health Statistics; Series 11, Number 245. Centers for Disease Control and Prevention. National Center for Health Statistics, Hyattsville, Maryland, DHHA Publication No. (PHS) (2002): 1695.

[14] Looker, AC, Dallman, PR et al. Prevalence of iron deficiency in the United States. *JAMA* 277.12 (1997): 973-976.

[15] Centers for Disease Control and Prevention. Iron Deficiency – United States, 1999-2000. *MMWR* 51 (2002): 897-899.

[16] Lieu, PT, Heiskala, M et al. The roles of iron in health and disease. *Mol Aspects Med* 22.1-2 (2001): 1-87.

[17] Ross, EM. Evaluation and treatment of iron deficiency in adults. *Nutr Clin Care* 5.5 (2002): 220-224.

[18] Golden, NH. A review of the female athlete triad (amenorrhea, osteoporosis and disordered eating). *Int J Adolesc Med Health* 14.1 (2002): 9-17.

[19] Sabatini, S. The female athlete triad. *Am J Med Sci* 322.4 (2001): 193-195.

[20] Hobart, HA and Smucker, DR. The female athlete triad. *Am Fam Physician* 61.11 (2000): 3357-3364, 3367.

[21] Sanborn, CF, Horea, M et al. Disordered eating and the female athlete triad. *Clin Sports Med* 19.2 (2000): 199-213.

[22] Malczewska, J, Raczynski, G and Stupnicki, R. Iron status in female endurance athletes and in non-atheletes. *Int J Sport Nutr Exerc Metab* 10.3 (2000): 260-276.

[23] Kim, SH, Kim, HY et al. Nutritional status, iron-deficiency-related indices, and immunity of female athletes. *Nutrition* 18.1: 86-90.

[24] Nichols, DL, Bonnick, SL and Sanborn, CF. Bone health and osteoporosis. *Clin Sports Med* 19.2 (2000): 233-249.

[25] Fujita, T. Calcium paradox: consequences of calcium deficiency manifested by a wide variety of diseases. *J Bone Miner Metab* 18.4 (2000): 234-236.

[26] Dwyer, JT. Nutritional consequences of vegetarianism. *Annu Rev Nutr* 11 (1991): 61-91.

[27] Lowik, MR, Schrijver, J et al. Long-term effects of a vegetarian diet on the nutritional status of elderly people (Dutch Nutrition Surveillance System). *J Am Coll Nutr* 9.6 (1990): 600-609.

[28] Madar, Z and Thorne, R. Dietary Fiber. *Prog Food Nutr Sci* 11.2 (1987): 153-174.

[29] Torre, M, Rodriquez, AR and Saura-Calixto, F. Effects of dietary fiber and phytic acid on mineral availability. *Crit Rev Food Sci Nutr* 30.1 (1991): 1-22.

[30] Rehrer, NJ. Fluid and electrolyte balance in ultra-endurance sport. *Sports Med* 31.10 (2001): 701-715.

[31] Maughan, RJ. Fluid and electrolyte loss and replacement in exercise. *J Sports Sci* (Summer) 9 (1991): 117-142.

[32] Norman, AW and Ziegler, EE, Filer, LJ Jr. eds. Vitamin D. In: *Present Knowledge in Nutrition* (Seventh edition) (ILSI Press, 1996) pg. 120-129.

[33] Bentley, R and Meganathan, R. Biosynthesis of vitamin K (menaquinone) in bacteria. *Microbiol Rev* 46.3 (1982): 241-280.

[34] Binkley, NC and Suttie, JW. Vitamin K nutrition and osteoporosis. *J Nutr* 125 (1995): 1812-1821.

[35] Gibaldi, M. Antioxidant vitamins and health. *J Clin Pharmacol* 36.12 (1996): 1093-1099.

[36] Haulica, I, Boisteanu, D and Bild, W. Free radicals between health and disease. *Rom J Physiol* 37.1-4 (2000): 15-22.

[37] Raha, S and Robinson, BH. Mitochondira, oxygen free radicals, disease and ageing. *Trends Biochem Sci* 25.10 (2000): 502-508.

[38] Knight, JA. Free radicals: their history and current status in aging and disease. *Ann Clin Lab Sci* 28.6 (1998): 331-346.

[39] Irshad, M and Chaudhuri, PS. Oxidant-antioxidant system: role and significance in human body. *Indian J Exp Biol* 40.11: 1233-1239.

[40] Bannister, WH and Bannister, JV. Evolutionary aspects of superoxide dismutase: the copper/zinc enzyme. *Free Radical Res Commun* 12-13.Pt 1 (1991): 349-361.

[41] Michelson, AM. Selenium glutathione peroxidase: some aspects in man. *J Environ Pathol Toxicol Oncol* 17.3-4 (1998): 233-239.

[42] McDermott, JH. Antioxidant nutrients: current dietary recommendations and research update. *J Am Pharm Assoc (Wash)* 40.6 (2000): 785-799.

[43] Sonksen, P and Sonksen, J. Insulin: understanding its action in health and disease. *Br J Anaesth* 85.1 (2000): 69-79.

[44] Taft, P. The action and uses of insulin. *Aust Fam Physician* 5.10 (1976): 1429-1431.

[45] Suda, T, Ueno, Y et al. Vitamin D and bone. *J Cell Biochem* 88.2 (2003): 259-266.

[46] Weber, P. Vitamin K and Bone Health. *Nutrition* 17.10 (2001): 880-887.

[47] Advani, S and Wimalawansa, SJ. Bones and nutrition: common sense supplementation for osteoporosis. *Curr Womens Health Rep* 3.3 (2003): 187-192.

[48] Eastell, R and Lambert, H. Strategies for skeletal health in the elderly. *Proc Nutr Soc* 61.2 (2002): 173-180.

[49] Love, C. Dietary needs for bone health and prevention of osteoporosis. *Br J Nutr* 12.1 (2003): 12-21.

[50] Rodriguez-Martinez, MA and Garcia-Cohen, EC. Role of Ca(2+) and vitamin D in the prevention and treatment of osteoporosis (2002).

[51] Meunier, PJ. Calcium, vitamin D and vitamin K in the prevention of fractures due to osteoporosis. *Osteoporosis Int* 9.Suppl 2 (1999): S48-S52.

3 WATER

Essentials of Hydration and Balancing Fluids for Performance

By Kelly James-Enger

Water: A Critical Nutritional Component

When you think about good nutrition, the thoughts that come to mind may be of consuming the right balance of macronutrients like protein, carbohydrates and fat, or of getting plenty of essential micronutrients like vitamins and minerals. But did you think of water?

If you haven't considered the importance of water as part of your overall nutrition plan, you're not alone. Everyday exercisers and athletes alike sometimes downplay, or worse yet, ignore the importance of this essential nutrient. Yet maintaining optimal hydration levels can play an important role in your performance in the gym, on the court and on the field, whether you're giving an all-out effort or simply playing for fun.

In the pages that follow, you'll learn why water is the most essential of all nutrients; how it helps you perform at your best, both in life and in fitness; and how to determine and ingest the appropriate amounts of fluid for your lifestyle and training program.

The Whys of Water

Think about it. You may be able to recall what you ate yesterday, but can you remember what—and how much—you *drank*? While there are countless books devoted to proper nutrition and effective exercise regimens, water is sometimes downplayed as an integral part of any fitness program. Part of the reason is that many people don't realize water's importance for good health, says Kristine L. Clark, Ph.D., director of the sports nutrition department at Penn State University. "People don't realize that water is one of the six classes of nutrients," says Clark. "The average person thinks of water as an insignificant beverage but it's very significant. It's like a vitamin or mineral—if you don't get enough of it, you're really missing out."

There are both health and physical performance reasons that make proper hydration important to all adults and children, agrees Larry Armstrong, Ph.D., professor of environmental and exercise physiology at the University of Connecticut. "Our bodies are made up of 60 percent water by weight, and we need to maintain that water for proper functioning of our cells and our body organs," says Armstrong. "For example, the circulatory system includes blood which is primarily water and the inside of our cells contains primarily water; thus, it's important to replace the water each day."

Our bodies also use water to convert food into energy, remove waste, regulate body temperature and carry nutrients and oxygen throughout our bodies. In fact, every system in your body—from reproduction to energy production to toxin elimination to thermoregulation—requires water to function properly.[15,16]

Consuming enough water can have long-term health consequences as well. Research suggests that appropriate fluid consumption—particularly water consumption—can have a positive effect on your risk of developing health problems including urinary stone disease; breast, colon and urinary tract cancer; and mitral valve prolapse. Drinking enough water may also help reduce rates of childhood obesity and help older people protect their health.[16]

Yet most of us walk around chronically dehydrated—and athletes aren't immune to this problem. It's easy to be dehydrated and not even realize it. "We have the ability to mask our thirst mechanism," explains Clark. "And when we do feel thirsty, we're already about 2 percent dehydrated. The feeling of thirstiness is actually a symptom of dehydration." (Dehydration is measured in percentages relating to body weight—for example, a 150-pound person who is 1 percent dehydrated has lost 1.5 pounds in water weight.)

Yet while water is a vital nutrient, the majority of Americans don't consume the amount their bodies need—a survey conducted in 2000 found that over half drink less than eight 8-ounce glasses of water a day; however, this commonly cited figure is only an estimate. Your hydration needs may fall short or exceed that number, depending on your weight, activity level and even the climate you live in. Heinz Valtin, a physiologist at Dartmouth Medical School in Lebanon, N.H., recently debated the question of the accuracy of the "8 x 8" recommendation in a journal article published in 2002. He noted that after this recommendation became widespread, people were drinking more water and more fluids overall (674 milliliters of water and 1,696 milliliters of total fluids from 1977 to 1978 compared to 841 milliliters of water and 2,188 milliliters total from 1994 to 1996 and in 1998). After a comprehensive review of the published literature, Valtin concluded that there was no scientific basis for the 8 x 8 theory, and that the data suggested that most people, absent special circumstances, were probably drinking enough water.[23]

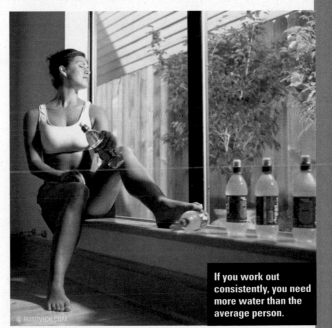

If you work out consistently, you need more water than the average person.

As a regular exerciser, you need more than the average person. Because our bodies need water to function normally, when you're dehydrated you may also feel tired, have trouble concentrating or wind up eating more than usual since it's common to misinterpret thirst as hunger. Shorting yourself on H_2O negatively affects your athletic performance, and taken to extremes, dehydration can have life-threatening consequences as well.[20]

How do you know you're dehydrated? The symptoms vary from person to person, but some of the most common include headache, loss of appetite, flushed skin, heat intolerance, light-headedness, dry mouth and eyes and a burning sensation. Your urine may be dark and scanty with a strong odor. (Tracking your urine output is an effective way of checking hydration levels that will be discussed later in this chapter.) If you're more severely dehydrated, you may experience muscle spasms, clumsiness, shriveled skin, difficulty swallowing, dim vision, painful urination and delirium.[20]

Water's Role in Athletic Performance

Since dehydration affects every system of the body, it's not surprising that it impacts athletic performance as well. If you're only minimally dehydrated, it may not be an issue, but once you lose more than that, you're likely to feel it. "From 0 percent to 2 percent of body weight loss, the responses of the body are mainly physiological, and you see few performance changes," says Armstrong. "If you lose 1 percent to 2 percent

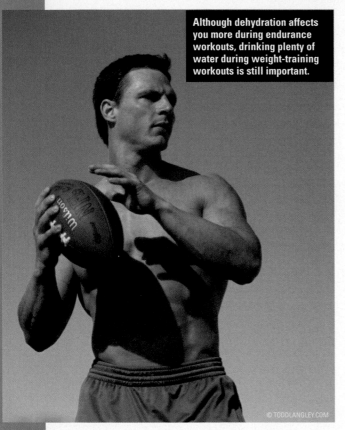

Although dehydration affects you more during endurance workouts, drinking plenty of water during weight-training workouts is still important.

© TODDLANGLEY.COM

of your body weight as water in sweat, you'll see an increased heart rate, an increased body temperature, a more concentrated blood plasma, and so forth."[8]

Lose more than 3 percent of your body weight as sweat, though, and your performance will suffer. Dozens of studies have found that performance suffers as dehydration levels increase. Dehydration results in physiological changes including increased heat strain, increased cardiovascular strain, altered central nervous system function and altered metabolic function.[2] These factors appear to interact together to affect performance, but the relative contribution of each factor depends on the event, weather conditions, athletic prowess and level of performance.[5,20]

"Lose beyond 3 percent of body weight loss as sweat, and you'll find that endurance performance is affected negatively," says Armstrong. For high-power strength performance activities—like jumping, throwing and lifting weights, the detrimental effects in performance kick in at about 5 percent. Dehydration affects endurance activities first because the loss of water affects circulation and reduces blood volume and is more important in endurance activities and less critical in high intensity events lasting less than 30 seconds, explains Armstrong.

Numerous studies have confirmed that dehydration has a more significant effect on endurance activities than on shorter-duration activities; for example, competitive runners who participated in running trials while dehydrated saw their performance suffer more at distances of 5,000 and 10,000 meters than a shorter race of 1,500 meters.[3] In another study involving endurance cyclists, the more dehydrated riders were, the higher their heart rates, the higher their core temperatures and the lower their stroke volumes or performances were.[24] Other research confirms that athletes who are dehydrated perform at significantly lower levels and report higher ratings of perceived exhaustion than when they're allowed to drink fluids during exercise.[17,20]

A review of recent studies reveals that dehydration of 2 percent to 7 percent of body weight decreases athletic performance, especially in hot environments, by as little as 7 percent to as much as 60 percent. Dehydration levels of only 1 percent to 2 percent did not affect performance in events of less than 90 minutes; however, even modest dehydration—2 percent of body weight—will affect performance in endurance events, especially if they last longer than 90 minutes. Exercising in a cooler environment can reduce this effect to some degree—an athlete who's 2 percent dehydrated will notice a decrease in performance of about 40 percent in a hot environment in a hot, dry climate and a reduction of performance of about 20 percent in a temperate one.[16]

In addition to increasing performance, proper hydration reduces your risk of heat-related illnesses. Other factors that can increase your risk of heat illness include taking diuretics, which are sometimes used to facilitate weight loss or "make weight" for sports like wrestling. Using diuretics creates a higher likelihood of becoming dehydrated and can lead to electrolyte imbalances as well. Dressing inappropriately—for example, wearing heavy clothes that don't allow sweat to wick away from the skin—can contribute to heat-related illness, and obesity can limit a person's ability to tolerate heat. Some medications and underlying conditions including diabetes, anorexia and gastrointestinal infection can also increase the risk of developing a heat illness.[22]

Heat cramps, or painful muscle contractions, are the most common heat-related illness and are caused by insufficient circulation to the cramping muscle due to dehydration. Proper hydration reduces the risk of heat cramps, and the more acclimated and fit an athlete is, the less likely he/she is to suffer from heat cramps. Heat exhaustion is another condition that can occur due to excessive sweating and can cause headache, muscle weakness, dizziness, nausea or blurred vision. Symptoms of heat exhaustion should be treated with re-hydration and rest to lower the body temperature.[22]

Heat stroke is the most serious heat-related illness and occurs when body temperature exceeds 42 degrees C. Athletes with heat stroke have elevated temperatures and may sweat profusely or have hot, pale, dry skin. This life-threatening condition should be suspected in anyone who collapses during physical activity, especially in hot weather. Treatment consists of lowering body temperature, re-hydration and immediate medical attention. If you suspect you or someone else has heat stroke, move the person to a cool place and call a doctor or ambulance right away.[22]

Staying well-hydrated will reduce the risk of heat-related illness, but other factors like body mass index (BMI) can play a role in susceptibility as well. One study of male Marine Corps recruits found that recruits with a BMI of 22 or greater and a timed 1.5 mile run of more than 12 minutes were eight times more likely to develop heat-related illness than those with a BMI of less than 22 and a 1.5-mile run time of less than 10 minutes. To help prevent heat-related illness, athletes can work toward heat acclimatization by exercising at low to moderate intensity in warm environments and gradually increasing both time spent exercising and intensity during the first 10 to 14 days of hot weather training.[11]

tip

Top Signs of Heat Stroke:
- Elevated temperature
- Profusive sweating
- Hot, pale, dry skin

The Role of Electrolytes

Proper hydration is essential not only because of your body's need for water but also to help it maintain its electrolyte balance as well. Electrolytes are dissolved substances in your body fluids. Sodium and chloride, which we commonly call table salt, account for over 80 percent of the dissolved compounds found in blood and cellular fluid. If you're lacking salt, your body water volume will be smaller because the salt and other electrolytes help your body retain the appropriate amount of fluid. That's why replacing electrolytes is important—they help maintain your body's water volume, especially in blood plasma and the fluid around your body's cells.[4,19]

How much electrolyte replacement do you need? One of the major factors is the amount of sweat produced, and the amount of electrolytes found in the sweat. For example, the amount of sodium and chloride in sweat varies widely depending on the degree of physical activity, heat exposure, how well someone is acclimated to heat and the amount of salt they consume in their diet. The amount of electrolytes in sweat is the most concentrated at the beginning of physical activity, but decreases with prolonged activity. When different types of sports were measured, researchers found that the concentration of electrolytes depended on the type of sport, level of training and duration of activity. In general, athletes who participated in high-endurance sports like cyclists and rowers had lower levels of electrolytes in their sweat than did other athletes. Fitter athletes also tend to have lower levels of sodium and chloride in their sweat.[12,22]

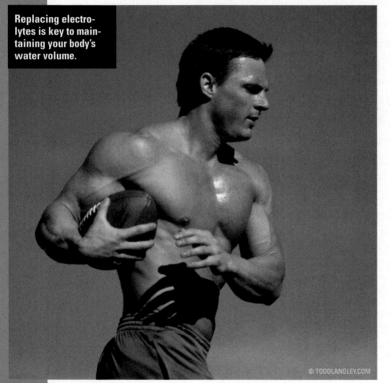

Replacing electrolytes is key to maintaining your body's water volume.

© TODDLANGLEY.COM

The mineral potassium is also lost in sweat, but its low concentration is usually fairly constant; however, some research suggests that low levels of potassium in the diet and excessive sweating could possibly lead to a potassium deficiency. And while a very small amount of magnesium is excreted in sweat, it appears that this is insufficient to cause any kind of magnesium deficiency.[4]

Usually, a healthy diet that includes some salt is sufficient to replace sufficient electrolytes that you lose from sweat, but endurance athletes like marathoners and long-distance bicyclists may benefit from drinking beverages that contain electrolytes. (See "Drinking During Exercise" later in this chapter for more.) If your electrolytes are out of balance, you run the risk of developing hyponutremia, in which your body's sodium levels are decreased to the point that you become ill and you begin to show clinical symptoms. This condition is relatively rare in all but endurance athletes, but if you drink excess water—say, 8 liters to 10 liters over the course of four to six hours—or exercise continuously for more than four hours without replacing electrolytes, you're at risk for this potentially life-threatening condition.[2]

Is Water the Best Option?

In recent years, a question has arisen as to whether water is the best fluid to maintain hydration levels, particularly for athletes training and competing at high levels. In response, a slew of enhanced beverages that contain electrolytes and/or carbohydrates have hit the market. Whether these beverages will make a difference on your performance depends on the length and intensity of exercise. The American College of Sports Medicine recommends that ingested fluids be at a cool temperature (between 59 and 72 degrees) to enhance absorption and flavored to enhance palatability and promote fluid replacement. According to a recent Position Stand on Exercise and Fluid Replacement, the ACSM says, the "Addition of proper amounts of carbohydrates and/or electrolytes to a fluid replacement solution is recommended for exercise events of duration greater than one hour since it does not significantly impair water delivery to the body and may enhance performance. During exercise lasting less than one hour, there is little evidence of physiological or physical performances differences between consuming a carbohydrate-electrolyte drink and plain water."[1] Other research supports the idea that a carbohydrate-electrolyte drink may maximize performance for activities that are longer than an hour. Other research shows the addition of protein to a carbohydrate-electrolyte drink may be beneficial. (See chapter 10 for more on this.)

In addition to sports drinks that contain electrolytes and/or carbohydrates, there are also a variety of other "designer" waters available. Some contain additional vitamins and minerals; others contain caffeine or other stimulants. The effect of these beverages isn't well studied, and it's doubtful that waters containing extra vitamins will affect your performance. However, some people find that drinking flavored water makes it more palatable, so if these designer beverages appeal to you, give them a try.

Drinking During Exercise—and Afterward

Drinking throughout the day is one thing. But drinking water before, during and after exercise is critical for athletes. The benefits of consuming fluids during exercise in particular should not be overlooked. Ingesting water or other fluids have been proven to help maintain blood volume, assist thermoregulation, reduce the risk of heat injury, provide energy and enhance performance during continuous exercise. It also appears that fluid consumption during intermittent exercise—activities like baseball, basketball, soccer and tennis—is beneficial as well.[25]

It's clear that ingesting water during exercise helps minimize the effects of dehydration and enhances exercise performance. One small study also found that consuming water during intense exercise may have metabolic consequences as well—five trained athletes who participated in a cycling exercise had higher levels

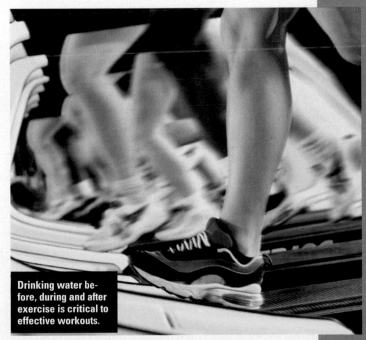

Drinking water before, during and after exercise is critical to effective workouts.

of muscle glycogen and lower levels of lactate when they consumed water during exercise than when they exercise without replacing their fluid levels; however, for activities of all but the shortest duration, adding carbohydrates can further enhance performance. The question is how much carbohydrate should be consumed, at what rate and when.

Taking in carbs during strenuous or prolonged exercise helps maintain blood glucose concentration, helping give you sustained energy levels as you work out. That

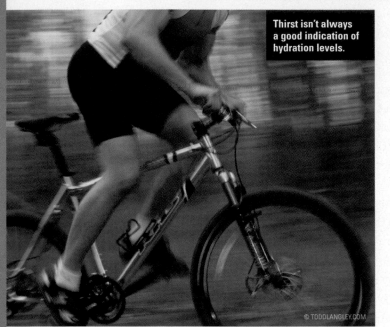

Thirst isn't always a good indication of hydration levels.

© TODDLANGLEY.COM

means you can exercise for a longer period of time and perform at a higher intensity at the end of a workout. After reviewing a number of studies, researchers at the Human Performance Laboratory at the University of Texas at Austin found that ingesting approximately 30 grams to 60 grams of carbohydrates during each hour of exercise was generally sufficient to maintain blood glucose oxidation late in exercise and delay fatigue. This translates to drinking 625 to 1,250 milliliters an hour of beverages containing 4 percent to 8 percent carbohydrate.[10]

However, taking in this amount of fluid can be easier said than done. Cyclists, for example, may find it easier to drink fluid while competing than

distance runners, who experience more stomach "sloshing" as they run.[9] For athletes who struggle with consuming enough fluids during exercise, the post-exercise period is particularly important. Unless they drink steadily to compensate for fluid losses, most athletes will be dehydrated after a workout. In fact, athletes replace only about 30 percent to 70 percent of sweat losses incurred through exercise, regardless of activity. Ideally the remaining sweat loss will be replaced post-exercise, but factors such as taste and temperature of the beverage affect how much will be consumed. In one study with dehydrated cyclists, those who drank water replaced 63 percent of their sweat losses; those who drank sweetened drinks consumed more fluids and replaced 79 percent of their fluid losses.[6]

The amount of electrolyte content may also affect hydration levels post-exercise as electrolytes can help retain fluid and reduce the amount lost through urination. In one study, exercisers who were approximately 2 percent dehydrated consumed 150 percent of their fluid losses with drinks containing varying levels of sodium. The drinks with higher levels of salt led to retaining optimal amounts of fluid while the beverages with less salt failed to completely replace the body weight loss due to sweat. The appropriate amount of electrolytes may depend on the amount of sodium lost in sweat, which on average ranges from 20 to 80 millimoles a liter; however, sports drinks like Gatorade® and POWERade® contain more moderate levels of sodium—10 to 25 millimoles a liter.[7,21]

In another study, six endurance-trained competitive male cyclists and triathletes cycled to exhaustion in a hot environment at high intensity after an hour of moderate

tip

Fluid-Loss Facts:
- Most athletes replace only 30 percent to 70 percent of sweat lost through exercise.
- Athletes report higher levels of exhaustion in a dehydrated state.
- When hydrated, athletes can exercise at high intensity almost four minutes longer.

exercise. During one attempt, they drank 400 milliliters of an artificially flavored electrolyte solution immediately before the event began; then they drank 120 milliliters every 10 minutes during the first hour of the 60-minute ride. On the other attempt, they didn't take in any fluid, resulting in loss of about 1.8 percent of their body weight in sweat. During the no-fluid attempt, each athlete performed at significantly lower levels than when she/he ingested an electrolyte-containing solution. On average, they were able to exercise at high intensity almost four minutes longer (14 minutes on average) than when they were dehydrated (10 minutes on average). They also reported higher ratings of perceived exhaustion in a dehydrated state.[24]

To promote post-exercise hydration, athletes should have a plan in place to replenish fluids and realize that they may need to consume as much as 1.5 to 2 times the volume of sweat loss to fully restore fluid balance. Replacing sodium with sports drinks or eating salty foods can help retain fluid, especially for endurance athletes, while caffeine-containing beverages and alcohol should be avoided because they may increase urine loss. To replace significant sweat losses, it appears that sports drinks may be more effective than plain water because the electrolytes they contain help retain fluids post-exercise.[2,13,25]

Water: The Basics

1. Water is an essential nutrient, and drinking too little can significantly affect how you feel and perform at home, at work and in the gym.
2. While minimal levels of dehydration (less than 2 percent) probably won't impact performance, higher levels of dehydration have a significant negative impact on exercise performance, particularly for endurance athletes. High levels of dehydration also increase an athlete's risk of heat-related illness.
3. For everyday exercisers, water is the best beverage to consume before, during and after exercise. Endurance athletes and others training at high levels may benefit from the addition of carbohydrate and electrolyte containing beverages during and post-exercise to maintain optimal levels of hydration.
4. The amount of fluid you should consume varies from person to person and depends on a number of factors including level of fitness, weather conditions, activity and sweat rate.

Fluid Recommendations:

The "eight 8-ounce glasses of water a day" idea may be a myth, but it's a decent place to start. In general, you should drink enough fluid during the day so your urine is a light yellow color. (Dark or scanty urine often indicates dehydration.) In addition, follow the ACSM's guidelines, which recommend that athletes:

- **Drink 14 to 22 ounces of fluid two to three hours before exercise**
- **Drink six to 12 ounces of fluid every 15 to 20 minutes during exercise**
- **Drink 16 to 24 ounces of fluid for every pound of body weight lost during exercise**

During and after exercise, drink enough fluid to replace all the water lost through sweating—and err on the side of consuming more than enough to ensure proper hydration. If you exercise for more than an hour at a time, you may also want to consume sports drinks to help replenish lost electrolyte stores as well.

Meeting Your Daily Water Needs

While it might seem logical that if you simply drink when you're thirsty, you'll have no hydration problems, the fact is that thirst isn't always a good indicator of hydration levels. First you have to understand how the body's thirst mechanism works. Your brain reads the concentration of your blood constantly, and when your body water level has been reduced by about 1 percent or 2 percent, you'll feel thirsty and presumably drink something. The problem is that people often don't drink *enough* to make up the difference and maintain that 1 percent to 2 percent level of dehydration over time. This so-called "involuntary dehydration" often occurs when people face a variety of stresses including exercise, hot or cold environments, altitude and water immersion, all of which increase the body's fluid needs.[14]

So how much water should you be drinking? It's probably more than you think—the average sedentary person loses about 2.5 quarts of water a day through ordinary activity alone. And if you exercise, you lose between .8 and 1.5 quarts of fluid each hour in addition to that. All of this fluid must be replaced to maintain optimal hydration.

Earlier we discussed the 8 x 8 recommendation, but recall that your water needs are probably higher than this baseline. In its Position Stand on Exercise and Fluid Replacement, the American College of Sports Medicine recommends that people drink 14 to 22 ounces of fluid two to three hours before exercise; 6 to 12 ounces of fluid every 15 to 20 minutes during exercise; and 16 to 24 ounces of fluid for every pound of body weight lost during exercise. The ACSM also recommends that athletes drink at regular intervals during exercise "at a rate sufficient to replace all the water lost through sweating (i.e., body weight loss), or consume the maximum amount that can be tolerated."[1] (The National Athletic Trainers' Association's Position Statement on Fluid Replacement for Athletes makes similar recommendations.)[18]

Complicating matters is that different people sweat at different rates, and the type of activity, weather, level of conditioning and even clothing choices can all significantly affect sweat rates. Experimenting with the appropriate water intake before competitive events will help you determine your optimal hydration levels. "When we're talking about hot environments, the sweat rate increases," says Armstrong. "Be sure to realize that your sweat rate is different under different conditions, so try to simulate an event or competition several weeks beforehand, to learn what your needs are. The average person may not be aware that they are dehydrated."

For serious athletes or competitors, weighing yourself before and after exercise is an easy, effective way to maintain proper hydration. "For every pound of body weight a person uses, it's essentially all water loss," says Armstrong. "They should replace each pound of body weight with one pint of fluid. People should also watch urine volume and urine color. If it's a pale color it means that the body is releasing fluid. If it's dark in color—dark yellow or even brown—the body is conserving water severely because it's dehydrated."

While water is always a good bet, you needn't rely only on H_2O to satisfy your fluid needs. Beverages like juice contribute to your daily total as do foods like soup, fruits and vegetables that are naturally high in water content. Because beverages that contain caffeine or alcohol can be dehydrating, however, you'll want to make sure that you drink plenty of water to offset your coffee or beer consumption. You can up your intake by having a big glass of water first thing in the morning; keeping a bottle of water on your desk at work; drinking a glass at mid-morning and mid-afternoon; and being sure to drink before, during and after exercise.

Make it one of your fitness priorities to aim for optimal hydration. If you've been drinking too little, you may notice a marked improvement in the way you feel and perform when you increase your water intake. Even if you don't notice a difference, by drinking more water you'll also be helping your body function at its best.

The Latest Research

While it's clear that proper hydration is critical for good health and athletic performance, researchers are continuing to study the unique fluid needs of different athletes participating in different types of activities. One of the areas of greatest interest is enhanced beverages—like fluids that contain carbohydrates and or electrolytes—and how they can assist athletes to maximize their performance. As the literature continues to grow, athletes will face more information and more choices about how to tweak their beverage choices, and what to drink, how much and when. For the time being, though, water is the classic and proven choice.

REFERENCES CITED:

[1] Kleiner, SM. Water: an essential but overlooked nutrient. *Journal of the American Dietetic Association* 99.2 (1999): 200-206.

[2] Horswill, CA. Effective fluid replacement. *International Journal of Sports Nutrition* 8 (1998):175-195.

[3] Valtin, H. Drink at least eight glasses of water a day. Really? Is there scientific evidence for "8x8"? *American Journal of Regulatory, Integrated and Comparative Physiology* 283 (2002): R993-R1004.

[4] Sawka, MN, Pandolf, KB. Effects of body water loss on physiological function and exercise performance. *Perspectives in Exercise Science and Sports Medicine* (1990): 1-38.

[5] Cheuvront, SN et al. Fluid balance and endurance exercise performance. *Current Sports Medicine Reports* 2 (2003): 202-208.

[6] American Dietetic Association. Position on nutrition and athletic performance. *Journal of the American Dietetic Association* 100 (2000): 1543-1556.

[7] Armstrong, LE and Maresh, CM. The induction and decay of heat acclimatization in trained athletes. *Sports Medicine* 12.5 (1991): 302-12.

[8] Armstrong, LE et al. Influence of diuretic-induced hydration on competitive running performance. *Medicine and Science in Sports and Exercise* 17.4 (1985): 456-461.

[9] Walsh, RM et al. Impaired high-intensity cycling performance time at low levels of dehydration. *International Journal of Sports Medicine* 15 (1994): 392-398.

[10] Montain, SJ and Coyle, EF. Influence of graded dehydration on hyperthermia and cardiovascular drift during exercise. *Journal of Applied Physiology* 73.4 (1992): 1340-1350.

[11] Squire, DL. Heat illness: fluid and electrolyte issues for pediatric and adolescent athletes. *Pediatric Clinics of North America* 37.5 (1990): 1085-1109.

[12] Gardner, JW et al. Risk factors predicting exertional heat illness in male Marine Corps recruits. *Medicine and Science in Sports and Exercise* 28.8 (1996): 939-944.

[13] Sawka, MN. Physiological consequences of hypohydration: exercise performance and thermoregulation. *Medicine and Science in Sports and Exercise* 24.6 (1992): 657-670.

[14] Armstrong, LE, Costill, DL and Fink, WJ. Changes in body water and electrolytes during heat acclimation: effects on dietary sodium. *Aviation, Space and Environmental Medicine* 58 (1987): 143-148.

[15] Gisolfi, CV and Duchman, SM. Guidelines for optimal replacement beverages for different athletic events. *Medicine and Science in Sports and Exercise* 24.6 (1992): 679-687.

[16] American College of Sports Medicine (ACSM). Position stand on exercise and fluid replacement. *Medicine and Science in Sports and Exercise* 28.1 (1996): i-vii.

[17] Xiaocai, S and Gisolfi, CV. Fluid and carbohydrate replacement during intermittent exercise. *Sports Medicine* 25.3 (1998): 157-172.

[18] Coyle, EF and Montain, SJ. Carbohydrate and fluid ingestion during exercise: are there trade-offs? *Medicine and Science in Sports and Exercise* 24.6 (1992): 671-670.

[19] Coyle, EF and Montain, SJ. Benefits of fluid replacement with carbohydrate during exercise. *Medicine and Science in Sports and Exercise* 24.9 (1992): S324-S330.

[20] Brouns, F et al. The effect of different re-hydration drinks on post-exercise electrolyte excretion in trained athletes. *International Journal of Sports Medicine* 19 (1998): 56-60.

[21] Shirreffs, SM et al. Post-exercise re-hydration in man: effects of volume consumed and drink sodium content. *Medicine and Science in Sports and Exercise* 28.10 (1996): 1260-1271.

[22] Burke, LM. Nutrition for post-exercise recovery. *The Australian Journal of Science and Medicine in Sport* 29.1 (1996): 3-10.

[23] Gonzalez-Alonso, J et al. Re-hydration after exercise with common beverages and water. *International Journal of Sports Medicine* 13.5 (1992): 399-406.

[24] Greenleaf, JE. Problem: thirst, drinking behavior, and involuntary dehydration. *Medicine and Science in Sports and Exercise* 24.6 (1992): 645-656.

[25] National Athletic Trainers Association. Position statement on fluid replacement for athletes. *Journal of Athletic Training* 35.2 (2000): 212-224.

4 THE PERFORMANCE NUTRITION PYRAMID
An Update of the USDA's Food Guide Pyramid

By Brett Hall, R.D.

Let's take a closer look at USDA's Food Guide Pyramid—who built it, how it was built, why it was built and what it recommends. In its place we'll suggest a Performance Nutrition Pyramid based on solid dietary principles for active individuals interested in optimal nutrition.

The Food Guide Pyramid in a Nutshell

The concept of a governmentally derived nutrition guidance document is not a new one. The first simple governmental nutrition guide was produced over a hundred years ago and is actually the same document upon which our modern FGP is based; however, over the years the USDA has tweaked their recommendations to (supposedly) keep up with new research and changing dietary habits. And just over a decade ago they created the graphic summary of their nutritional guidelines in the form of a pyramid. Their thought was that this pictorial form of advice would be the easiest for people to understand and follow.

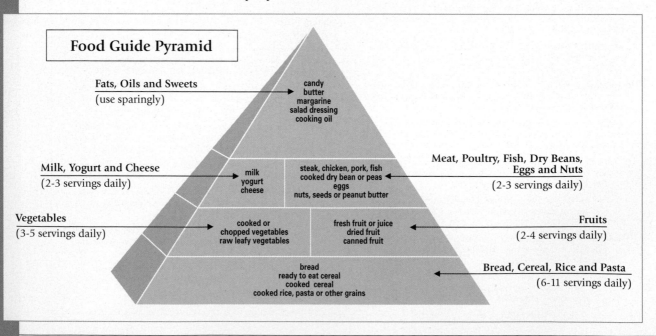

Food Guide Pyramid

Fats, Oils and Sweets
(use sparingly)

candy
butter
margarine
salad dressing
cooking oil

Milk, Yogurt and Cheese
(2-3 servings daily)

milk
yogurt
cheese

steak, chicken, pork, fish
cooked dry bean or peas
eggs
nuts, seeds or peanut butter

Meat, Poultry, Fish, Dry Beans, Eggs and Nuts
(2-3 servings daily)

Vegetables
(3-5 servings daily)

cooked or
chopped vegetables
raw leafy vegetables

fresh fruit or juice
dried fruit
canned fruit

Fruits
(2-4 servings daily)

bread
ready to eat cereal
cooked cereal
cooked rice, pasta or other grains

Bread, Cereal, Rice and Pasta
(6-11 servings daily)

Today, the definition of the modern FGP—straight from the official FGP booklet—is "The Pyramid illustrates the research-based food guidance system developed by USDA and supported by the Department of Health and Human Services. The Pyramid is based on USDA's research on what foods Americans eat, what nutrients are in these foods and how to make the best food choices for you. The Pyramid is an outline of what to eat each day. It's not a rigid prescription, but a general guide that let's you choose a healthful diet that's right for you."[1] In essence, they looked at what Americans were already eating and then made recommendations within those dietary parameters to help people make healthier food choices—a baby step toward helping Americans eat and feel better, but truly only a baby step.

They base their dietary recommendations within the pyramid on the seven *Dietary Guidelines for Americans*, also created and published by the USDA.[2] In their words, "These guidelines are the best, most up-to-date advice from nutritional scientists ..." These guidelines are as follows:

- Eat a variety of foods.
- Balance the food you eat with physical activity—maintain or improve your weight.
- Choose a diet with plenty of grain products, vegetables and fruits.
- Choose a diet low in fat, saturated fat and cholesterol.
- Choose a diet moderate in sugars.
- Choose a diet moderate in salt and sodium.
- If you drink alcoholic beverages, do so in moderation.

Now, it's hard to argue with these guidelines. It's all good advice. The trick is creating a single, one-size-fits-all plan, in the form of a picture that tells you exactly how to attain these goals—a dubious task indeed. And the FGP was the USDA's best answer. They designed the pyramid simplistically, using a recommended number of daily servings from each of the five food groups as the basis for their guide. Check out the pyramid graphic above.

You'll notice that bread, cereals, rice and pasta form the base of the pyramid, with fruits and veggies next up the ladder. Clearly the emphasis is heavy on the carbohydrates. And it's really not so much that they think you should eat a ton of carbs. It has more to do with the fact that these foods are low in fat, and cutting fat is one of the prime directives of the FGP.

You see, the current FGP was developed over 10 years ago. And the main nutritional dogma of that time was the need to cut fat from the diet of Americans. The average American at the time was consuming 42 percent of his or her calories as fat. The pyramid guides people to cut that to 30 percent (still far too high). And because most available protein sources at that time tended to come laden with fat, recommending carbs was the easy and logical answer. Hence a FGP weighted heavily toward carb-rich foods.

did you know?

The Food Guide Pyramid promotes carb-rich, low-fat foods.

Another goal of the FGP is to help people control their overall caloric intake. To this end they give you three calorie levels to choose from: 1,600 calories for "sedentary women and older adults"; 2,200 calories for "most children, teenage girls, active women and many sedentary men"; and 2,800 calories for "teenage boys, active men and some very active women." An exact number of servings from each food group are then recommended for each calorie level.

For "young children" (those under 2 years old), this is what the pyramid booklet has to say about calories: "It is hard to know how much food children need to grow normally. If you're unsure, check with your doctor." Clearly there is a need for better guidance in terms of caloric requirements. More on this later.

Next, it is important to know what a "serving" is for each food in the various food groups. The USDA has created this little table to help guide you. However, they are not all that uptight about you actually sticking with these recommended serving sizes.

And that's the FGP in a nutshell. Basically it recommends how many daily servings to eat from each food group, end of story. Is it simple? Absolutely. Is it effective at promoting optimal nutrition? Not a chance. Here's why.

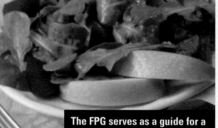
The FPG serves as a guide for a healthier way of eating, but not necessarily optimal nutrition.

© SOUDERSSTUDIOS.COM

Renovating the Pyramid

First and foremost, it's important to understand that the FGP was never meant to be everything to everyone. It was created to help guide the American masses toward a more healthy way of eating. It speaks mainly to those who have virtually no knowledge of nutrition. It gives them a stepping stone upon which to start moving in the right direction; however, for those of you who are more interested and educated in nutrition—who already have a basic knowledge of what it means to truly eat well—that stepping stone is behind you. For you, reverting to the FGP would be like deciding you're tired of walking and deciding to drop down on your hands and knees and start crawling again; not a good idea.

Ancient Knowledge

One of the main reasons the FGP just doesn't work today is that it is over 10 years old. It was introduced in 1992 and hasn't changed since. What the USDA refers to as the "best and most up-to-date advice from nutritional scientists" is actually ancient history. During the past decade we have seen more research on optimizing human nutrition than in any previous period. Literally thousands of new studies have been published. New discoveries are being made every month. And none of this new knowledge is included in the FGP. It simply wasn't available when it was created.

This being the case, many of the assumptions upon which they base their recommendations are simply no longer true, including assumptions such as the fact that 60 grams of protein is sufficient to meet the needs of all adults, or that 30 percent of calories as fat is a healthy level, or that beans and nuts are a good stand-alone protein source.

The FGP is based on outdated knowledge and thus provides faulty advice. But the new and improved Performance Nutrition Pyramid (PNP) takes all of the latest research into account: everything from the Glycemic Index of carbs, to proper nutrient timing and combining, to the underappreciated value of essential fatty acids.

Manageable vs. Optimal

As mentioned earlier, the FGP is really not a document describing what optimal nutrition is, but more of a document outlining how to take the first step away from a bad diet, toward a more healthy way of eating. Even with the antiquated research knowledge they possessed 10 years ago, they could have created a more aggressive guide—something that sets a standard for optimal nutrient intake, not just for general health, but for extraordinary health. But they didn't do this. Why?

There are two main reasons: First, one of the broad-scope goals of the FGP is to help prevent various lifestyle diseases (e.g., heart disease, high blood pressure, diabetes, etc.) through improving people's nutrition. This being the case, the main focus of the recommendations was to cut down dietary risk factors such as saturated fat, sodium and sugar consumption. They figured that by addressing these specific issues they could lower disease rates, thus improving the overall health of the population. But the simple lack of disease isn't the best definition for optimal health. Optimal health is about abundant energy, fitness, strength and stamina. And these things are just not really considered in the FGP.

The next reason the FGP was developed as it was is because governmental scientists figured it would be much too hard for most Americans to ever adopt a regimen of truly optimal nutrient intake. Starting from a staple diet of Big Gulps and Doritos, drafters of the FGP simply didn't think people could make the jump. So they set the bar much lower. They created a goal that they believed would be attainable for virtually everyone. But in so doing they have set a standard that is not optimal, thus providing no guidance or goal to people who might be inclined to achieve the highest level of nutritional health possible.

But the PNP changes all of that. It gives you the recommendations that allow you to achieve peak nutrition. If you fall short, so be it. At least you will know where you ultimately want to go.

Achieve peak nutrition with the Performance Nutrition Pyramid.

The Food Guide Pyramid: Macronutrient Mayhem

What level of nutrition does the pyramid provide? When you break it down into the nitty gritty of macronutrient makeup, here is what you get by following the FGP:

PERCENT OF CALORIES FROM:
Protein = 14 percent
Carbohydrates = 56 percent
Fat = 30 percent

This is truly old-school thinking. One of the stated objectives of the FGP pyramid is to help people "Balance the food you eat with physical activity and maintain or improve your weight." But how can a diet composed mainly of carbs and fats possibly help anyone improve their weight? All of the latest research shows that our country's carb addiction, combined with an overabundance of fat intake, is what is making us all fatter by the day.[3,4,5] A more balanced ratio of carbs to protein and a lower fat intake is really what we should be focusing on. This is what would help control blood sugar, boost overall metabolism and avoid fat storage.

And as far as providing proper support for physical activity, 14 percent of calories from protein is far from optimal. It is well established in the research that people who are physically active on a consistent basis require more protein to optimize muscle metabolism, as well as other general metabolic processes.[6,7] And 14 percent of calories (or 76 grams on a 2,200-calorie diet) simply doesn't cut it. At this level your muscles will recuperate more slowly and less completely; therefore, in order to support both optimal body composition and muscular growth and function, a macronutrient ratio of 40 percent protein, 40 percent carbs and 20 percent fat is suggested. And this is exactly the ratio of macronutrients provided by the PNP.

To calculate your calorie needs, keep a food journal.

Calorie Confusion

The FGP offers very little guidance in terms of caloric intake. It provides a vague description (as listed above) of how many calories different types of people should consume. But this is clearly far too generalized to offer any real guidance or benefit; for instance, it lumps all "active men" into the same 2,800-calorie category—but what about the type, duration and frequency of the "activity?" What about differences in body mass? What about personal metabolic genetics? Does a 260-pound football player, working out four hours per day, six days a week really require the same level of calories as a 150-pound desk jockey whose exercise is walking the 1.5 miles to work every day?

For any nutrition plan to work, the first step is to accurately calculate calorie needs. For this reason, your first step in putting the PNP to work for you will be to assess your own personal calorie requirements. You can do this by keeping a food record for a week and analyzing the results. A detailed description of how to keep your food record, assess your results and choose your perfect calorie level is given in Chapter 8 of this book.

Once you have your personal calorie goal, you can decide exactly how best to use the PNP to help you meet your health and fitness goals. Serving recommendations for the PNP are arranged in 500-calorie intervals. Simply pick the calorie level that is closest to your desired intake and use the chart with the PNP to assess the number of servings per day per food group.

Serving Size

Knowing what is expected of you is absolutely crucial in helping you to perform any requested task right. But if the parameters or the goal of the task are not well understood, you are unlikely to be able to complete the task satisfactorily. And this is the way it is with the serving sizes outlined in the FGP. First of all, there are over a dozen different ways you are asked to measure serving sizes using the FGP. Unless you carry a cheat sheet with you wherever you go, you are unlikely to be able to remember all of the different serving size suggestions.

And another thing is that many of the FGP suggested serving sizes leave a lot of room for ambiguity that could greatly skew the outcome of your choices. Take the "Bread" serving recommendation for example. It states that a serving is "one slice of

bread." But what about different types of bread? One slice of wheat bread provides about 60 calories and 12 grams of carbs. While one plain bagel provides 195 calories and 38 grams of carbs, and a pita provides 170 calories and 35 grams of carbs. This ambiguity could easily lead to over-consumption.

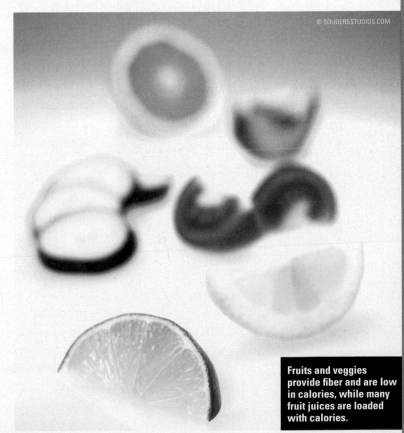

© SOUDERSSTUDIOS.COM

Fruits and veggies provide fiber and are low in calories, while many fruit juices are loaded with calories.

The FGP also makes the mistake of including fruit and vegetable "juices" in their respective food groups. This is a huge no-no. Because while whole fruits and veggies provide lots of fiber and have a low caloric density, juices are just the opposite— they are loaded with calories and devoid of fiber. And to top it off, the FGP suggests a cup of fresh veggies or three-fourths of a cup of juice as equivalent servings. If we take carrots as an example here, one serving of carrot juice would provide about 78 calories and 16 grams of carbs, with a serving of whole carrots coming in at 52 calories and only 12 grams of carbs.

The list of serving size transgressions goes on and on. But suffice it to say the FGP serving size system is ambiguous, misleading and creates the potential for massive variation within the guidelines. That is why we have simplified the serving size recommendations for the PNP. One serving for all food groups is as follows:

- A portion the size of a deck of playing cards, the size of your closed fist or the palm of your hand for all solid foods.
- One cup for all liquids.
- 4 grams for all fats.

It's that simple. It is possible to make the serving sizes this uniform and easy due to the way the food group categories have been changed in the PNP. Using these very clear and uniform serving sizes with the PNP, you can be assured that you are always consuming the proper level of calories and macronutrients.

What Goes With What?

Another little item that the FGP fails to address is food combining. It gives absolutely no guidance on what constitutes an optimal mix of foods for a meal. It only recommends daily servings for each individual food group. You could eat

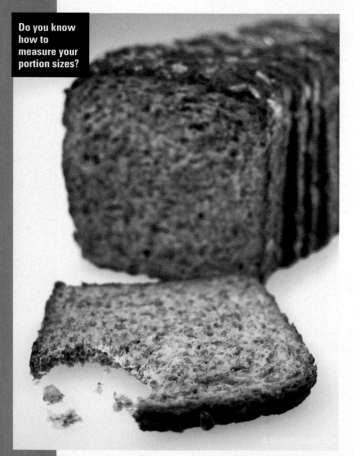

Do you know how to measure your portion sizes?

a bowl of plain spaghetti the size of your head, and chase it with two glasses of orange juice and a baked potato for lunch and still be in perfect compliance with the FGP. Of course, you would store about 3 pounds of fat over the two hours following your meal, then be in carb overload—but at least you managed to squeeze servings from three of the food groups into that meal.

This approach is clearly not optimal. We know that by combining various types of food within a meal you can dramatically affect the way your body handles and reacts to the meal; for instance, by simply adding a dose of healthy fats to a baked potato you can decrease the normally high Glycemic Index of that potato.[8] And by combining foods from the protein group with your carbs, you can increase the uptake of proteins into muscles.[9] There are a hundred other examples of how proper food combining is key to optimizing your nutritional intake. That's why the PNP takes the issue of food combining into consideration. Using the PNP, we suggest that you always include at least one serving from each of the three bottom levels of the pyramid in each meal. That way you are always receiving a balanced dose of protein, carbs and good fats with each meal and snack.

Timing Is Everything

Would it be OK for you to eat all of your recommended daily servings of every food group in one big meal? Well, according to the guidelines set out by the FGP that would be just fine, because there are no guidelines provided for food timing. The FGP completely neglects to discuss the value, and absolute necessity, of timing your food intake properly.

The typical American diet consists of two large meals per day, the largest being in the evening before bed. And it is this daily pattern of feast and famine that is partially responsible for our nation's growing obesity problem.[10] On the flip-side, consuming your daily calories in five or six small frequent meals is the healthiest way to eat (see more on this in Chapter 6). Not only does this pattern help to keep your metabolism humming and limit fat storage, it also provides the most consistent energy levels throughout the day.[11,12] The use of small frequent meals is a must in any complete nutrition plan.

There are also specialty situations in which proper timing of food intake is key, and after exercise is one of those times. Research shows that by consuming a meal combining protein and carbs within one hour after exercise you can greatly enhance muscular recuperation and growth (see Chapter 10 for even more on this).[13,14]

For these reasons we recommend the following meal pattern be used with the PNP:

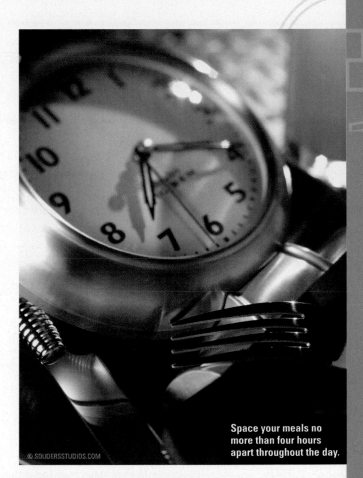

Space your meals no more than four hours apart throughout the day.

© SOUDERSSTUDIOS.COM

- For calorie levels 2,000 and below, split your daily calories up into at least five total meals per day—three main meals and two or three small snacks.
- For calorie levels above 2,000, split your daily calories up into six total meals per day—three main meals and three snacks.
- Space your meals no more than four hours apart throughout the day.
- Remember to include at least one serving from each of the lower three levels of the PNP in each meal.
- Consume one of your meals within one hour following your daily workout.

Where's the Water?

If you were asked which nutrient you thought was the most important of them all, what would you say? Most of you would probably go with protein or carbs, but really it's water that is the king of all nutrients. We can live without food for over a month, but if you go for a day or two without water, we dry up and die. Everything that happens in your body happens in a liquid medium. Water hydrates muscle cells to help them grow. It cleanses the blood and organs. It makes all those critical chemical reactions in your body possible. And yet water is not even mentioned in the FGP.

Of all the oversights of the FGP, this is the biggie. Water should be numero uno when it comes to nutrition recommendations. Statistics show that very few of us drink enough water to maintain proper hydration. And proper hydration is key to muscular performance. As a matter of fact, a mere 3 percent decrease in muscle hydration leads to a 10 percent loss of contractile strength, and an 8 percent loss of speed.[15,16]

Because of this, the PNP is purposefully depicted as floating in a sea of fresh, clean water, to emphasize the fact that the whole pyramid itself is supported by water at the very base. If the water dries up, the pyramid falls apart. Therefore the water intake recommended by the PNP is:

- ⊞ A base intake of 1 gallon of pure water per day for everyone.
- ⊞ Additionally, if exercising hard, measure your body weight before you exercise and after. Replace every pound of weight lost during your exercise with 16 ounces of water.

All Proteins, Carbohydrates and Fats Are Not Created Equal

While there is some mention in the FGP of the preferred use of fiber-rich grains and breads and staying away from saturated fats, there is very little guidance in terms of other qualitative aspects of the different macronutrients; for example, starchy vegetables

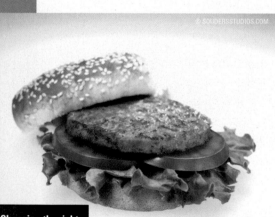

Choosing the right proteins, carbs and fats is essential to any nutrition plan.

(like potatoes) are included with more fibrous veggies (like celery) in the general category of vegetables. But these two vegetables couldn't be more different. A half-cup serving of potato provides about 60 calories, with virtually no fiber, while a half-cup serving of celery contains only 6 calories and over a gram of fiber.

And it's not just the quantity of calories or carbs that can be misconstrued due to poor categorizing. The Glycemic Index of carbs is not considered or discussed at all in the FGP. The reason for this is that the use of the GI to assess the affect of carbs on blood sugar is fairly new. It just wasn't part of the nutritional dogma when the FGP was created. But now we know how important it is to both athletic performance and physique management. It absolutely needs to be considered in any complete food plan.

In terms of fats, the FGP spends so much time warning you off of saturated fats that it forgets to mention the value of essential fatty acids—not just the value of these fats, but the absolute necessity of having them in your diet. These are fats we must eat in order to maintain health—to survive. They are not readily available in our modern processed diet, and many of you are probably not getting as much as you need.[17] But nowhere is the necessity of this vital nutrient mentioned.

Proteins are also treated indiscriminately. The FGP booklet talks a little about trying to focus on lean meats versus fatty meats, but then turns around and uses fat- and nitrosamine-laden lunch meats in their examples. They have also included beans and legumes in the "meat" category. But it is well-known that, by themselves, these are incomplete proteins and only minimally valuable as a protein source.[18] On top of that, beans pack a 3-to-1 carb-to-protein ratio, making them much more of a "starchy vegetable" versus a "meat."

The PNP takes all of these qualitative differences into consideration. You will notice that the levels of the pyramid each represent a macronutrient versus a specific food group. Also, carbs have been separated by the Glycemic Index and meats are divided into high- and low-fat categories. Additionally, vegetables have been segregated according to their caloric density (starchy vs. fibrous). By creating these macronutrient levels and greater delineation among the food groups, the PNP is a much more realistic and effective nutritional tool.

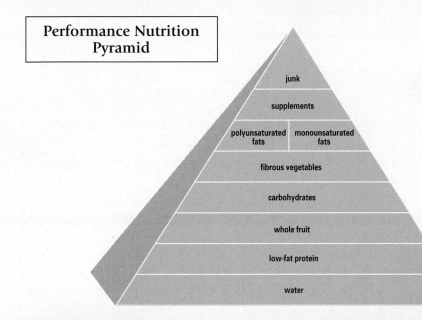

Performance Nutrition Pyramid

THE PERFORMANCE NUTRITION PYRAMID

Serving Recommendations By Calorie Level

Food Group	1,000	1,500	2,000	2,500	3,000	3,500	4,000
Low-fat protein	4	6	8	10	12	14	16
Whole fruit	2	3	4	5	6	7	8
High-fiber, low-GI carbs	2	3	4	5	6	7	8
Fibrous veggies	4	6	8	10	12	14	16
Polyunsaturated fats	4	6	8	10	12	14	16
Monounsaturated fats	2	3	4	5	6	7	8
Nutritional supplements	AS NEEDED OR DESIRED						
Junk	½	¾	1	1 ¼	1 ½	1 ¾	2

Serving Sizes

- A portion the size of a deck of playing cards, your closed fist or the palm of your hand for all solid foods.
- One cup for all liquids.
- 4 grams for all fats.

Water

- A base intake of 1 gallon of pure water per day for everyone.
- Additionally, if exercising hard measure your body weight before your exercise and after. Replace every pound of weight lost during your exercise with 16 ounces of water.

Meal Timing

- For calorie levels below 2,000, split your daily calories up into at least five total meals per day—three main meals and two or three small snacks.
- For calorie levels above 2,000, split your daily calories up into six total meals per day—three main meals and three snacks.
- Space your meals no more than four hours apart throughout the day.
- Remember to include at least one serving from each of the lower three levels of the PNP in each meal.
- Consume one of your meals within one hour following your daily exercise.

Food Combining

- Always include at least one serving from each of the three bottom levels of the pyramid in each meal.

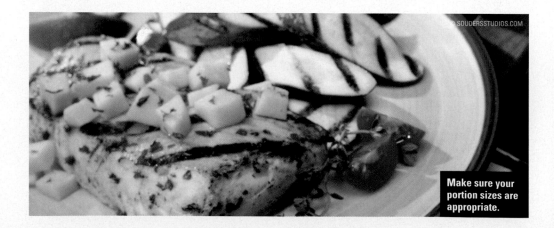

© SOUDERSSTUDIOS.COM

Make sure your portion sizes are appropriate.

Sample Foods in Each Food Group

This is only a sample listing of the foods in these categories. For a more extensive listing, you can purchase a booklet entitled "Exchange Lists for Meal Planning" for $1.95 at www.diabetes.org.

Low-Fat Protein (5 grams of fat or less per serving)

** It is assumed that all meats are cooked without added fat—such as baking, broiling or roasting.***

- Tuna, salmon or other cold water fish
- Skinless chicken or turkey breast
- Lean cuts of beef, including:
  - Round
  - Sirloin
  - Loin
- Lean cuts of pork, including:
  - Tenderloin
  - Center loin
  - Ham
- Lean cuts of lamb, including:
  - Leg
  - Loin
  - Fore Shank
- Non-fat milk
- Non-fat cottage cheese
- Non-fat, sugar-free yogurt
- Egg whites
- Pure protein powder supplements

Whole Fruit

- Any and all fresh fruits
- If using canned fruit, make sure it is packed in its own juice and not heavy syrup
- Fruit juices are not included in this food group
- If using dried fruits, cut the serving size in half

High-Fiber, Low-GI Carbs (GI of less than 70 and at least 2 grams of fiber per serving)

- All beans, including but not limited to:
  - Kidney
  - Navy
  - Black
  - Red
  - Garbanzo
  - Lentils
  - Pinto
  - Soy
- Slow-cooked brown rice
- Wild rice
- Yams
- Most whole grains, including:
  - Barley
    Buckwheat
  - Corn
  - Rye
  - Oats
- Cereals, including:
  - All-Bran
  - Whole-Wheat Mini-Wheats
  - Muesli
  - Slow-cooked oatmeal
  - Raisin Bran
- Whole-wheat pasta
- All whole-wheat and multi-grain breads. Only breads with whole grains in them, and/or with nuts and seeds.

Fibrous Vegetables

- ⊞ All non-starchy vegetables, including:
  - Carrots
  - Celery
  - Broccoli
  - Cauliflower
  - All leafy veggies
  - Cabbage
  - Asparagus
- ⊞ Starchy veggies are *not* included in this food group, and include:
  - Potatoes
  - Corn
  - Peas
  - Yams

Polyunsaturated Fats

- ⊞ Flax seed oil
- ⊞ Hemp seed oil
- ⊞ Soybean oil
- ⊞ Fish oil
- ⊞ Walnuts
- ⊞ Pumpkin seeds
- ⊞ Sunflower seeds
- ⊞ Essential fatty acids (can be purchased at any specialty nutrition store or health food store)

Monounsaturated Fats

- ⊞ Olive oil
- ⊞ Canola oil
- ⊞ Peanut oil
- ⊞ Avocado
- ⊞ Olives
- ⊞ Peanuts and peanut butter
- ⊞ Almonds
- ⊞ Pecans
- ⊞ Pistachios
- ⊞ Cashews

Nutritional Supplements

- ⊞ This could include virtually any supplement you want to use; however, some that may work well to round out your optimal nutrition plan are:
  - Pure protein powders (such as EAS® Precision Protein™)
  - Essential fatty acids
  - Multivitamins and multi-minerals
  - Antioxidants
  - Fiber powder

Junk

- ⊞ In general this group contains every food that does not fall under any of the other groups. Some of the main offenders are
  - Ice cream
  - Candy
  - Chocolate
  - Alcoholic beverages
  - Pastries
  - Cakes
  - Processed white-flour bakery products
  - Pizza
  - Sugary cereals
  - Fried foods
  - Soda
  - Cheese
  - Whole-fat dairy foods
  - High-fat meats like bacon, sausage, lunch meat, hot dogs, etc.
  - Chips

A Plethora of Pyramids

Noting the ethnocentricity of the USDA-derived FGP for the American population, a variety of groups have created adaptations of the original FGP to create their own, more ethnically applicable pyramids. Here is a quick overview of the different pyramid guides available.

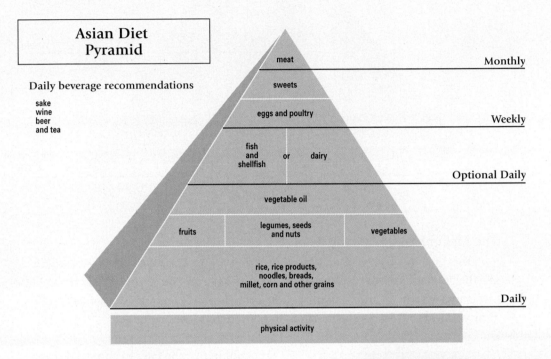

Asian Diet Pyramid

Daily beverage recommendations

sake
wine
beer
and tea

meat — Monthly

sweets

eggs and poultry — Weekly

fish and shellfish — or — dairy — Optional Daily

vegetable oil

fruits — legumes, seeds and nuts — vegetables

rice, rice products, noodles, breads, millet, corn and other grains — Daily

physical activity

The Asian Diet Pyramid

The Asian Diet Pyramid reflects the traditional, plant-based rural diets of Asia. It emphasizes a wide base of rice, rice products, noodles, breads and grains, preferably whole-grain and minimally processed foods, topped by another large band of fruits, vegetables, legumes, nuts and seeds. Daily physical exercise, a small amount of vegetable oil and a moderate consumption of plant-based beverages, including tea (especially black and green), sake, beer and wine also are recommended daily. Small daily servings of dairy products (low-fat) or fish are optional; sweets, eggs and poultry are recommended no more than weekly, and red meat no more than monthly.

It was developed by specialists from the Cornell-China-Oxford Project on Nutrition, Health and Environment based at Cornell University; the Harvard School of Public Health; and the Oldways Preservation and Exchange Trust, which issued the Mediterranean Diet Pyramid three years ago.

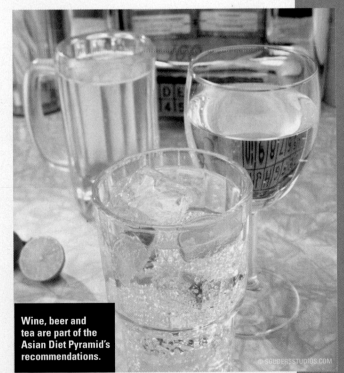

Wine, beer and tea are part of the Asian Diet Pyramid's recommendations.

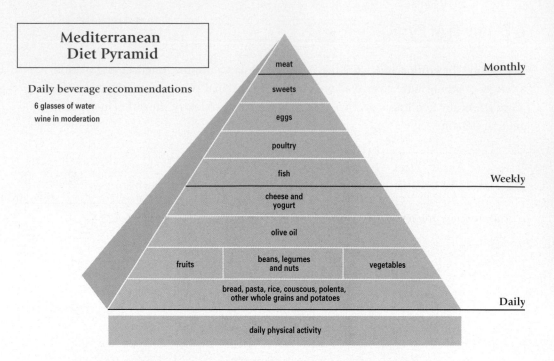

Mediterranean Diet Pyramid

Daily beverage recommendations

6 glasses of water
wine in moderation

meat	Monthly
sweets	
eggs	
poultry	
fish	Weekly
cheese and yogurt	
olive oil	
fruits — beans, legumes and nuts — vegetables	
bread, pasta, rice, couscous, polenta, other whole grains and potatoes	Daily
daily physical activity	

The Mediterranean Diet Pyramid

This pyramid, representing a healthy, traditional Mediterranean diet, is based on the dietary traditions of Crete, much of the rest of Greece and southern Italy circa 1960, structured in light of current nutrition research. The selection of these regions and this time period as a basis for the design follows from three considerations:

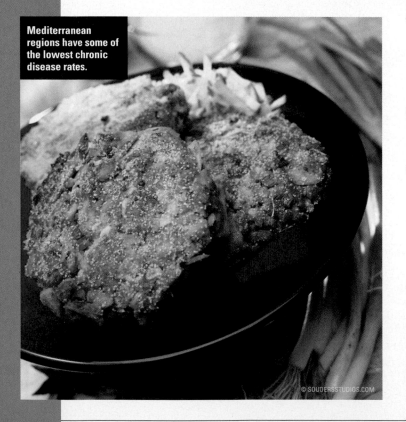

Mediterranean regions have some of the lowest chronic disease rates.

© SOUDERSSTUDIOS.COM

- Recognition that the rates of chronic diseases were among the lowest in the world and adult life expectancy was among the highest for these populations at that time, even though medical services were limited.
- Availability of data describing the character of food consumption patterns of the areas at that time.
- The convergence of the dietary patterns revealed by these data and current understanding of optimal nutrition based on epidemiological studies and clinical trials worldwide.

The design of the pyramid is not based solely on either the weight or the percentage of energy (calories) that foods account for in the diet, but on a blend of these that is meant to give relative proportions and a general sense of frequency of servings, as well as an indication of which foods to favor in a healthy Mediterranean-style diet.

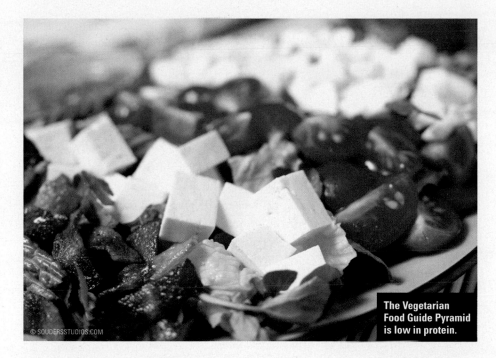

The Vegetarian Food Guide Pyramid is low in protein.

© SOUDERSSTUDIOS.COM

Vegetarian Food Guide Pyramid

Based directly off of the original FGP, this derivation was developed in 1997 by the American Dietetic Association. The only notable change is that soy milk and tofu have been added to the "meat" food group in place of meat. All of the serving recommendations and other food groups remain unchanged.

This adaptation for vegetarians is very low in protein. And there is no discussion of combining legumes and grains to create complete proteins. Also, there is no discussion of supplementing the vegetarian diet with vitamin B_{12} or iron, which both can (and would, with this pyramid) be in short supply in a vegetarian diet.

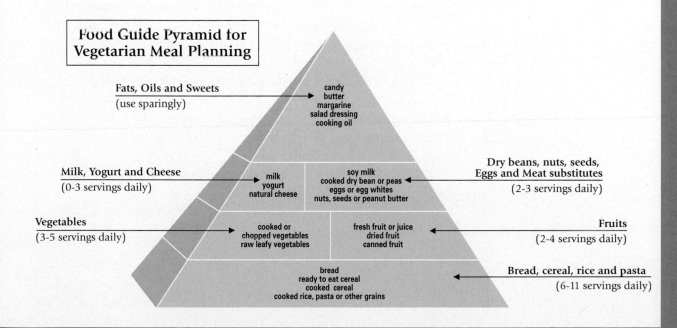

Food Guide Pyramid for Vegetarian Meal Planning

Fats, Oils and Sweets (use sparingly)

candy
butter
margarine
salad dressing
cooking oil

Milk, Yogurt and Cheese (0-3 servings daily)

milk
yogurt
natural cheese

soy milk
cooked dry bean or peas
eggs or egg whites
nuts, seeds or peanut butter

Dry beans, nuts, seeds, Eggs and Meat substitutes (2-3 servings daily)

Vegetables (3-5 servings daily)

cooked or chopped vegetables
raw leafy vegetables

fresh fruit or juice
dried fruit
canned fruit

Fruits (2-4 servings daily)

bread
ready to eat cereal
cooked cereal
cooked rice, pasta or other grains

Bread, cereal, rice and pasta (6-11 servings daily)

Calculating Your 40/40/20 Balance

There has been a lot of discussion of the 40/40/20 macronutrient balance for optimal sports performance in this book. But what does it mean exactly, and how can you calculate your daily nutrient intake using this ratio? Here's the scoop.

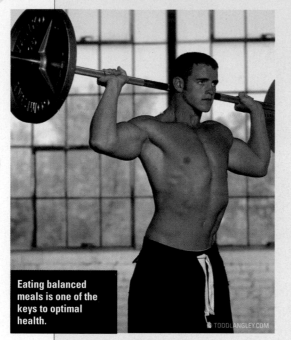

Eating balanced meals is one of the keys to optimal health.

© TODDLANGLEY.COM

40/40/20 is shorthand for "40 percent protein, 40 percent carbohydrates, 20 percent fat." Meaning that 40 percent of your daily caloric intake will come from protein, 40 percent from carbs and 20 percent from fat. That's pretty easy. But calculating the actual calorie and gram level for each of these nutrients can be a bit trickier. Here's how you do it:

First, figure out your overall daily calorie goal. Let's say, for example, that it's 2,000 calories per day. To figure how many calories each nutrient will provide under the 40/40/20 plan, simply multiply your total calories by the percentage of calories for that nutrient. As follows:

For protein: 2,000 x .40 = 800 calories from protein
For carbs: 2,000 x .40 = 800 calories from carbs
For fat: 2,000 x .20 = 400 calories for fat

To calculate how many grams this represents for each nutrient, you have to divide the calories for each separate nutrient by the number of calories that specific nutrient contains per gram. Protein and carbs both contain 4 calories per gram. And fat contains 9 calories per gram. So you can calculate the grams for each nutrient as follows:

For protein: 800 protein calories / 4 calories per protein gram = 200 grams of protein
For carbs: 800 carb calories / 4 calories per carb gram = 200 grams of carbs
For fat: 400 fat calories / 9 calories per fat gram = 44 grams of fat

That's it: A 2,000-calorie diet with a 40/40/20 profile will consist of 200 grams of protein, 200 grams of carbs and 44 grams of fat.

REFERENCES CITED:

1 US Department of Agriculture. *The Food Guide Pyramid* (Center for Nutrition Policy and Promotion, Home and Garden Bulletin, 1992: 252) pg. 1-29.

2 US Department of Agriculture. *Dietary Guidelines for Americans* (Department of Health and Human Services, Home and Garden Bulletin, 1995: 232).

3 Astrup, AL et al. The role of dietary fat in body fatness: evidence from a preliminary meta-analysis of ad libitum low-fat dietary intervention studies. *Br J Nutr* 83.Supp 1 (2000): S25-32.

4 Saris, WH et al. Randomized controlled trial of changes in dietary carbohydrate/fat ratio and simple vs. complex carbohydrates on body weight and blood lipids: the CARMEN study. *Int J Obes Relat Metab Disord* 24.10 (2000): 1310-1318.

5 Robinson, SM et al. Protein turnover and Thermogenesis in response to high-protein and high-carbohydrate feeding in men. *Am J Clin Nutr* 52 (1990): 72-80.

6 Friedman, JE and Lemon, PWR. Effect of chronic endurance exercise on the retention of dietary protein. *Int J Sports Med* 10 (1989): 118-123.

7 Lemon, PWR and Nagle, FJ. Effects of exercise on protein and amino acid metabolism. *Med Sci Sports Exer* 13 (1981): 141-149.

8 Wu, CL, Nicholas, C, Williams, C, Took, A and Hardy, L. The influence of high-carbohydrate meals with different glycemic indices on substrate utilization during subsequent exercise. *Br J Nutr* 90.6 (2003): 1049-56.

9 Suzuki, M. Glycemic carbohydrates consumed with amino acids or protein right after exercise enhance muscle formation. *Nutr Rev* 61.5 Pt 2 (2003): S88-94.

10 Antoine, JM, Rohr, R, Gagey, MJ, Bleyer, RE and Debry, G. Feeding frequency and nitrogen balance in weight-reducing obese women. *Hum Nutr Clin Nutr* 38.1 (1984): 31-8.

11 Bertelsen, J et al. Effect of meal frequency on blood glucose, insulin, and free fatty acids in NIDDM subjects. *Diabetes Care* 16.1 (1993): 4-7.

12 Iwao, S, Mori, K and Sato, Y. Effects of meal frequency on body composition during weight control in boxers. *Scand J Med Sci Sports* 6.5 (1996): 265-72.

13 Williams, MB, Raven, PB, Fogt, DL and Ivy, JL. Effects of recovery beverages on glycogen restoration and endurance exercise performance. *J Strength Cond Res* 17.1 (2003): 12-9.

14 Esmarck, B et al. Timing of postexercise protein intake is important for muscle hypertrophy with resistance training in elderly humans. *J Physiol* 535.1 (2001): 301-11.

15 Sawka, MN et al. Influences of hydration level and body fluids on exercise performance in the heat. *J Am Med Assoc* 252 (1984): 1165-1169.

16 Armstrong, LE, Costill, DL and Fink, WJ. Influences on diuretic-induced dehydration on competitive running performance. *Med Sci Sports Exer* 17 (1985): 456-461.

17 Meyer, BJ et al. Dietary intakes and food sources of omega-6 and omega-3 polyunsaturated fatty acids. *Lipids* 38.4 (2003): 391-8.

18 Groff, JL, Gropper, SS and Hunt, SM. *Advanced Nutrition and Human Metabolism* (Second Edition) (West Publishing Company, 1990) pg. 189.

5 EATING ON THE RUN
Out of Time? Learn How to Make the Best Nutrition Choices

By Hale Deniz-Venturi, R.D., and Kelly James-Enger

The Challenge

In a perfect world, you'd have time to prepare healthy, nutritious meals designed to help you increase your athletic performance or achieve the body you're striving for—and plenty of time to consume those meals, too. In the real world, however, eating often takes a back seat to other priorities like work, family obligations, errands, socializing and finding time to get a workout in. But skipping meals, making poor choices or relying on fast foods often result in extra pounds, an increased risk of heart disease, cancer and other medical problems, add pounds and a lack of energy. If you tend to eat on the run without thinking about what's on your plate, you may be sacrificing performance on the job, at the gym and hurting your health as well.

That's the bad news. The good news is that it *is* possible to eat well when you don't have a lot of time—once you make it a priority. Planning ahead, preparing quick but healthy meals and educating yourself about smart nutrition options when you're on the go can help you improve your nutritional profile, have more energy and lose fat while maintaining lean muscle mass. In the pages that follow, you'll learn how to create a healthy "eat on the run" plan that will provide you with adequate nutrients and calories to fuel your lifestyle and your workouts in a minimum amount of time. By the chapter's end, you'll have a concrete idea of how to eat healthfully whether you're preparing a meal at home, dining at a sit-down restaurant or hitting the drive-through window at your favorite fast food place.

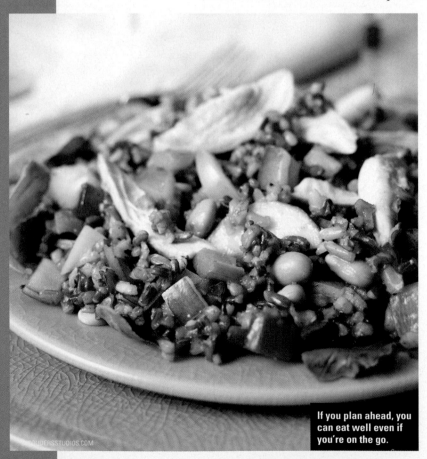

If you plan ahead, you can eat well even if you're on the go.

NUTRITION ESSENTIALS

The Importance of Planning Ahead

Smart eating starts with smart planning. An athlete wouldn't dream of a slipshod approach to training and a businessperson wouldn't launch a new company without researching the market, yet many of us want to lose weight or perform better but don't spend enough time *planning* how we'll do it. To begin, take a look at your current eating style. Knowing your typical eating pattern will help you identify strengths and weaknesses in your nutritional habits and determine how you can improve upon them.

The simplest way to do this is to keep a food diary for a week. Write down everything you eat and drink, how much you consumed, when you ate and where you were when you ate. Take a look at your diary after you're done to answer these basic nutrition questions:

1. Do you eat at least five servings of fruits and vegetables daily?
2. Do you eat a snack before and after working out?
3. Do you drink at least eight glasses (64 ounces) of water daily?
4. Do you eat out often, and if you do, do you choose healthy foods at fast food places and restaurants?
5. Do you eat at least six servings of whole-grain foods (such as whole-grain cereals, breads, crackers, rice, pasta) each day?
6. Do you eat at least two servings of low-fat dairy products and choose lean or low-fat meat/protein choices over fattier ones?
7. Do you eat fatty foods (like chips, fries, dressings, large meat servings, fried foods and cheese) often?
8. Do you skip meals or go longer than four hours without eating?
9. Do you travel frequently or find yourself on the go without healthy food choices nearby?
10. Do you forget or forgo eating for work, chores, sleep, socializing or exercising?
11. Do you keep healthful snacks on hand at home and at work?
12. Do you tend to wait until you're ravenous to eat?

Reviewing your journal and answering these questions will give you an idea of your eating patterns. You may notice that you tend to skip breakfast, and then overeat at lunch. You might discover that you're relying on fast food for lunch everyday because you never seem to have time to bring something from home. Or you may be surprised to discover that you're drinking four cans of cola a day but only four glasses of water. Keeping this food journal can be a powerful tool because it makes you more aware of the choices you're making rather than simply eating out of habit. It also lets you track the positive changes you're making in your diet. If you like, keep track of your workouts and how you feel throughout the day as well. Seeing the difference you're making in your eating habits—and the positive results—in black and white is a powerful motivator for most people.

The Basics of Good Nutrition

Consider the way you're eating today as your starting point. Good nutrition can help you improve your health, athletic performance and even your mood, and it needn't be complicated or radical. Remember, there's no such thing as a "good" or "bad" food. Sure, some foods are more nutrient-dense than others, but any food can fit into your diet—in moderation. Remember, eating a piece of chocolate cake won't make or break you nutritionally, upset your weight balance or affect the way your body stores and accesses glycogen—the fuel stored in muscle—which your body uses for energy throughout the day.

Most experts agree that the healthiest diet is one that contains a balance of complex carbohydrates and moderate amounts of protein and fat, but little saturated fat (the kind that's found in animal products). People who eat carbohydrate-rich diets tend to consume more low-fat foods, grain products and fruits and are less likely to be obese than people who consume more protein and fat.[1] Use the recommendations at the end of this section to help determine how many servings of the major food groups (breads, vegetables, fruits, dairy and meat/protein) you should aim for while limiting fats, oils and sweets.

Consistency is the most important factor when it comes to nutrition. When you're often on the run, you need a plan that you can easily adopt—not a diet so difficult to follow that you'll continually slip off of it. If you focus on developing a meal plan that features a foundation of healthy foods, you'll have room in your diet for occasional treats without feeling guilty or affecting your performance. In general, you should aim for progress, not perfection with your eating habits.

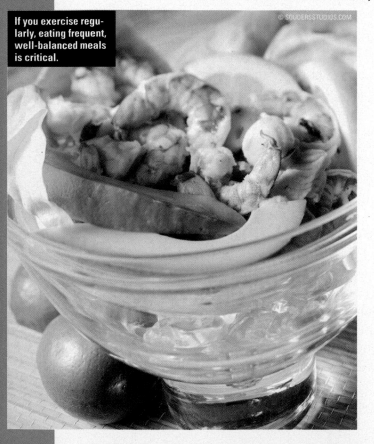

If you exercise regularly, eating frequent, well-balanced meals is critical.

© SOUDERSSTUDIOS.COM

Eating frequent, well-balanced meals is essential for anyone who wants to lose or maintain weight, have energy during the day and improve focus and concentration. It's even more critical for athletes and regular exercisers. Good nutrition will help your body develop sufficient glycogen (muscle fuel) storage, provide energy for workouts, promote post-exercise recovery, maintain hydration and prevent injury. In fact, when you eat may be as important as what you eat. Researchers have been studying the optimal times to eat before and after exercise; for example, a recent study found that eating a high-carb, low-protein, low-fat meal three hours before intense exercise improves athletic performance.[2] Other studies have shown that eating carbohydrates immediately after exercise—as opposed to ingesting carbs two or more hours later—results in higher levels of muscle glycogen storage.[3,4] For more on pre- and post-exercise nutrition recommendations, please go to Chapter 10.

If you're on the go, it helps to keep things simple. Employ these strategies when developing a meal plan, and you'll wind up eating, feeling and performing better:

- Learn how many calories you need and what proportion of carbs/fat/protein you should aim for, and use this to determine how much to eat during the day. You don't want to eat more calories than you need, but you don't want to skimp on calories or nutrients, either.

- Create an eating program that consists primarily of balanced, healthy choices but leaves room for treats throughout the week. Depending on your lifestyle and goals, you may want to plan for three meals and two snacks or five or six "mini-meals" of similar amounts of calories.

- When you eat a meal, make sure to include complex carbohydrates, lean protein and healthy fats. Even small snacks should include these food groups.

- Don't skip meals. While this is often a result of lack of time, skipping meals can cause a drop in blood sugar, which can result in fatigue, loss of concentration and a tendency to overeat at your next meal. You should plan to eat every three to four hours, especially if losing weight is one of your dietary goals. Research shows that eating frequently helps with appetite control and weight loss.[5,6]

- If you're in training or want to increase athletic performance, remember that meal timing is critical. Plan for pre- and post-workout snacks to give you energy to work out and replenish glycogen stores afterwards.[7,8]

- Get in the breakfast habit. Research shows that people who eat breakfast perform better on cognitive tasks and are more likely to maintain a healthy weight over time than those who skip this important meal.[9]

- Always be prepared to eat on the run. Keep a snack or mini-meal nearby whenever you're away from home even if it means having to eat during your commute, at your desk or between appointments.

- Plan for a mid-afternoon snack. This means you won't arrive home ravenous and will be able to take time to make a healthy dinner instead of inhaling the contents of the refrigerator when you walk in the door.

- Choose low-fat foods when possible, but remember that low-fat and no-fat foods still have calories. Sometimes a smaller serving of a full-fat version is a better bet.

- Keep track of your progress with your food diary. It will help you create new habits.

- Set aside one day a week to grocery shop (see next section). Having healthy food at hand makes it much easier to forgo junk food in favor of nutritious meals and snacks.

The Grocery Store

So, you've taken a look at the way you're eating and understand the basic principles of eating for improved performance. The next step is a well-planned trip to the grocery store, and that means starting with a list. Head to the store without a list and you're likely to waste time—and be overwhelmed by the variety of eye-catching, high-sugar, high-fat processed foods that will do your diet in. Use the Smart Shopping Tips section to help create your list before hitting the store.

Oh, and another thing—don't shop hungry! Shopping on an empty stomach is dangerous; everything looks appealing. Instead, go after a meal, preferably during the evening or on an early weekend morning, when the stores are less crowded and you can get in and out in little time. Plan to spend most of your time on the perimeters of the store. The basics of a healthy diet—produce, lean protein sources, dairy products and whole-grains—are usually found on the edges of the store. Often the produce section will be the first section of the store, which should encourage you to load up your cart with vitamin-packed fruits and vegetables.

While most of us fall short in getting the recommended minimum of five servings of fruits and vegetables a day, research shows that a diet high in produce protects against cancer and heart disease.[10] Consuming plenty of fruits and vegetables also helps ensure that you get plenty of fiber, helping you feel satisfied and full while maintaining a healthy digestive system.[11] A high-fiber diet also helps with weight loss and maintenance.[12,13]

Read All About It

Pay attention to food labels as you shop; for example, in the meat section, look for packaging that says "higher than 90 percent lean" or "95 percent extra lean." Those are the lowest-fat meat choices. If the label doesn't have a "lean" designation, it's probably high in fat. (Also examine the cut of meat itself—the more marbling you see in the meat, the higher the fat content.) Good lean meat choices include sirloin steak, skirt steak, pork tenderloin, chicken and turkey (but check the label as ground turkey can be higher in fat than you might think). In the dairy section, look for ways to cut back on fat by choosing low-fat options.

When checking labels, don't be distracted by the claims on the front, which can be misleading. Turn to the nutritional information first; for example, you might think that ramen noodles would make a cheap, healthy snack, right? A close look at the label reveals that the cup contains 310 calories, of which 44 percent is from fat, and a whopping 1,750 grams of sodium! (The National Academy of Sciences recommends a daily limit of 2,400 milligrams of sodium each day.) Look for entrees that have fewer than 500 milligrams of sodium. Canned goods and soups also tend to be high in sodium, so check the labels—foods that contain fewer than 140 milligrams per serving are considered low-sodium foods.

Make sure to check the fat content—choosing low-fat foods will help ensure that you can provide your muscles with sufficient carbohydrates to restore glycogen stores, while consuming high-fat foods provides lots of calories but may interfere with the

NUTRITION ESSENTIALS

storage of glycogen. With packaged foods, look for items that have 3 grams of fat or fewer for every 100 calories. This formula will help you maintain a low-fat diet.

Also, check the label for the food's fiber content—foods that contain 3 grams or more of dietary fiber per serving are considered good fiber sources. Look for fiber content when choosing whole-grain foods, cereals, breads and crackers. Fruits and vegetables are automatically good fiber sources and provide numerous other health benefits as well.[14,15]

You may also want to double-check the sugar content of your favorite foods. While a little sugar in your diet is fine, you're better off with natural sugars like those found in fruit than the sugar found in processed foods, which has few nutrients. In general, fewer than 5 grams to 8 grams of sugar (1 to 1½ teaspoons) per serving is acceptable.

Finally, look for convenience foods at the store that can make cooking faster and easier. There are a variety of new items that you can use to create easy, energy-producing meals by pairing them with vegetables, whole grains and fruits. Look for meals that are low in fat, moderate in calories and high in fiber, and check how the protein compares to the calories. If it's your primary protein source for that meal, it should have at least 20 grams of protein.

SMART SHOPPING TIPS

In the produce section:
- Stock up—the more the better. Aim for a variety of colors in your cart to ensure a variety of nutrients.
- Try pre-washed, pre-cut veggies and pre-bagged salads for quick snacks and side dishes.
- Buy walnuts, almonds and other nuts for a high-protein addition to a meal or snack.

At the dairy case:
- Skim milk and yogurt: choose low-fat (1 percent or 2 percent) or non-fat (skim) products.
- Cheese: choose the 2 percent type (usually "part-skim"), which contains 5 grams of fat or fewer per serving. Or try fat-free cheese, although it differs in consistency and taste.
- Cottage cheese: choose low-fat or non-fat (1 percent fat or fewer).
- Margarine: choose the lowest-fat soft versions or liquid or spray varieties.
- Fresh pastas: choose the lower-fat filled pastas like ravioli and tortellini for a quick dinner; you can also find these in the freezer section.

In the meat/deli section:
- Beef: choose lean cuts like eye of round, top round and round tip or loin cuts. Look for 90 percent or 95 percent lean labels.
- Chicken: buy skinless, or remove the skin at home. Boneless, skinless chicken breasts are fast and easy to prepare, and many deli sections offer pre-roasted chicken as well.
- Turkey: remove the skin before eating. Check the label on ground turkey before buying—it's usually high in fat.

- Pork: choose tenderloin or other loin cuts and Canadian bacon over regular bacon.
- Luncheon meats: choose meats that have 2 grams of fat or fewer per serving and are low in sodium. Read the labels on hot dogs—most are high in fat.
- Fresh fish: most is low in fat.
- Salads, pre-packaged sandwiches and other convenience foods: you can pick up a quick meal at the store's deli, but look for lower-fat versions and avoid mayonnaise-heavy dressings.

In the grocery section:
- Bread: choose whole-grain type, with a whole grain as the first ingredient and 2 or more grams of fiber per slice. Look for bagels, pita bread and English muffins, but avoid higher-fat bread products like muffins, croissants and pastries.
- Cereals: choose whole-grain types with at least 4 to 5 grams of fiber and fewer than 10 grams of sugar per serving.
- Crackers: choose low-fat crackers and whole-grain varieties.
- Pastas and rice: look for whole-grain or whole-wheat versions.
- Canned soups: bean-based soups are often good choices. Choose broth-based type soups like minestrone, chicken noodle or chicken/rice and vegetable, which are lower in fat than cream-based soups. Look for lower sodium varieties.
- Fruit and vegetable juices: choose 100 percent fruit juices. Select lower-sodium vegetable juices. Look for canned fruits packed in their own juice for less sugar and fewer calories and lower-sodium versions of canned vegetables.
- Canned chicken and tuna: choose packed in water, not oil.
- Canned Italian tomatoes, tomato paste, tomato sauce: these low-fat sauces make whipping up a meal of pasta a cinch.
- Peanut butter: choose a lower-fat or natural brand (pour off the oil) to lower the fat content.
- Dried fruit: a great portable snack.

In the frozen food section:
- "Skillet meals" and frozen entrees: choose those that are low in sodium and fat.
- Frozen soups: look for broth- and bean-based versions.
- Frozen rice bowls: a healthy choice, but watch the salt content.
- Low-fat frozen breakfast items: double-check the labels for fat content.
- Frozen mashed potatoes and frozen vegetables: check the salt content.
- Frozen fruit like strawberries, raspberries and blueberries: look for fruit-only versions— they're great for quick smoothies.
- Frozen stir-fry rice or pasta and veggies: look for low-sodium varieties.
- Frozen desserts: look for fruit juice bars, frozen fruit, sorbet, frozen yogurt and low-fat ice creams with fewer than 5 grams of fat per serving.

Eating In: Quick Meals

Now that you've got a pantry, refrigerator and freezer filled with healthful choices, a simple, healthy meal is closer than you might think. With the right foods at hand, you can pull together a meal in a matter of minutes that's probably a healthier version than something you'd buy at a store or restaurant. Takeout pizza, for example, is usually laden with cheese and meat toppings, making it a high-fat, high-calorie food. If you make your own pizza at home, though, you can control the amount and type of cheese you use, and load it up with fresh vegetables for added nutrition.

If you're not keen on cooking, focus on putting together simple meals from easy-to-prepare items, including three of the food groups (dairy, whole-grains and protein, for example). Instead of having just a frozen entrée which might include some protein and carbs, you could add some cooked frozen vegetables; pre-washed cut veggies with a low-fat dip; fresh fruit; whole-grain bread or a whole-grain roll; simple green salad; or a glass of low-fat skim milk to provide additional nutrients, calories and satisfaction.

Create your own low-fat pizza at home and load it with vegatables for added nutrition.

Keeping a list of simple, easy meals on hand can make shopping and cooking much easier. These "stand-by" dinners should be things that take little time and can be made from what's usually in your kitchen. Good choices include whole-wheat pasta with chunky tomato sauce and extra vegetables thrown in; stir-fried frozen vegetables and chicken breasts over wild rice; hearty beef and vegetable soup or chili served with whole-grain bread; corn tortillas with refried beans, cheese and salsa; and omelets with low-fat cheese and a variety of vegetables. Here are some other suggestions for quick, easy meals:

- Start with a low-fat skillet meal and add sliced chicken and frozen vegetables for more fiber and protein. Add a roll, a glass of skim milk and fruit for dessert, and you've got a satisfying, hearty meal in fewer than 20 minutes.
- Bake a potato in the microwave and top with low-fat cottage cheese and broccoli for a fast lunch.
- Wrap a piece of meat or chicken in aluminum foil, add some sliced vegetables and spices, and bake in the oven until food is done. Add a glass of skim milk and some hearty bread for a wholesome dinner.
- Grill or microwave a low-fat veggie burger and serve on a whole-wheat roll along with fruit or salad.

If you're stumped at what to make, pick up a cookbook that focuses on fast, healthy meals, and start experimenting. (See the Cookbook List in Appendix D.) Or take a few minutes during the day to think about what sounds good to make for dinner. Another great strategy is to plan to cook up big batches of your favorites on a particular day of the month—like making a big pot of chili or cooking up several pounds' worth of chicken breasts. Then you can freeze or refrigerate the food and use it for a quick meal when needed—just add a vegetable, salad, whole-grain bread or fruit to round out the meal.

Look for creative ways to reuse leftovers as well. If you pick up a roasted chicken at the grocery store and have it for dinner that night with quick-baked potatoes and frozen vegetables, the next night you can make chicken tacos or BBQ chicken sandwiches with the left-over chicken. A large skillet dinner can serve as dinner one night, lunch to reheat in the microwave the next.

Eating on the Road: Healthy Snacking

As you can see, once you have a well-stocked kitchen, it's easy to eat well at home. But what about when you leave the house? Your secret weapon is being prepared with simple, portable snacks that you can easily slip into your gym bag, purse or briefcase. High-energy, healthy snacks help keep your energy levels high, maintain glycogen levels and better performance. Regular snacking not only gives you the energy you need to get through even your most harried day or demanding workout, it also helps keep your spirits—and your motivation—high.

Snacking between meals provides your body with the calories it needs throughout the day and helps keep your blood sugar levels stable. Going too long without eating makes your blood sugar fall, making you feel lightheaded, tired or just plain cranky—not to mention ravenous. A healthy snack can give you a boost before a workout, aid in exercise recovery, replace a meal you would otherwise miss and help you manage your hunger to offset overeating at the next meal.

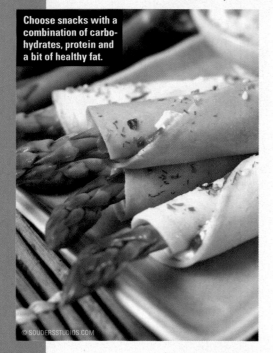

Choose snacks with a combination of carbohydrates, protein and a bit of healthy fat.

© SOUDERSSTUDIOS.COM

If, like many of us, you're trying to lose fat or maintain your weight, you might think the fewer calories a snack has, the better. But while a handful of carrot sticks may take the edge off your hunger, they won't keep you going for very long. Snacks that include a combination of carbohydrates and protein and/or fat will give you sustained energy for hours. So instead of having a piece of fruit or a bagel (both of which contain primarily carbohydrates), put a little peanut butter on your apple slices or add some turkey to your bagel. Another key to satisfying snacking is choosing foods high in fiber. Opt for a piece of fruit rather than fruit juice—the fiber helps fill you up and makes you feel more satisfied, and dietitians recommend consuming between 25 grams and 35 grams of fiber a day. As we mentioned, fruits, veggies and whole-grain breads and crackers are all good sources of fiber.

Besides preventing you from overeating, consuming snacks throughout the day can boost your mood and performance as well.[16] One study suggests that people who consume high-carbohydrate snacks before taking on stressful tasks experience fewer feelings of depression and fatigue.[17] Since your brain runs on glucose, which your body produces from carbohydrates and retrieves from its glycogen stores, keeping it well-fueled will improve your thinking abilities and help you feel calmer and less irritable.

Eating well throughout the day can also stave off the nighttime munchies. If you take in too few calories during the day, you may be so hungry by the time you get home that you'll wind up polishing off hundreds of extra calories.[18] Spread out your nutrients and calories throughout your day, and your hunger won't rage out of control at night. We've provided a list of possible healthy snacks below.

One more thing: if you're looking for easily portable snacks, you may also want to consider the growing number of "meal replacement" options. These are usually products sold in bars or ready-made or powdered liquids. Many companies offer meal replacement options, which are usually whey- or soy-based and include other ingredients along with vitamins and minerals. Some are carbohydrate-based while others are higher in protein, and they usually range in calories from 170 to 290 a serving. The advantage to these products, especially nutrition bars, is that they make a quick, tasty snack and can be tossed into a gym bag or desk until you're hungry.

Snack Ideas

Remember, creating snacks that include at least two food groups will help you increase nutrients and feel satisfied longer. Use this list to create snack combinations of your own:

- Dry cereals (whole-grain cereals are easy to eat by hand—look for those with 3 grams of fiber or more per serving.)
- Granola bars, nutrition bars or breakfast bars
- Whole-grain, whole-wheat or rye crackers or bread sticks
- Whole-grain bagels, breads, rolls
- Whole-wheat pitas
- Fresh fruit
- Baby carrots, cherry tomatoes, celery, red or green peppers, zucchini
- Baked potato (white or sweet)
- Dried fruit like raisins, apricots, prunes, apples
- Peanut butter for bagels, crackers or fruit (look for small tube containers)
- Foil-packed or single-serve cans of chicken and tuna
- Soup cups
- Ready-to-eat soup
- Nuts, soy nuts, seeds
- Air-popped popcorn
- Whole-wheat pretzels
- Low-fat cottage cheese and yogurt cups/squeezable yogurt
- Low-fat sliced cheese, small wrapped cheese wedges or string cheese
- Hard-boiled eggs
- Low-fat frozen meals (with fewer than 10 grams of fat and 500 milligrams of sodium per serving)
- Hummus
- Low-fat salad dressing cups for veggies
- Meal-replacement drinks, ready-to-drink shakes

Eating Out

Whether it's a fast-food sandwich, a meal in the cafeteria or a formal dinner, Americans love to eat out—according to the National Restaurant Association, we consume nearly 54 billion meals in restaurants and cafeterias every year. And on an average day, four out of 10 of us eat at least one meal away from home. Of all weekly meals consumed in 2000, 68.2 percent were prepared at home, 11.8 percent were skipped and 19.9 percent were prepared at a restaurant or school/work cafeteria.[19]

But restaurants often feature high-fat, high-calorie choices, and their portions are growing in size along with Americans' waistlines. A recent study found that portion sizes of foods like hamburgers and French fries are two- to five-times larger than their original sizes. And the average cookie sold in restaurants is *700 percent* larger than the U.S.D.A.'s recommended serving size of half an ounce.[20]

With the calorie-laden choices and overly large portions most restaurants feature, eating healthfully while eating out may seem to be an oxymoron. But it needn't be if you arm yourself with some smart eating strategies first: First, consider the restaurant you're choosing, and select ones with a varied menu where you're likely to find healthy

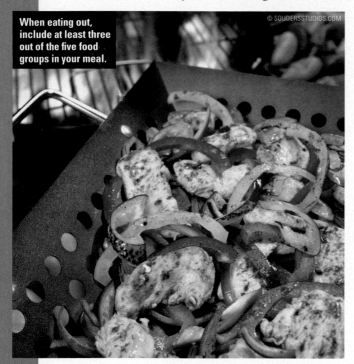

When eating out, include at least three out of the five food groups in your meal.

© SOUDERSSTUDIOS.COM

choices. Some buffets and cafeterias have a selection of low-fat choices, but you may want to skip the barbecue joint or all-you-can-eat restaurant.

Next, make sure you're not overly hungry when you head out the door. If you're starving when you get to the restaurant, it will be harder to make healthy choices. Have a piece of fruit and a big glass of water before you leave so you don't inhale the bread basket as soon as you get there.

If you're dining at a sit-down restaurant, take a careful look at the menu before you order. (Or decide before you sit down what you'll have to avoid temptation!) Many restaurants offer "lite" choices that feature meals that are lower in fat. Look at what types of foods are offered and how they're prepared— foods that start out healthy may not be smart choices; for example, a broiled chicken breast is naturally low in fat, but if it's breaded and served in a heavy sauce, it may not be the smartest choice. Pasta can be an excellent option if you get it with marinara sauce, but when it's swimming in carbonara (a white sauce with bacon and peas) or Alfredo sauce, it's loaded with fat.

In general, you'll also want to avoid fried foods and those that are sautéed in butter or oil. Even "salads" like potato salad and macaroni salad tend to be high in fat because they're mayonnaise-based. Stay away from creamy sauces, heavy sugar glazes, thick gravies and other fat-laden toppings.

Aim to include at least three out of the five food groups in your meal, just as you would at home. Some smart, low-fat choices include clear, broth-based soups; shrimp

NUTRITION ESSENTIALS

cocktail; lean meats, poultry or fish that are braised, broiled, grilled or baked; and "au jus" sauces rather than gravies or cream sauces. Words like "broiled" or "stir fried" or "steamed" usually denote healthy choices.

Look for side dishes like vegetables, and ask if they can be steamed or grilled instead of sautéed in butter. Ask for a plain baked potato with butter served on the side rather than mashed potatoes that have cream and butter added, and request whole-grain rolls. Also request that salad dressings always be served on the side, and ask whether sauces and gravies can be left off of foods.

If you've never asked questions about the way food is prepared or requested a special dish in a restaurant, you may be nervous the first couple times you do it. If you're polite and friendly, you can have almost any request granted. Be assertive—don't hesitate to ask questions or make special requests. Most servers are more than happy to accommodate you, and the people working there want you to be happy with your meal. If you don't have any say in how your food is prepared, simply make the best of it—scrape off any fatty sauces, and concentrate on what you can enjoy. Carrying complex carbohydrate snacks like pretzels, fig bars, whole-grain crackers, nutrition bars or juice boxes can help you round out an otherwise unsatisfying or too-fatty meal.

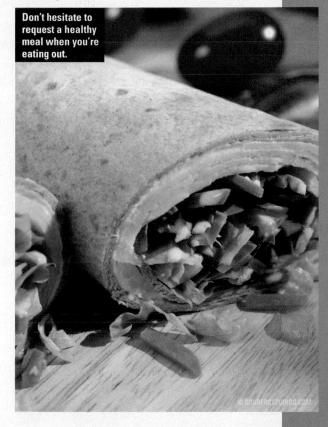

Don't hesitate to request a healthy meal when you're eating out.

Eating out is a great time to make sure you're staying hydrated. Keep a big glass of water in front of you, and shoot for drinking several glasses during your meal. It can also help prevent you from eating too much of the overly large portions most restaurants serve. One way to combat this is to ask for a half-portion of the dish, or simply divide your dinner in half (or thirds, if necessary) when it's served and plan on taking the leftovers home. Have your waitperson clear your plate as soon as you're finished—it's easy to keep eating another bite here and there after we're no longer hungry.

Finally, go easy on the alcohol—the calories add up quickly and you're more likely to abandon your good eating intentions when you drink. Remember that eating out doesn't give you carte blanche—it's OK to splurge occasionally but you can't do it every time. Plan ahead, choose your options carefully and don't be afraid to speak up, and you'll find that eating out can enhance your diet rather than derailing it.

Fast Food

Of course much of our eating out is on a "grab-and-go" basis, whether it's at a fast food restaurant or deli counter. Even the most dedicated of athletes will sometimes find themselves looking for a quick, easy meal during a typical day or while traveling.

The key to survival here is not to "supersize" your meal, even if you can get double the amount of food for a few pennies more. Go for normal portions; for example, if you order a hamburger, small fries and a diet Coke at McDonald's, you'll consume 480 calories, including 21.5 grams of fat. But opt for a Big Mac and large fries instead and you'll take in a whopping 960 calories and 54 grams of fat!

There's no question that fast food offers convenience, quick service and lower prices than traditional restaurants. The drawback is that most of the things on the menu, while low in price, are usually high in fat and calories, with few complex carbohydrate foods available. It's not surprising that a study found that the greater the more people at fast food restaurants, the more likely they were to take in more calories, more fat and less fiber and fruit.[21] However, today some fast food chains are expanding their menus to incorporate a greater variety of lower-fat and nutritious foods like baked potatoes, grilled meat items and salads. You may pay a bit more for these healthier choices, but it's worth it. Eating higher-fat foods after a workout can delay or slow glycogen reloading, and eating high-fat foods before exercise can cause feelings of heaviness, sluggishness or stomach upset. Fast foods also tend to be higher in salt as well.

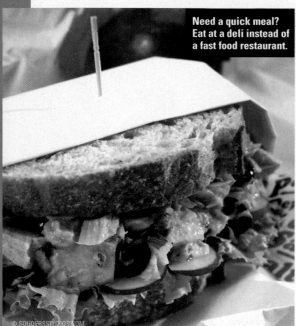

Need a quick meal? Eat at a deli instead of a fast food restaurant.

© SOUDERSSTUDIOS.COM

In addition to looking for healthy choices and ordering smaller portions, skip the carbonated beverages that are full of empty calories, in favor of water, low-fat milk or juice. Choose a fast food restaurant with a varied menu where you're more likely to find leaner choices like delis, sub shops or pizza places. Skip the fried foods, or limit your choice to only one—if you get fried chicken, for example, opt for a salad over French fries instead. (Removing the skin from fried chicken will save you lots of unnecessary fat calories.) Choosing pizza with thin crust, and loading it with vegetables but going light on the cheese is better than downing a deep dish sausage and pepperoni pie, and if you have a craving for beef, choose a roast beef or Italian beef sandwich, both of which are lower in fat than hamburger. Skip the mayonnaise and other high-fat sauces in favor of mustard and/or ketchup, and if you have any questions, ask for nutritional information at the restaurant.

When searching for a quick meal, don't overlook delis, which usually offer fresh meat or deli meat sandwich options, few fried foods and a variety of side dishes like salads, coleslaw, soups and chips. Other menu options depend on the type of deli, but there are a number of fast food "deli" chains including Subway, Quiznos, Schlotzky's and Blimpie.

At the deli, opt for low-fat meats like turkey or chicken breast, and avoid higher-fat meats like ham, pastrami and salami. As with any fast food, watch the size of your sandwich—many delis serve large portions. Choose whole-grain bread over white, and ask for a 3-ounce to 4-ounce meat sandwich rather than a 6-ounce to 8-ounce version. Skip the cheese in favor of lots of vegetables like green peppers, tomatoes, onions, lettuce and pickles. Stuffing your sandwich with vegetables will help fill you up and boost your nutrient intake, but remember that olives and avocados are also high in fat.

Use mustard, ketchup or vinegar but skip the mayonnaise, "special sauce" and oil. When choosing salads, choose a green salad over tuna, seafood or crab salad, which are usually very high in fat. Or look for vinaigrette versions of coleslaw, bean or pasta salad, which are lower in fat than the mayonnaise-based kinds. Broth-based soups are a healthy option, and if you prefer a bag of chips, buy the one-serving bag and choose low-fat chips or pretzels to save some fat grams.

The Latest Research

It's clear that the way you eat affects your performance, whether you're an exerciser or a competitive athlete. While researchers agree that spreading calories out through the day is the most effective way to ensure consistent energy levels and maintain a healthy weight, the newest area of research in this area focuses on the appropriate composition of pre- and post-workout meals. Researchers are trying to determine the appropriate balance of carbohydrates, protein and fat for athletes involved in different sports (endurance activities versus weight lifting, for example) and what combinations of fuels can help increase strength and endurance gains. Look for more emphasis on these factors in future sports nutrition research.

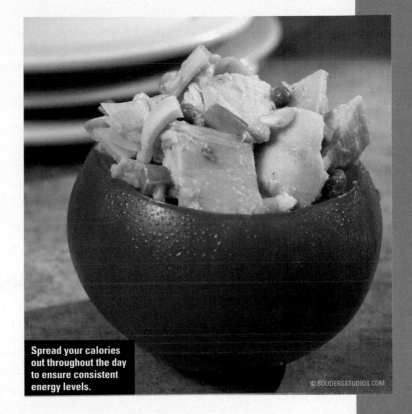

Spread your calories out throughout the day to ensure consistent energy levels.

© SOUDERSSTUDIOS.COM

Conclusion

Eating healthfully on the run does take a little bit of planning and extra effort at first, but once it's a healthy habit, you may be surprised at how much better you feel and perform. Making a commitment to eating regularly throughout the day, choosing lower-fat foods and eating a variety of foods will help you optimize your training program. Looking for the best options while dining out can help any exerciser maintain good nutrition. While snacking is recommended, particularly important are pre- and post-workout meals or snacks, which can help you perform at your peak and reload your muscles' glycogen stores. The information in this chapter applies to anyone wanting to make the most of their fitness program, but serious athletes may want to learn more about meal timing and its effect on performance by reading further on the subject (please see Chapter 10) or working with a registered dietitian who specializes in sports nutrition.

THE ULTIMATE "FAST FOOD" By Ryan Mattingly

The Scoop on Meal-Replacement Powders, Ready-to-Drink Shakes and Nutrition Bars

Many of us find ourselves giving into temptation in the name of convenience: we grab a bag of chips on our way to the big meeting, or scarf down a handful of cookies as we bolt out the door. There's so little time to spare during the day that we don't give ourselves enough time to eat balanced "mini-meals" that fuel our bodies with the right kinds of protein, carbs and healthy fats. And this isn't just the couch potatoes, either—regular gym-goers have fallen into the junk food trap as well, as they hustle from the health club to pick up the kids.

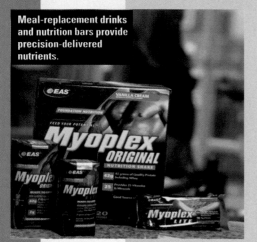

Meal-replacement drinks and nutrition bars provide precision-delivered nutrients.

We often don't realize that these daily nutrition pitfalls can sabotage all of the gains we have made in our workouts, and in our overall health. Fortunately, though, there are options for those who want a satisfying and balanced meal without the hassle of spending an hour preparing a full-course meal. Meal-replacement powders, ready-to-drink shakes and nutrition bars represent a new way to feed ourselves, with the correct blend of precision-delivered nutrients we need to make our bodies perform at peak levels. Here is a brief rundown of the benefits of these nutrition shakes and bars and how they can fit into your busy lifestyle. You'll also find out how to choose one to best suit your needs.

MEAL-REPLACEMENT SHAKES

Meal-replacement shakes (MRPs) often come in ready-to-drink (RTD) form, or as a mixable powder. Serving sizes will vary depending on the goals of the person using them. For people looking to increase size and strength, an MRP—like EAS' popular Myoplex® powders and RTDs—offers up to 42 grams of protein and 28 vitamins and minerals at 290 calories.

For those who want the benefits of a balanced nutrition product without the added calories, a product like EAS Myoplex® Lite may be the product for you. It offers 25 grams of quality protein and fiber, but with only 190 calories. Either product will give you a substantial amount of protein and a balance of carbohydrates and "good" fats that will keep your metabolism going between your main meals of the day.

Just as there are different types of meal-replacement shakes, there are different types of protein. You should look for blends of protein sources that are of high quality:

Whey protein
- Supports immune function
- Offers branched-chain amino acids (BCAAs) to aid the muscle-building process
- Is easily absorbed and utilized by the body

Casein

- Lowers insulin response of whey protein to avoid insulin spikes
- Contains glutamine, which can aid in post-workout recovery
- In studies, casein has resulted in lean-muscle gains and fat loss

Soy protein isolate

- Numerous health benefits may include lowered cholesterol and triglycerides
- Contains BCAAs

Egg albumin

- A cheap and easy source of protein (though difficult to gain benefits on its own)

You should also be looking for a blend of these nutrients:

Quality dietary fiber

- Increasing fiber may help your body process carbohydrates and sugar, a major factor in controlling insulin spikes; furthermore, scientists have found that fiber consumption is valuable in changing body fat percentages.

Essential fatty acids
(including borage, sunflower, flax seed and primrose oils)

- Essential fatty acids (EFAs) are added to many MRPs, and they have incredible benefits that include growth hormone secretion, liver support and increased metabolism. Remember, not all fats are created equal; quality EFAs can have a positive impact on your training and overall health.

Vitamins and minerals

- A major function of MRPs—like the Myoplex® family of products—is their inclusion of a major percentage of the recommended daily allowance of vitamins and minerals. Consuming these fortified MRPs can deliver a precise dose of the micronutrients you need on a daily basis.

NUTRITION BARS

Like shakes, nutrition bars come in many forms and fulfill the same function: They can provide important nutrients, and though they are not a total substitute for food, they can be a great source of protein and carbohydrates. Be aware, however, of false label claims and bars that seem to good to be true. Here are three tips for choosing a good bar:

1) Buy from reputable companies
2) Look for a quality protein blend (as mentioned before)
3) Look for minimal fat amounts

RECOMMENDED SHAKES AND BARS

Meal-Replacement Powders and Ready-to-Drinks

Weight-training and high-performance athletes

- Myoplex® Deluxe—EAS®
- Myoplex® Sport—EAS®

Change-seekers and fitness enthusiasts looking for better nutrition

- Myoplex® Ready-To-Drink Nutrition Shake—EAS®
- Myoplex® Carb Sense® Ready-To-Drink—EAS®
- Myoplex® Lite—EAS®
- Myoplex® Original—EAS®
- AdvantEdge® Protein Drink—EAS®

Nutrition Bars

Weight-training and high-performance athletes

- Myoplex® Deluxe Bar—EAS®

Change-seekers and fitness enthusiasts looking for better nutrition

- Myoplex™ Storm™—EAS®
- Myoplex® Carb Sense®—EAS®

Eating on the Run: The Basics

Key Concepts:

1. Your diet is an essential component of any fitness program, and you won't have optimal results unless you make it a priority.

2. The first step to creating an eat-on-the-run program is to understand why it's important to eat regular, nutritious meals, and create a plan for how you will do that. You should plan to eat three meals and two snacks or six mini-meals a day.

3. Regular grocery shopping helps keep your kitchen stocked with the food choices you need to make quick, healthy meals and prepare snacks for the road.

4. Carrying healthy snacks with you is one of the best ways to ensure that you fuel your body with healthy foods throughout the day.

5. Eating out need not derail your healthy eating program if you make smart menu choices and limit your portions. Fast food restaurants and delis also offer lower-fat options that athletes can choose for maximum nutrition on the road.

Recommendations:

❶ Write down how you eat over a week to get an idea of what your biggest eating challenges are.

❷ Create a basic framework for healthy eating based on either three meals and two snacks or six mini-meals a day. Select from at least three food groups for each meal and from at least two for each snack.

❸ Stock your kitchen with healthy foods, and learn how to create quick, nutritious meals and snacks. Carry healthy snacks with you so you're prepared to eat when hungry.

❹ Look for sit-down restaurants, fast food chains and delis that offer healthy choices.

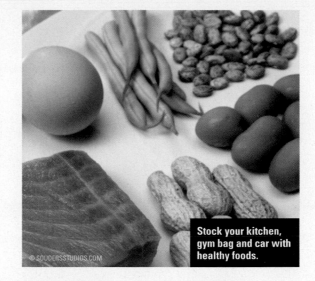

Stock your kitchen, gym bag and car with healthy foods.

© SOUDERSSTUDIOS.COM

REFERENCES CITED:

[1] Bowman, SA, Spence, JT. A comparison of low-carbohydrate vs. high-carbohydrate diets: energy restriction, nutrient quality and correlation to body mass index. *Journal of the American College of Nutrition* 21.3 (2002): 268-274.

[2] Maffucci, DM, McMurray, RG. Towards optimizing the timing of the pre-exercise meal. *International Journal of Sports Nutrition and Exercise Metabolism* 10 (2000): 103-113.

[3] Lemon, PWR, Berardi, JM, Noreen, EE. The role of protein and amino acid supplements in the athlete's diet: does type or timing of ingestion matter? *Current Sports Medicine Reports* 4 (2002): 14-221.

[4] Jentjens, R, Jeukendrup, AE. Determinants of post-exercise glycogen synthesis during short-term recovery. *Sports Medicine* 33.2 (2003): 117-144.

[5] Speechly, DP, Buffenstein, R. Greater appetite control associated with an increased frequency of eating in lean males. *Appetite* (1999): 285-297.

[6] Garrow, JS et al. The effect of meal frequency and protein concentration on the composition of the weight lost by obese subjects. *British Journal of Nutrition* 45 (1981): 5-15.

[7] Fairchild, TJ et al. Rapid carbohydrate loading after a short bout of near maximal-intensity exercise. *Medicine & Science in Sports & Exercise* 34.6 (2002): 980-986.

[8] Hargreaves, M. Pre-exercise nutritional strategies: effects on metabolism and performance. Canadian Journal of Applied Physiology 26(Supp) (2001): S64-S70.

[8] Haff GG, Lehmkuhl MJ, McCoy LB, Stone MH. Carbohydrate supplementation and resistance training. *Journal of Strength and Conditioning Research* 17.1 (2003): 187-196.

[9] Wyatt, HR, et al. Long-term weight loss and breakfast in subjects in the National Weight Control Registry. *Obesity Research* 10.2 (2002): 78-82.

[9] Benton, D, Parker, PY. Breakfast, blood glucose, and cognition. *American Journal of Clinical Nutrition* 67 (Supp) (1988): S772-S778.

[10] Craig, WJ. Phytochemicals: guardians of our health. *Journal of the American Dietetic Association* 97.10 (1997): S199-205.

[11] Van Duyn, MS. Overview of the health benefits of fruits and vegetable consumption for the dietetics professional: selected literature. *Journal of the American Dietetic Association* 100.12 (2000): 1511-1521.

[12] Howarth, NC, Saltzman, MD. Roberts S.B. Dietary fiber and weight regulation. *Nutrition Reviews* 59.5 (2001): 129-139.

[13] Yao, M, Roberts, SB. Dietary energy density and weight regulation. *Nutrition Reviews* 59.8 (2001): 247-258.

[14] Craig, WJ. Phytochemicals: guardians of our health. *Journal of the American Dietetic Association* 97.10 (1997): S199-205.

[15] Van Duyn, MS. Overview of the health benefits of fruits and vegetable consumption for the dietetics professional: selected literature. *Journal of the American Dietetic Association* 100.12 (2000): 1511-1521.

[16] Kanarek, R. Psychological effects of snacks and altered meal frequency. *British Journal of Nutrition* 77.S1 (1997): S105-S120.

[17] Markus, CR et al. Does carbohydrate-rich, protein-poor food prevent a deterioration of mood and cognitive performance of stress-prone subjects when subjected to a stressful task? *Appetite* 31 (1998): 49-65.

[18] Kanarek, R. Psychological effects of snacks and altered meal frequency. *British Journal of Nutrition* 77.S1 (1997): S105-S120.

[19] National Restaurant Association. *Frequently asked questions.* www.restaurant.org/faq.cfm.

[20] Young, LR, Nestle, M. The contribution of expanding portion sizes to the US obesity epidemic. *American Journal of Public Health* 92.2 (2002): 246-249.

[21] French, SA, Harnack, L, Jeffery, RW. Fast food restaurant use among women in the Pound of Prevention study: dietary, behavioral and demographic correlates. *International Journal of Obesity* 24 (2000): 1353-1359.

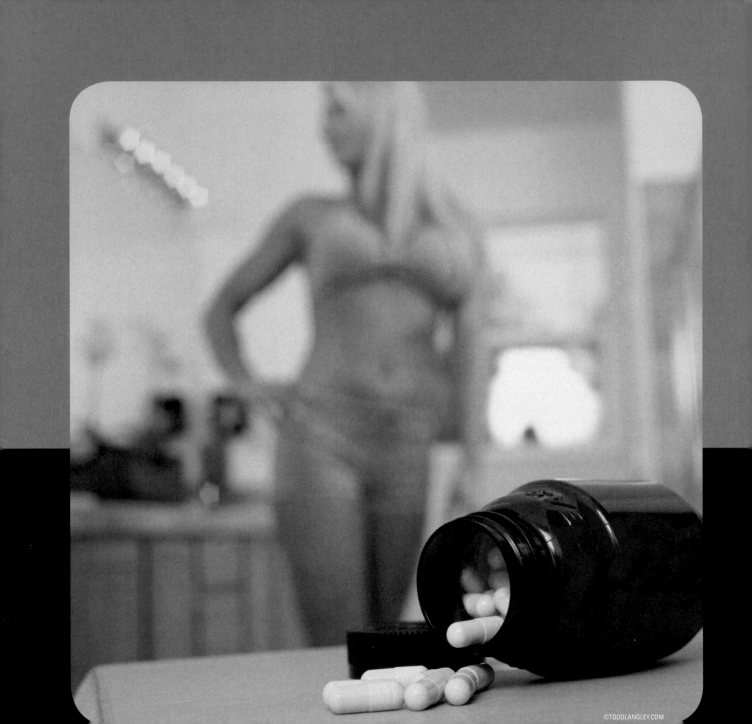

WEIGHT LOSS & WEIGHT MANAGEMENT

part two

6 NUTRITION FOR FAT LOSS

A Balanced Nutrition Plan for Losing Fat

By Brett Hall, R.D.

Losing fat not only improves your health and energy levels, but the simple act of losing excess body fat can affect every facet of your ability to perform at peak levels. By shaving off unproductive pounds, your body becomes much more efficient. The lighter you are—the better your muscle-to-fat ratio—the more nimble you'll be, the faster your body will accelerate, stop, cut, twist and turn. Not to mention that your strength to body-weight ratio will also increase dramatically. You'll feel stronger and more in control of your body.

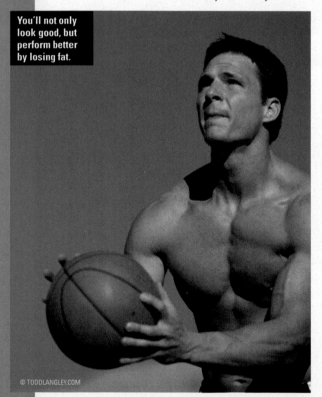

You'll not only look good, but perform better by losing fat.

© TODDLANGLEY.COM

And endurance enhancement goes hand in hand with this increase in strength and agility. The very fact that your muscles have to move less body mass allows them to work longer and move your body more quickly over greater distances. That's simple physics, and it's research-proven. Subjects in two recent studies who lost a substantial percentage of body fat also significantly increased their aerobic endurance, anaerobic capacity, 5-mile run times and even muscular strength, with little or no exercise.[1,2]

Physiologically speaking, you are also increasing your cardiovascular efficiency. For every pound of body fat you carry, you force your blood to detour through an extra *mile* of capillaries. By shedding fat, you decrease the distance and time it takes to deliver oxygen- and energy-rich blood to hungry muscles. This not only feeds muscles more efficiently, it also decreases the workload on your heart; allowing your muscles to work harder while keeping your heart rate lower.

Another dramatic physiological effect of fat loss is an improvement of glucose (blood sugar) handling. Recent research shows that by losing just 15 percent of your body fat, you can literally *double* the rate at which your body burns up and clears glucose from your blood stream.[3] This means your muscles are converting glucose more efficiently into energy, and your chances of storing excess blood sugar as fat are dramatically reduced. More muscular energy, less fat storage. This is good.

The Road to Fat Loss: Where Are You Now?

In order to know how much fat you would like to (or need to) lose and how much muscle you'd like to gain as you get going on your plan, you need to know what your current body composition is. You can get an accurate body composition test done at your local gym or hospital. One of the simplest and easiest ways to determine your fat-to-muscle ratio is by getting a five- to six-point fat caliper test performed by an experienced individual. To best judge your progress, you should use the same method (and person) to test your body fat each time.

Now that you know exactly where your physical starting point is, it's time to assess your dietary starting point. This is one of the most important aspects of your fat-loss program planning. In order to build a plan that works specifically for you, you have to know how your particular body handles calories. Not all bodies are the same, and that's why so many of those "cookie cutter" diet plans fail so often.

Everyone has a distinctive metabolism, meaning you handle calories differently; for instance, you may be able to pack down 3,000 calories a day and not gain an ounce of fat, while your workout partner skimps along on 1,500 calories a day and has a hard time keeping the fat off. Is it fair? Well, not for your partner.

The first thing you need to do is to see where you fall along this metabolic continuum. And the best way to do that is to assess your current calorie consumption by keeping a detailed account of everything you eat for an entire week. This is your "Food Record."

You may think you already have a pretty good idea of what your daily caloric intake is, but you may be surprised. While we tend to remember our habitual food items and the main meals, we often leave out the snacks we grab on the run, the M&Ms® we sneak off our co-worker's desk, as well as drinks, condiments, side dishes, etc. And they all add up.

did you know?

The Benefits of Fat Loss
- Increased energy
- More endurance
- More strength
- Better health
- A smaller waistline

Keeping Your Food Record

This is one of those tasks that is simple—but not necessarily easy. It's simple because all you do is keep track of every morsel of food and drink you consume for seven days. But it takes a great amount of diligence and attention to detail to do it, and do it right. And doing it right is very important. Because if you don't—if you just jot down guesstimates—you'll get an inaccurate picture of your intake, leading to an imperfect plan and poor results. This needs to be a precise record.

Here is a quick step-by-step breakdown of exactly how to keep your food record:
- First, buy a small, pocket-sized note pad. Carry this and a pen with you at all times (or as often as you can).
- On the first page of your notebook, write down your starting weight, your body fat percentage and the date and time you are starting and ending your food diary (i.e., Start upon waking: Monday, January 4, 2004. End when going to bed: Sunday, January 10, 2004).

tip

IMPORTANT: Please do not alter your typical eating habits while keeping this record. The goal isn't to see how good you can be for a week but to get a clear picture of what your current habits are like and how they have been affecting your body over time. This is where the value lies.

- Make sure to record every bit of food you eat.
- For every food item you enter make sure to include the following:
    - Type of food (ham sandwich)
    - How it was cooked, prepared or served (cold)
    - All the various components of the food (ham, whole-wheat bread, mayonnaise, tomato, mustard, Swiss cheese)
    - Exact amounts (or close guesses) of each food or food component. Use weight or volume measurements (ounces, cups, tablespoons, etc.) (Example: 3 ounces of lean ham, 1 ounce of Swiss cheese, 1 tablespoon mayonnaise, 1 teaspoon mustard, two slices of tomato, on two slices of whole-wheat bread)
    - All condiments, side dishes, etc. (Example: 1 tablespoon mayonnaise, 1 teaspoon mustard)
    - All drinks, even coffee, tea or sodas, as well as the stuff you put in them—sugar, cream, etc. It's easy to forget these, and they can make up a substantial portion of your caloric intake
    - The exact time of day each food is eaten
- Write down a sentence or two about how you are feeling a few times throughout the day. (i.e., 2 p.m.: Feel tired and groggy. 7 p.m.: Strong and alert.) Being able to pinpoint how different meals make you feel at different times can be invaluable.

Analyzing Your Food Record: You Are What You Eat

First, you need to figure out your overall daily caloric intake from this record. You'll use this to calculate your personalized calorie intake. Here's what you need to do.

There are two different ways you can go about assessing your calories. You can buy a calorie-counting book or you can go online and use a diet analyzing program, such as www.nutri-facts.com. This program pulls from the USDA database of over 12,000 foods. It's easy to use, fast and accurate. If you choose to use a book, try *The Most Complete Food Counter*, by Annette B. Natow, Ph.D., R.D., and Jo-Ann Heslin, M.A., R.D. (Pocket Books, 1999).

Whatever method you choose to use, here's what you do:
- Get an accurate calorie count for each and every food on your list. Make sure to find the food that most closely matches your food (i.e., broiled, skinless chicken breast versus just chicken breast).
- Be sure to use your quantity measurements and be as accurate as possible when matching them to the choices in your analysis tool.
- Total up all of the calories for each food item for each day. Obtain a calorie total for each day separately (notice how your caloric intake bounces around from day to day).

- Next, add all of the daily totals together to get a total weekly calorie count.
- Then divide the total weekly calorie count by seven.
- This will give you your average daily calorie intake.

And this is the magic number. This is what you'll use to calculate the calorie level around which you'll build your personal program.

Calculating Your Maintenance Calorie Level

Now that you know how many calories you typically eat per day, you have to know how those calories have been affecting your body. First, ask yourself if your current eating and exercise patterns have been fairly consistent over the past six months. Hopefully (and more than likely) the answer will be yes. (If not we'll deal with that later.) Next, take stock of how your body may or may not have changed within that same six-month period of time. Have you lost fat? Gained fat? Stayed the same?

For example, if you have gained 6 pounds of fat over the course of the last six months, and your average daily caloric intake is about 2,400 calories, then you know, at your current level of activity and consumption, that you are in positive calorie balance; therefore, your maintenance calorie level (MCL)—the calorie level you would need to just keep your weight constant—lies somewhere below 2,400 calories a day.

Now let's get a bit more technical and pinpoint exactly what your MCL is. Each pound of body fat represents 3,500 calories of stored energy. And if, in this example, you gained an average of 1 pound of fat per month over the last six months, that's 3,500 excess calories you were consuming each month. All you have to do is divide 3,500 calories by 30 days in the month, and you get your daily average excess calorie intake, which would be 117. Meaning that on average you were consuming 117 more calories each day than you were burning—leading to fat storage. With this information, you can

CALCULATING YOUR MAINTENANCE CALORIE LEVEL

- **Average daily caloric intake:**
  - (Example: 2,400 calories)

- **Weight lost or gained over the last six months:**
  - (Example: Gained 6 pounds = 3,500 extra calories each month)
  - (Example: Lost 6 pounds = 3,500 fewer calories each month)
  - (Example: No weight lost or gained: 2,400 average daily caloric intake is your maintenance calorie level)

- **Excess or negative calories consumed over the last six months:**
  - (Example: Gained 6 pounds = 3,500 extra calories/30 days = 117 extra calories each day)
  - (Example: Lost 6 pounds = 3,500 fewer calories/30 days = 117 too few calories a day if weight loss is not desired)

- **Maintenance caloric level: Average daily caloric intake minus excess calories or plus negative calories**
  - (Example: 2,400 average daily caloric intake – 117 excess calories = 2,283 calories = maintenance calorie level)
  - (Example: 2,400 average daily caloric intake + 117 negative calories = 2,517 calories = maintenance calorie level)

then calculate your rough MCL as 2,400 calories − 117 calories = 2,283 calories. And this is the "magic" number you need to create all your meal plans around. More on that later.

The Treacherous Trail to Fat Loss

Here's a look at the possible obstacles you might encounter along the way and how you can effectively and efficiently navigate past challenges.

How many times have you been derailed on your fat-loss journey by the insidious effects of constant hunger? Hunger is your body's first metabolic line of defense when it senses a lack of caloric intake. Through a complex and multi-faceted series of physiological mechanisms, when you drop below the caloric intake to which your body has become accustomed, it sends signals to your brain letting it know that it must eat, now. Hence the gnawing in your gut, the sense of emptiness and the overwhelming urge to eat. Hunger, and the sense of deprivation it induces, is one of the main reasons people fail on calorie-restricted diets.[4,5]

And hunger is by no means the only metabolic challenge you will face. Others include:

- Suppression of thyroid hormone production, which strongly influences metabolic rate[6,7]
- Direct suppression of Resting Metabolic Rate (RMR—the number of calories your body burns at rest). This leads to a decrease in overall metabolic rate, forcing you to drop your caloric intake even lower in order to continue to lose fat[8,9]
- Decrease in energy level due to low blood sugar levels and compromised glycogen stores[10]
- Increase in catabolic hormone production—namely glucagon and cortisol—which stimulates muscle catabolism (breakdown) and loss[10]
- Suppression of the immune system.[11] This puts you at risk for becoming sick and further enhancing your catabolic state, causing serious muscle loss[12]
- In low-carb diets, due to a severe lack of carbs for blood sugar support, there is a further stimulation of muscle catabolism. Muscles are broken down because amino acids (which make up muscle protein) are a source for gluconeogenesis (creation of blood sugar)[10]

So that's the bad news. Want some good news? Every one of these challenges can be overcome or completely avoided. You can lose fat *and* maintain all your muscle. You can reach your fat-loss goal without compromising your metabolism or your energy levels. Here's the secret.

The Metabolic Master Switch

Leptin is a protein-based hormone secreted primarily from fat cells, and it holds the key to lasting fat loss. Leptin (from the Greek "leptos," meaning "thin") is what you might call a master control hormone. It sits atop a large chemical bureaucracy in your body, meaning that it has the ability to control a wide variety of other hormones that sit below it, and they in turn affect the function of a huge array of metabolic functions. These functions include everything from appetite control, to lipolysis (fat burning), to metabolic rate, to muscle maintenance and even the production of testosterone and growth hormone.[13] Anything and everything having to do with the shedding of fat stores is at least partially controlled by this one master hormone.

Where did leptin come from, and why is it so dead set on keeping us fat? To answer this question, we have to step back in time about 10,000 years or so. Before the industrial revolution, before farming, even before the domestication of animals, humans were hunters and gatherers. They existed, for thousands of years, by living off what the land provided from day to day. Food availability was often sporadic—it was heavily dependent upon seasons, weather, animal migration, etc. This scarcity of food availability led to a "feast or famine" type of existence. At times, after a big kill or finding a fertile valley, people would have more food than they knew what to do with. And then there would be times during the winter or drought when there would be very little food available for long periods of time. This pattern of feast or famine made it necessary for humans to become very efficient at storing energy reserves during the times of feast in order to make it through the famine. Those who couldn't, died off, leaving those who could to propagate the species.

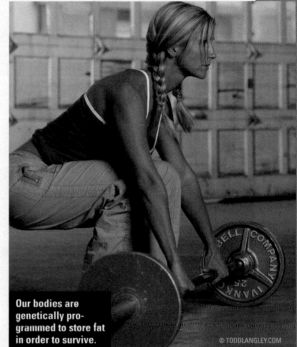

Our bodies are genetically programmed to store fat in order to survive.

© TODDLANGLEY.COM

This concept is perfect Darwinian evolution, in which it's a matter of survival of the fittest. And in this case, the "fittest" were the fattest. Those who were genetically predisposed to store the most fat survived, passing this fat-storing genetic trait on. And the main gene that was selected for this evolutionary process was what scientists call the "fat gene." And it's this gene that is responsible for producing leptin.

As you can see, our bodies are literally programmed by thousands of years of evolution to be very efficient energy conservers. The sole purpose of leptin is to keep us from starving to death. That's why whenever your body senses a nutritional threat—a lack of sufficient intake—it shuts down leptin production, which in turn affects every aspect of your metabolism, from metabolic rate to hunger. Anything and everything it can to decrease energy expenditure, increase energy storage and convince you that you really need to be eating more.

Let's take a quick look at exactly what leptin does and how it does it in order to help you understand how you can work with this genetic coding in order to create fitness versus fatness.

The Leptin Effect

First and foremost, leptin is a potent regulator of both long- and short-term appetite. Its short-term effects have to do with its ability to potentiate the appetite- suppressing effects of other hormones such as cholecystokinin (CCK). After you eat a meal, the gut sends out messengers to the brain to tell you when to stop eating. One such messenger is CCK. But research has shown that when leptin is low, CCK doesn't produce its normal appetite-suppressing effect, and could therefore fail to inhibit further food intake.[14] Basically, when leptin levels are low, you have a hard time eating enough to feel full. Not good.

While this short-term effect is an issue, it's leptin's long-term effects on appetite that are truly important. Leptin is produced in fat cells, and this production is stimulated in the fat cell when the cell expands. The more fat your fat cells are storing, the more leptin they will produce.[15] Once produced, leptin is shuttled in the blood stream to the brain where it acts on the hypothalamus and other areas of the brain. It stimulates the hypothalamus to produce a variety of other peptides (protein messengers) that are distributed throughout the body and reduce hunger on the neurological level.[16] In other words, when you carry excess fat, your chronic hunger levels are low. But when you lose fat and leptin production drops off, chronic hunger kicks in.

Leptin is also a powerful regulator of metabolism. It has the ability to modulate the secretion of a variety of hormones—including thyroid hormone, cortisol and testosterone.[17,18] All of these hormones can dramatically affect energy balance, metabolic rate and fat loss; for instance, when leptin levels drop, it brings thyroid and testosterone levels down with it, while stimulating cortisol production. The end result is that your metabolic rate slows down, muscle growth is halted and muscle catabolism is increased. A lose-lose situation for fat loss (so to speak) if ever there were one.

Leptin Regulators

So, how is leptin controlled in the body? What determines the levels of this potent hormone? On the highest level, there are two main things that affect your body's production of leptin—body fat and food intake. This makes sense because leptin's whole purpose is to act as a body weight regulator, to help keep your body at a certain level of fatness to "protect" you from starvation. Here's how it works.

As stated above, much of the leptin in your body is produced in fat cells. When the fat cell expands (as you store more fat) more leptin is produced. When it shrinks (as you

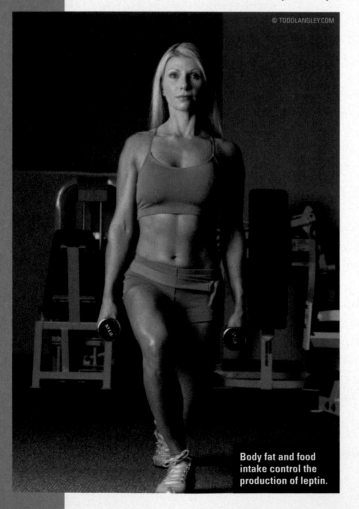

© TODDLANGLEY.COM

Body fat and food intake control the production of leptin.

lose fat) leptin production is sharply diminished.[19] This is the main mechanism by which leptin keeps your body at a "set point" of fatness. As you get leaner, it becomes harder to keep the fat loss going. Because as your fat levels decrease, so do your leptin levels, which in turn stimulate intense hunger, slows your metabolism, slows muscle growth, and speeds muscle breakdown. Your body is doing everything it can to convince you that this fat loss is not a good thing.

Your level of food intake is the other major piece to the leptin production puzzle. Leptin production is stimulated by eating. Every time you eat your leptin levels increase by as much as 40 percent.[20] Research shows that insulin is the mechanism by which eating stimulates leptin production. Every time you eat, your body produces insulin in order to handle the influx of blood sugar. This same insulin effectively stimulates leptin production.

On the flip side of the coin, a lack of food intake (either long periods with no food or very small doses of food) will suppress your circulating insulin levels, thus suppressing leptin production.[20] This is the main reason that traditional calorie-restricted diets just don't work in the long run—and why our American habit of eating as little as two meals per day has led us down the road to obesity.

A recent study puts this all in perspective. Overweight subjects were all put on a sensible diet which was 500 calories below their calculated daily maintenance calorie level. Half of the subjects received injections of tiny doses of pure leptin each day, and the other half received a placebo. After 24 weeks, the group receiving leptin lost an average of 14 pounds while the placebo group only lost about 3 pounds.[21] And what's more impressive is that almost all of the weight lost in the leptin group was from fat (95 percent), with vir-

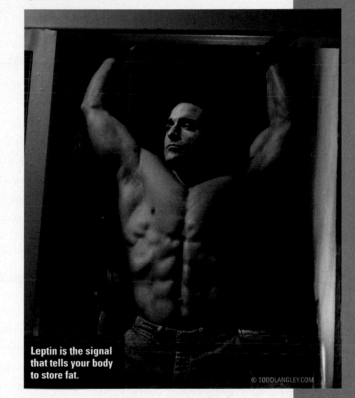

Leptin is the signal that tells your body to store fat.

© TODDLANGLEY.COM

tually no loss of muscle mass. Under normal situations in which calories are restricted, both muscle and fat are lost at about a 50:50 ratio.[2] Losing so much muscle during weight loss is clearly not optimal and can contribute to rebound weight gain. Studies have demonstrated as much as a 6.5 percent drop in resting metabolic rate after losing just 4 pounds of muscle on a calorie-restricted diet.[22]

Leptin is the latest and greatest discovery in the fight against fat, and on the following pages you'll see how you can make it work for you.

The Fat-Loss Plan

Now you know that leptin is the signal that tells your body to protect its energy reserves—its fat stores. And you know that it is very sensitive to any changes in diet or body composition that would make it think it's at risk of starvation. What you have to do is convince your body that it's not at risk; that there is plenty of food for survival. And you have to do this while putting your body in a slightly negative calorie balance to stimulate fat loss—in other words, inducing a state of slow, steady starvation. Sound tricky? It is, but it's doable.

But first and foremost, this plan is not about crash dieting. It's not about slashing off 10 pounds per week. It's not a quick fix. If you try and go that route, you will be fighting evolution, and you will lose. This plan is about working *with* your body, not against it. It's designed to put you on the path to lifelong leanness. It's a slow and steady path that's about modifying habits and molding your metabolism. But be patient. It took you many months or years to shape your body as it is today. And it may take some time to get it where you want it to be. But in the end it will be well worth the wait.

Picking Your Calorie Level

Have you ever heard anyone espouse the philosophy that "calories don't count?" In the absolute end analysis of fat loss, calories are the *only* things that truly count. The number of calories that end up in your blood stream minus the number of calories your body burns each day will determine how much excess energy there is for your body to store. That said, the number of calories that go in your mouth represent only one factor in the energy balance equation. The number of those calories that eventually end up in your blood stream, how many of *those* then end up as excess, and where those excess calories end up (in fat or muscle glycogen stores) can be manipulated and depend on a variety of other dietary factors, which we will be addressing. So, while the number of calories you eat is key, it's not everything.

This being the case, you need to take a conservative approach to your calorie cutting. You have seen how damaging drastic calorie deprivation can be to your metabolism and fat-loss efforts. And you know that cutting calories too far will stimulate your body's defense mechanisms and crush leptin levels. It's simply not necessary, healthy or effective to do so. Therefore, you'll only be cutting calories by 15 percent; that is 85 percent of your calculated MCL.

One more quick thing about calories: If you decide to increase your typical exercise output as you begin your fat-loss plan (which will likely be the case) you'll need to adjust your caloric intake to accommodate that increase in caloric output. It's very important that your calorie intake doesn't drop too far below your overall caloric output each day, or you know what happens. If you add in some more exercise, account for it by calculating the number of calories you're likely to burn with the added activity. Then add those calories back into your meal plan in order to keep your DCG at 85 percent of your MCL. You can calculate the calories you expend by checking out any number of Web sites that can show you typical calories expended during just about any activity you can think of. One site to try is www.primusweb.com/fitnesspartner/jumpsite/ calculat.htm.

Calculate your calorie goal as follows:

- Let's assume your MCL is 2,200 calories. (Turn back to "Calculating Your Maintenance Calorie Level" to calculate your MCL.)

- Multiply your MCL by 85 percent to get your calorie goal: $2,200 \times 0.85 = 1,870$.

- Your daily calorie goal (DCG) is 1,870 calories.

- Summary equation: $MCL \times 0.85 = DCG$.

Macronutrient Makeup

Now that you know how much you're going to eat, let's look at what these calories should consist of and why. This isn't a low-carb diet. (Check out the sidebar "Balanced Is Best" to find out why.) The nutrient composition of your plan needs to be balanced in order to be sustainable, such as a 40/40/20 ratio of protein, carbs and fat. Here's why:

⊖ Carbs Are King

Carbs are king when it comes to supporting optimal energy levels and leptin production. They are responsible for filling up glycogen stores, and a solid dose of carbs following a strenuous workout is the surest way to replenish depleted glycogen stores,[23] thus assuring you have the energy reserves available for your next bout of exercise. Carbs also create an anabolic environment in your body by stimulating insulin production and suppressing cortisol.[24] Consumed at the proper time of day (i.e., first thing in the morning or after exercise), especially in combination with protein, this anabolic stimulation significantly upgrades amino acid uptake into and repair of muscle tissue. This means faster recovery and more muscle growth.

Carbs also stimulate the production and maintenance of robust leptin levels. This carb-induced stimulation of leptin is mediated by insulin. As insulin levels increase in response to carb intake, glucose metabolism within fat cells is enhanced, triggering leptin production.[25] Leptin levels then stay elevated for the next four to five hours.[26] And when you're eating small meals every three to four hours, as you will be on this plan, your leptin levels will remain constantly elevated—exactly what you want. The key here is to include just the right amount and type of carbs with each meal in order to induce a large-enough insulin response to instigate leptin production without stimulating fat storage. You'll find out how to do this shortly.

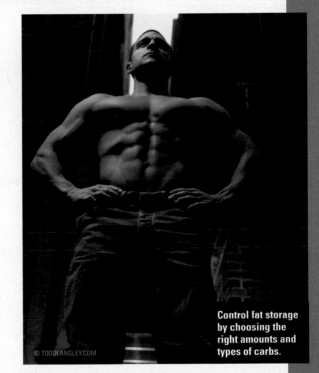

Control fat storage by choosing the right amounts and types of carbs.

© TODDLANGLEY.COM

⊖ The Power of Protein

As far as fat-loss nutrition planning is concerned, protein serves many purposes. If you want to preserve or enhance your muscle mass as you lose fat, and you'll also be exercising, having plenty of protein around is very important. Research indicates that exercise increases the need for protein in the diet.[27] Further studies have shown that the anabolic effects of intense training are increased with a high-protein diet.[28,29]

One study tested the effect of two different levels of protein head-to-head in weight-lifting men on low-calorie diets. One group received 1.6 grams of protein per kilogram of body weight (128 grams for a 180-pound guy), while the other group received half that. They were both fed the same number of calories (1,440 calories for a 180-pound guy). And both groups did the same exercise regimen. The findings were impressive. The high-protein group actually gained about a half pound of muscle in one week while losing fat, while the low protein group lost a half pound of muscle.[29]

Another effect protein has on fat loss is that it is far more thermogenic (heat producing, i.e., calorie burning) than carbs or fat. Every food we eat has what's called a thermic effect. This thermic effect is the amount of energy it takes to digest, process and metabolize that specific food. And protein has the highest thermic effect of all the macronutrients; in other words, if you eat 100 calories of pure fat in one meal and 100 calories of pure protein in an-

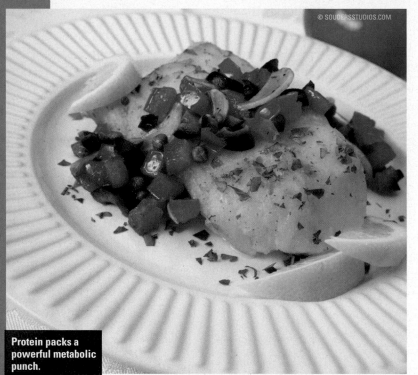

© SOUDERSSTUDIOS.COM

Protein packs a powerful metabolic punch.

other meal, because protein's thermic effect is about 30 percent versus about 7 percent for fat, 93 net calories end up in your body from fat, whereas only about 70 calories for protein.[30]

And this effect carries over to mixed meals as well. A recent study demonstrated that a meal consisting of 29 percent protein produced a dietary induced thermogenesis (DIT) of 14 percent, while the 9 percent protein meal produced a 10 percent DIT.[31] This is a 40 percent increase in DIT due to the higher level of protein.

Over the long run this can make a difference in fat loss—as is evidenced by another recent study where subjects lost more fat while consuming a higher protein diet compared to a control group who was on a high-carb diet.[32]

Suffice it to say, protein packs a powerful metabolic punch when it comes to fat loss and that's why it accounts for up to 40 percent of your total caloric intake on this recommended fat-loss plan.

The Functions of Fat

Fat is probably the trickiest of the nutrients in terms of fat loss. There is a fine line between too much and too little fat. Too much fat (more than 30 percent) and research shows that fat storage increases and obesity becomes much more prevelant.[33] Too little fat and you compromise the ability of your muscles to recuperate and can even significantly suppress vital hormone production. One study found that free testosterone dropped by 22 percent when dietary fat intake was cut from 36 percent of calories to 7 percent.[34] You need just the right amount of fat to support the multiple vital functions necessary to support fat loss and muscle growth, without overdoing it. And that amount is 20 percent of your total caloric intake.

The proper intake of fat in the right forms (i.e., essential fatty acids [EFAs]) will support all of the following metabolic actions:

- EFA intake is necessary for production of prostaglandins (PGE). Research has demonstrated that PGE is a potent stimulator of growth hormone (GH).[35] If PGE levels are supported by proper EFA intake, GH levels will also remain strong. And the power of GH to create fat loss and support muscle growth is well-known.
- EFA levels in the blood and as components of muscles have a dramatic effect on both the secretion and action of insulin. The higher the ratio of EFAs, the more efficiently insulin is produced and the more sensitive muscle cells are to its action.[36,37] This means a greater anabolic ability in muscle cells and a greater ability to support strong leptin levels.
- The specialty fat, conjugated linoleic acid (CLA), has been shown to not only decrease fat stores in the body, but to actually kill fat cells in the process.[38,39] For more on CLA and the role of it and other fat-loss supplements in your fat-loss plan, go to Chapter 7.
- And finally, dietary fat of any kind slows gastric emptying (the rate at which food moves out of the stomach into the intestine). This slowing effect increases the length of satiety after a meal and helps regulate food absorption and blood sugar fluctuations. The key here is including the right amount of fat in the right meals to create the desired effect.

How Much of What Goes Where, When and Why

This is where all of the theory we have been discussing comes together to create your actual meal plan—what percentage of your DCG goes in each meal, exact ratios of carbs, protein and fat in each meal and precise timing for when each meal should be eaten.

Your body has very different metabolic needs at different times of day and under differing circumstances. And if you just eat the same type of meal at all hours of the day, without regard to your body's needs, you'll be frustrated and probably fail in your goal. But by supplying the right combo of nutrients in the right amounts, at exactly the right times of day, you can cruise to a new body with very little pain involved.

Here's a breakdown of what is going on in your body at different times of the day, what your body needs at that time and what food combinations will address those needs. For purposes of this example, let's assume you have a "typical" office working lifestyle. Wake up at 6:30 a.m. Work all day at the office. Work out after work. To bed by 10 p.m. or so. If your lifestyle differs dramatically from this, just use the concepts discussed to tailor your program to your schedule.

BREAKFAST

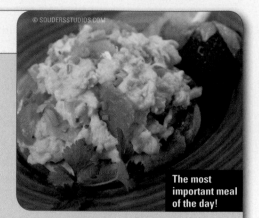

© SOUDERSSTUDIOS.COM

The most important meal of the day!

⊖ **Metabolic State**

Having been without any caloric input for somewhere between eight and 12 hours, your body is more or less in a "fasted" state. Hence the word for the first meal of the day: "break-fast." This being the case:

- Your glycogen reserves are a bit low.
- Your muscles are in a mild catabolic state.
- Fat stores are also slowly being mobilized and burned.
- Your cortisol levels are elevated.
- Your blood leptin level is falling. (Leptin levels are on a natural diurnal cycle. Without any external influences, they peak in the evening between midnight and about 3 a.m., then begin to decline until they hit a low in the early afternoon.[40])

⊖ **Metabolic Goals**

- With these metabolic issues in mind, your goals for this meal are as follows:
- Halt the muscle catabolism
- Support ongoing fat burning
- Replenish carbohydrate energy reserves (glycogen)
- Help boost falling leptin levels

⊖ **Meal Solutions**

This will be your biggest meal of the day. By providing a full 33 percent of your total carb calories for the day, as well as a powerful protein punch and a solid dose of fat, you are purposefully shocking your system into an anabolic state. Because your glycogen reserves are already low, and your fat cells are in a catabolic state, there is little to no risk of creating a fat-storage environment with this meal. All of the calories will go toward replacing glycogen reserves and halting the catabolic activities in your body.

By kicking the anabolic mechanisms into gear you will achieve the above stated goals through the following mechanisms:

➤ The large dose of carbs, especially in combination with the protein in this meal, will stimulate a fairly strong insulin response. This insulin will serve a number of purposes, including:
  - Stimulation of glycogen synthesis and replacement[23]
  - Support of leptin secretion, which in turn will help support ongoing fat utilization
  - Suppression of cortisol and glucagon secretion[24]

- Halting of muscle catabolism, and maybe even instigation of mild muscle anabolism

➤ The fat in this meal will also serve a number of purposes. It will:
  - Help create a longer satiety effect and even out and extend the blood sugar and insulin response by slowing gastric emptying
  - Provide EFAs to support vital hormone production

Nutrient Composition

Along with the amount, the specific types of protein, carbs and fat you include in this meal are important and will have an impact on the strength and effectiveness of the metabolic response created. Try the following:

➤ **Protein:** Use a fast-acting protein that will absorb easily and quickly, providing available amino acids to work with the insulin. Whey or egg protein are both good options.

➤ **Carbs:** This is probably the one time during the day where a simple, fast-acting dose of carbs is OK. Try a mix of simple and complex (high- and low-glycemic) carbs. A combination of fruit and slow-cooked whole-grain oatmeal would work well. (You can check out the GI values for many foods in Appendix J of this book.)

➤ **Fat:** It is important to get a good dose of EFAs in this meal. EFA levels have been mildly depleted overnight and replacing them sooner rather than later is a good idea. You can use flax seed oil to cook in or add to any of your other foods. You can also try any number of supplements for a more designer approach to your fat intake instead. Try using about 3 grams to 5 grams of an EFA supplement, and 1 gram of EAS CLA.

MORNING SNACK

Metabolic State

At this point your body will be rebounding a bit from its morning anabolic kick start.

- Blood sugar levels are probably trailing off.
- Insulin levels are falling.
- Muscle and fat metabolism are more or less at equilibrium.
- Your blood leptin level is probably still fairly strong but beginning to fall.

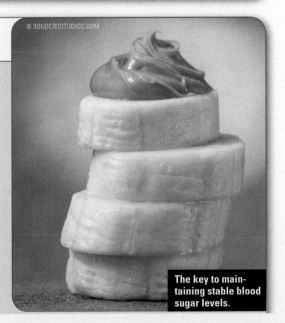

The key to maintaining stable blood sugar levels.

Metabolic Goals
- Provide muscles with enough energy and sufficient protein to keep them out of catabolism.
- Support a moderate and even blood sugar level.
- Help support leptin levels.

Meal Solutions
This is a small, balanced snack that focuses on simply providing enough fuel to keep your muscles fed and your blood sugar well balanced. The combination of moderate doses of protein and carbs, with a small dose of fat, will stimulate a gentle insulin response, which in turn will stimulate leptin.

Nutrient Composition
➤ Protein: Try a mixed protein source that will provide some quick amino acids and additional ones over two to three hours. Milk is a good choice, as it contains both casein and whey. Or you can try a balanced meal-replacement shake providing a mixture of proteins, preferably casein, whey and soy. EAS Myoplex® Lite would be a good choice.
➤ Carbs: Focus on low GI carbs. We don't want to or need to create a big insulin spike. If you do, your blood sugar will be crashing by lunch time, and you'll likely over-indulge. The meal-replacement or milk will provide the carbs you need.
➤ Fat: Your fat source isn't all that important here and will probably just come naturally with whatever food you choose.

LUNCH

Metabolic State
If you have followed your meal plan up to this point, your whole body should be pretty well in equilibrium by now; however:
- Your metabolism is in the process of slowing down.
- Muscles may be going slightly catabolic due to inactivity (if you have a desk job).
- Your blood leptin level is slipping again due to its natural cycle of being low in the early afternoon.

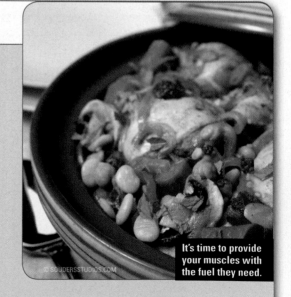

It's time to provide your muscles with the fuel they need.

© SOUDERSSTUDIOS.COM

Metabolic Goals
- Provide muscles with enough energy and sufficient protein to keep them out of catabolism.
- Continue to support a moderate and even blood sugar level.
- Provide strong caloric support for slumping leptin.

Meal Solutions

This is your second largest meal of the day. Your main goal here is to give your leptin production a kick in the pants. That's why you'll be hitting the carbs fairly hard. Combined with the protein, you'll get a decent insulin response and leptin surge. The protein will also serve to help support muscle metabolism, with the aim of preventing catabolism.

Nutrient Composition

- ➤ **Protein:** Try a mixed protein source with more emphasis on the fast-acting proteins like chicken, fish, whey or egg. You need to get a solid dose of amino acids to feed wilting muscles. But you also want to have some to carry you until your next snack. A skinless, grilled chicken breast with a side of low-fat cottage cheese would work well.
- ➤ **Carbs:** A quick hit of insulin will help spike leptin, but too much will crash you out. So try and use a blend of moderate-GI carbs. A fruit plate or fruit smoothie might work well.
- ➤ **Fat:** This is another opportunity to get in a good dose of EFAs and CLA. If you eat fish at this meal, you will naturally get some EFAs. If not, supplement with EFA and CLA again, just like at breakfast.

AFTERNOON SNACK

Metabolic State

At this time in the afternoon there is a good chance you are experiencing an energy slump. This will be the result of a combination of the following:

- Blood sugar levels have gotten a bit low in a rebound response to the calorie dose at lunch.
- Leptin has dropped to its lowest point of the day, suppressing metabolism and energy expenditure.
- Muscles are likely to be slightly catabolic.

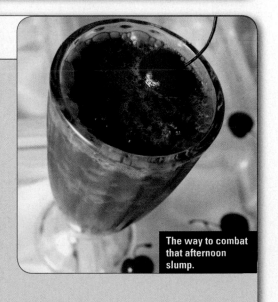

The way to combat that afternoon slump.

Metabolic Goals
- Ease blood sugar levels back up.
- Halt muscle catabolism.
- Prepare your body for exercise after work.

Meal Solutions

Just like in the morning, a small, balanced snack that focuses on simply providing enough fuel to keep your muscles fed and get your blood sugar back on track is in order. It's important to get your blood sugar back up in order to supply you with the energy you need for your after-work workout. Also, by supplying a decent dose of protein, you will help stimulate muscle recovery and growth following your workout. New research shows that protein taken before your workout is twice as effective at stimulating protein uptake into muscle cells as is protein taken after your workout.[41]

Nutrient Composition
- ➤ **Protein:** You should use a fairly slow-acting protein. Casein is a good choice because of its gel-forming properties. There are many nutrition bars that are casein-based that would work well.
- ➤ **Carbs:** Try moderate-GI carbs—something that will get your blood sugar up fairly quickly without spiking insulin levels and crashing your blood sugar in the middle of your workout. Look for a nutrition bar with a low "sugar" content and chances are it will be moderate on the GI scale.
- ➤ **Fat:** Again, your fat source isn't all that important here and will probably just come naturally with whatever bar or food you choose.

DINNER

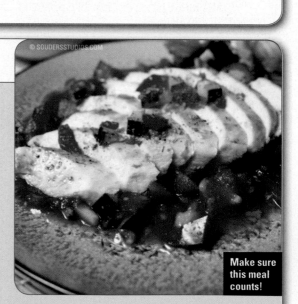

© SOUDERSSTUDIOS.COM

Make sure this meal counts!

Metabolic State

This is a key meal in your plan. Not only is it your post-workout meal, but also your last food for the next 12 hours or so. So you need to make this one count. Here's what's happening, and will be happening overnight, in your body:
- You've burned up some of your glycogen reserves working out, so they are slightly depleted.
- Blood sugar has been used up and is low.
- Insulin levels are down and cortisol levels are up.

- Muscles are in a highly active state, on the verge of catabolism, but very ready to soak up nutrients and turn anabolic.
- Leptin levels are sometimes decreased by intense exercise.[42] Combine that effect with low blood sugar and insulin and leptin levels are probably pretty low; however, due to its natural cycle, leptin will rebound overnight.
- Overnight your body will be mostly anabolic up until about midnight to 2 a.m. Then it typically turns catabolic, burning glycogen, muscle and fat.

Metabolic Goals

- Turn muscles from catabolic to anabolic.
- Sustain the overnight anabolic state as long as possible.
- Help your body focus on using fat versus muscle or glycogen during the catabolic stage of sleep.

Meal Solutions

This is when it pays to keep the carbs low and pack in the protein. By supplying just enough carbs combined with the protein to stimulate a bit of insulin and promote protein uptake in the muscle, without having excess blood sugar left over, you can avoid replenishing your glycogen stores that were depleted during your workout. This is a good thing as it will then help your body focus on utilizing either fat as its fuel source during overnight catabolism. And the combination of naturally increased leptin levels after 3 a.m. and the big dose of protein you are tossing in at night will protect your muscle mass.

You will also include a moderate dose of fat in this meal. This will not only help to slow gastric emptying, thus feeding nutrients into your body longer into the night, but will also support hormone production. Most of your hormone production for the day takes place at night.

Nutrient Composition

➤ Protein: You want to use a slow-acting protein combined with a fast-acting form. In order to help fuel muscles all night, you want a protein that will release amino acids into your blood stream throughout the night. And to help instigate post-workout protein absorption into muscles, you want a dose of fast-acting protein. Two good choices for the slow-acting protein are lean red meat and casein, and whey is the fast-acting protein of choice. If a meal-replacement is more convenient, try a serving of EAS Carb Sense® powder.

➤ Carbs: Because we have such a small dose of carbs, what type you use is not an issue. Just eat whatever carbs are convenient and filling.

➤ Fat: If at all possible, virtually every gram of this fat dose is composed of EFAs. Because most of your hormone production takes place overnight, it would be very helpful to supply your body with what it needs to make this happen. Also toss in a gram of CLA to help focus calorie burning on fat versus muscle.

Plugging In the Numbers

Now it's time to lay out the specific numbers for your plan. You will be calculating the specific number of calories and grams of carbs, protein and fat for each of your meals based on your personal DCG.

Remember, you are building a plan that provides a 40/40/20 profile carbs, protein and fat. Because building a personalized plan based on your specific needs is a bit complex, a worksheet is included for you to use. All you need to do is start with your MCL and calculate your exact personalized plan from there. (You can also go to www.eas.com and download a spreadsheet that will do all the calculating for you.)

Building Your Meal Plan

Meal planning can be a fairly time-consuming task. But once you've built yourself a meal plan for the week, you're set. All you have to do is eat what's on your plan every day, and you can't fail. A sample meal plan is included to help get you started.

When building your meals around your personalized plan, be sure to do the following:

- Include foods you like to eat, not just those you think you *should* eat. If you don't enjoy the food on your plan, you won't stick with it.
- Use your calorie-counting book or the nutrient analysis Web site to help you plug in the proper types and amounts of foods needed to match your plan as closely as possible.
- Use meal-replacement shakes and nutrition bars. They will go a long way toward making this plan convenient and successful.
- Remember to pay attention to the types of protein, carbs and fat outlined previously for each meal.
- Check out the Glycemic Index in Appendix J to help you choose which carbs to use and when.
- Plan out your whole week before you start.
- Make a shopping list from your completed meal plan and hit the store to stock up for the week. (See the "Sample Shopping List" to give you ideas and get you started.)

Sample Fat-Loss Meal Plan

* Based on a DCG of 1,700 (2,000 MCL).

	When	Goal		Sample Meal	Supplements***
BREAKFAST	7:00 a.m.	Calories: Protein: Carbs: Fat:	510 39 grams 56 grams 11 grams	• ¾ cup scrambled Egg Beaters™ (210 calories, 30/2/8 protein/carbs/fat ratio) • 1 piece multi-grain toast with 1 teaspoon natural peanut butter (100 calories, 4/14/4) • 1 small apple (80 calories, 0/21/0) • 1 small banana (90 calories, 1/23/0)	• 3 grams of an Essential Fatty Acid blend and CLA • 10 grams of whey protein in water (Any whey protein consisting mainly of whey protein isolate is fine to use here.)
MID-MORNING SNACK	10:00 a.m.	Calories: Protein: Carbs: Fat:	221 22 grams 22 grams 3 grams	• Myoplex® Lite Ready-to-Drink nutrition shake	• Ephedra-free thermogenic fat-burner (Try EAS Thermo DynamX®) • 3 grams of L-glutamine (EAS L-Glutamine or any powdered glutamine from a reputable manufacturer)
LUNCH	1:00 p.m.	Calories: Protein: Carbs: Fat:	459 39 grams 48 grams 11 grams	• 2 ounces of fresh deli cut turkey breast (90 calories, 18/0/1) • 1 tablespoon regular mayonnaise (60 calories, 0/1/5) • 2 slices of multi-grain bread (150 calories, 6/26/2) • 1 cup fresh baby carrots (55 calories, 0/13/0) • ½ cup low-fat cottage cheese (80 calories, 14/3/1)	• 2 grams of an Essential Fatty Acid blend and CLA

Sample Fat-Loss Meal Plan continued

* Based on a DCG of 1,700 (2,000 MCL).

When	Goal		Sample Meal	Supplements
MID-AFTERNOON SNACK 4:00 p.m.	**Calories:** 221 **Protein:** 22 grams **Carbs:** 22 grams **Fat:** 3 grams		• 1 balanced nutrition bar (EAS Myoplex® Lite nutrition bar)	• Ephedra-free thermo-genic fat-burner (EAS Thermo DynamX®) • 3 grams of glutamine (EAS L-Glutamine)
DINNER 7:00 p.m.	**Calories:** 289 **Protein:** 48 grams **Carbs:** 22 grams **Fat:** 8 grams		• 1 medium roasted, skinless chicken breast (140 calories, 26/0/3) • 1 cup lentil soup (Progresso makes a good one) (125 calories, 8/20/1) • 2 celery sticks with non-fat cream cheese (basically calorie-free)	• 4 grams of an Essential Fatty Acid blend and CLA • 15 grams pure protein powder mixed with water* (EAS Myoplex® Carb Sense® powder) • 5 grams of creatine (EAS Phosphagen HP)**

*If you are following the Body-*for*-LIFE Program, which recommends six small meals a day, you can add one last small pre-bed meal, which should be lower in carbs. One option is to substitute the 15 grams of protein powder and water suggested for your 7 p.m. meal as your sixth meal.

**Take your 5 grams of creatine post-workout.

*** See Chapter 7 and Chapter 10 for additional nutritional supplement recommendations.

Sample Shopping List

⊖ FOOD

6 fresh, skinless chicken breasts

2 pounds fresh roasted sliced turkey breast

2 cans white albacore tuna in water

2 fresh or frozen salmon filets

1 box basmati rice or brown rice

1 bag semolina wheat pasta (protein-fortified if you can find it)

1 small bottle of olive oil

1 jar of natural spaghetti sauce with no added sugar

2 sweet potatoes

1 stalk of fresh broccoli

1 small bag of baby carrots

1 stalk of celery

1 bag frozen peas

1 medium bag of fresh cherries

2 packages of dried apricots

3 grapefruits

4 apples

4 bananas

1 container of Quaker Old-Fashioned Slow-Cooking Oatmeal

1 loaf of 7-grain bread

1 box of All Bran Extra Fiber cereal

1 bag of dried 15-bean mix

3 cans of Progresso lentil soup

1 jar all-natural peanut butter

1 16-ounce tub of low-fat cottage cheese

1 gallon of non-fat milk

1 box sugar-free Jell-O

4 individual servings of unsweetened, low-fat yogurt

8 ounces of roasted almonds

1 package of turkey jerky

⊖ SUPPLEMENTS

• EFA supplement (found at any specialty or health food store)

• Udo's Choice Perfected Oil Blend™ or any oil blend from a health food store

• EAS* CLA

• EAS Thermo DynamX®

• EAS Phosphagen HP™

• EAS L-Glutamine

• EAS Myoplex® Lite Bars

• EAS Precision Protein™ or MyoPro® Whey

• EAS Myoplex® powder or Myoplex® Carb Sense®

* EAS products can be found online at www.eas.com, by calling 1-800-297-9776 or by going to an authorized specialty retailer.

Eat More (Often), Lose More Fat

One of the main reasons we as a nation struggle so greatly with obesity is because of our habit of eating only two or three large meals per day. This sets up a sort of "feast or famine" pattern in your body that promotes fat deposition, fluctuating energy levels and even muscle loss. By focusing on ingesting small portions of well-combined protein, carbs and fat every three hours or so throughout the day, the feast or famine pattern can be alleviated.

A lot of research has been done on this concept of small, frequent meals (SFMs), especially in relation to fat loss. The main take-home message from these studies is that if you are on a reduced-calorie diet, and you eat five to six meals per day versus only two or three, you will lose more fat and (most dramatically) preserve or gain more muscle.[43,44,45] There are a variety of metabolic explanations for why this SFM pattern of eating is so effective for fat loss.

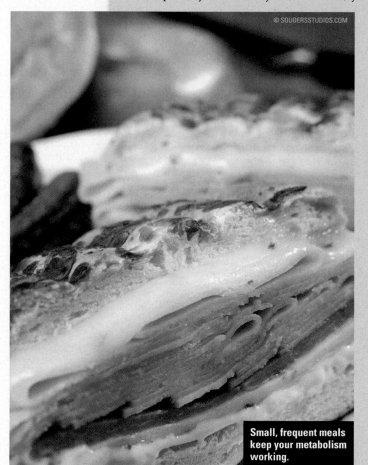

© SOUDERSSTUDIOS.COM

Small, frequent meals keep your metabolism working.

First, SFMs tend to stabilize both blood sugar and insulin levels throughout the day. In a recent study, two groups were fed the exact same foods for a day, differing only by the fact that one group consumed the food as two large meals and the other as six small meals. The blood sugar levels of the two-meal group spiked almost twice as high as that of those of the six-meal group throughout the day. Insulin levels were also more erratic.[46] These findings are important because blood sugar and insulin levels greatly effect fat storage, energy levels, metabolic rate and satiety.

When blood sugar levels spike, fat storage is strongly promoted because blood sugar must be kept under very tight control by the body. And if glycogen reserves are full, blood sugar must be stored as fat. These spikes will also cause an over production of insulin, usually leading to a rebound hypoglycemic (low blood sugar) effect a few hours after your meal. This can instigate hunger and cravings, cause your energy levels to crash and may slow your metabolism.

In contrast, keeping your blood sugar levels moderate and consistent smoothes out energy levels, keeps insulin levels more constant, helps keep your metabolism humming and enhances satiety levels. Part of this satiety effect is mediated by the effects of SFMs on leptin levels. By maintaining constant levels of insulin in your system, SFMs also tend to promote the consistent expression of leptin, which in turn helps decrease feelings of hunger.

Dietary induced thermogenesis (DIT) is another benefit of SFMs. As stated earlier, every time you have a meal your body burns energy in order to process the food eaten. This increase in energy, or DIT, lasts between three and four hours; therefore, if you are eating small meals every three hours or so, you keep your metabolic rate consistently at a higher level of activity.

Another important mechanism of the SFM effect is the consistency of nutrient availability it produces. By eating a mixed meal every few hours, you keep abundant doses of quality proteins circulating in your blood stream at all times. This constant protein availability means that it is not necessary for your body to break down muscles to supply amino acids for other vital functions in your body, such as enzyme production and organ maintenance. This supports an anabolic environment for your muscles throughout the day, preserving muscle mass even during low-calorie periods. This has been indicated in multiple studies.[43,45] One study in particular that examined boxers trying to make weight was quite convincing. Two groups of boxers consumed 1,200 calories per day in either two meals or six meals for a period of two weeks. They both lost the same amount of body weight, but the two-meal group lost almost twice the amount of muscle mass of the six-meal group.[45] Meaning not only did the six-meal group preserve more muscle, they actually lost more fat.

Finally, there are the emotional and mental benefits of SFMs. Simply stated, eating more often appears to make it much easier to stick to a reduced-calorie eating regimen. The reason being (apart from satiety effects and such) is that at any point during the day you know you are only a few hours from your next meal, as opposed to only eating twice a day and always being a full 12 hours from your next meal. With SFMs, no matter what your level of hunger or craving, it is easier to make it to your next feeding.

Even if you adopt none of the other ideas presented in this chapter, please break your daily calories down into five or six balanced meals. You'll love the way it makes you feel.

Guide To Acronyms

CLA—Conjugated Linoleic Acid
DCG—Daily Calorie Goal
DIT—Dietary Induced Thermogenesis
EFA—Essential Fatty Acids
GH—Growth Hormone
GI—Glycemic Index
HPLC—High-Protein/Low-Carb Diet
MCL—Maintenance Calorie Level
SFM—Small Frequent Meal

Balanced Is Better: Why Low-Carb Diets Are Only Quick Fixes

High-protein/low-carb (HPLC) fat-loss diets are quite popular, but in reality, the only thing a high-protein/low-carb diet is good for is a quick fix. If you've got a special event you're preparing for, and you have to lose weight fast, great, cut your carbs for a few weeks. But it is only a short-term fix and not a healthy sustainable answer to fat loss. You will gain most (or probably all) of the weight back as you unavoidably return to a "normal diet," and there will be a price to pay.

The best way to explain this is to give you a simple rundown of what happens in your body when you cut your carbs. Then you can make your own educated decisions about when, how, why and if this type of diet makes sense for you.

During the first three to five days (depending on exercise level) of a HPLC diet, the body slowly draws on, burns up and eventually depletes glycogen stores in the muscles and liver. Glycogen stores are burned first because they are the most readily available stored source of glucose energy for the brain and body. There is very little if any fat-burning going on during this time. The dramatic weight loss seen in the initial stages of the HPLC diet are almost exclusively from glycogen and water loss. The water loss is secondary to glycogen loss, because glycogen is stored with three times its own weight in water. And as glycogen is burned, water is released—you may recall how much you tend to urinate during the first few days of a HPLC diet.

This loss of glycogen will immediately produce some other effects beyond lost pounds—flattening of muscles, loss of endurance and strength, tiredness and irritability. The reason? Your body's number one energy source has just been depleted.

Now the real fun begins. With its glycogen now depleted, your body has to start pulling from fat stores. This is good, right? Well, yes and no. It does indeed begin to burn body fat and shed fat pounds. But fat is a funky fuel source, and your body's not used to relying on it exclusively. Doing so sends your body into a metabolic tizzy. Here's what happens:

- As fat is released, some is burned directly by muscles as fuel and some goes to the liver.
- Because the brain usually burns exclusively glucose for fuel (to the tune of 150 grams per day) and can't burn fat (it won't cross the blood/brain barrier), and fat can't be converted to glucose, the liver converts fat to "ketones," creating a state known as "ketosis." Ketones are a secondary fuel source the brain can use. But it can only use ketones for about 50 percent of its energy needs.[47] The other half must be glucose. Therefore,
  - Because there are no more direct glucose stores left, the body must create glucose from proteins.
  - Muscles are broken down to provide protein to create glucose for the brain (meaning you're losing muscle along with your fat).
  - Brain function suffers because ketones are not its preferred fuel source. Research shows that learning, memory, reaction time and mood are all compromised.
- Other side-effects of ketosis are:
  - Increased risk of dehydration due to lack of water stores in the body
  - Headaches
  - Lightheadedness

- Decrease in metabolic rate due to your body's perception of a starvation state
- Decrease in the number of muscle mitochondria (the little fat-burning plants inside muscle cells), which decreases the fat-burning efficiency of muscle cells
- Decreased exercise performance
- Kidney stress and possible long-term damage due to the increased protein metabolites in the blood stream
- Liver stress and possible long-term damage
- Aggravation or induction of gout attacks due to elevated ammonia levels
- Bone loss due to calcium leaching
- Risk of kidney stones due to increase uric acid and calcium oxalate levels

Beyond the physical nightmares are the lifestyle issues. It's simply not realistic to maintain a long-term HPLC diet, and you really wouldn't want to because of the physical side effects. Try following a balanced nutrition plan, as recommended in this book, featuring a combination of lean protein for muscle growth and strength, complex carbs to provide energy and fuel and healthy fats to support many of your body's essential functions.

Fiber Fires Up Fat Loss

Fiber: It's one of those words that calls to mind such things as "regularity" and Geritol®. Who would have thought that it would turn out to be one of the easiest, healthiest, cheapest and most effective fat-loss supplements ever? In recent research the following physiological effects of fiber on fat loss were elucidated. [48,49,50,51]

- When consuming a fixed number of calories (like on a structured 1,500-calorie diet) the addition of fiber to the diet:
  - Increases post meal satiety
  - Decreases subsequent hunger
- When caloric intake is not controlled, fiber added to the diet of over-weight subjects:
  - Decreased self-selected food and calorie intake by an average of 18 percent
  - Caused an average weight loss of over 5 pounds in a 3.8 month period with no other dietary changes
- In a review of multiple fiber studies it was found that "… weight loss was more than three times as great in individuals consuming diets both low in fat and high in fiber compared with diets only low in fat (a 7.5-pound loss versus a 2.2-pound loss)."
- In a study originally designed to assess the effects of fiber on blood lipids, it was found that healthy, normal weight adults all spontaneously lost body fat without any other dietary alterations. Average fat loss over

11 weeks was 3.5 pounds. No muscle mass was lost. And subjects with the initially lowest level of body fat actually gained muscle (1.3 pounds) while they lost fat mass.[52]

⊖ Soluble fiber (pectin in this study) decreases the absorption of both sugar and fat from the intestine.

As you can see, fiber is a formidable fat-fighting nutrient. It also has multiple other health benefits including cholesterol-lowering and colon-cleansing effects, as well as providing protection against some forms of cancer. It is an unsung nutritional hero and should be a part of your fat-loss plan.

There are two basic types of fiber—soluble and insoluble. As you may have guessed, soluble dissolves in water while insoluble doesn't. They tend to act a bit differently in the gut, with insoluble fibers soaking up water, creating bulk and a sense of fullness that lasts; while soluble fibers do a bit more of the fat and sugar binding. But as far as fat loss goes, it appears that a mixture of the two is optimal. And it has also been recognized that the effects of fiber are not really affected by whether you get it from food or a supplement.[52] Insoluble fiber sources include wheat bran, psyllium husk and any other whole-grain foods and fibrous veggies. Soluble fibers can be found in abundance in all types of beans and fruits.

The current fiber intake of the average American is 15 grams or less per day. The American Heart Association recommends 25 grams to 30 grams per day. For fat-loss purposes, try to have 40 grams a day. You can include 5 grams to 10 grams with each meal, but only use a few grams with your pre-workout meal, or your stomach could get a bit disturbed. Make sure to drink plenty of water with your meals, and between, as you increase your fiber intake. Fiber tends to soak up water and can cause some dehydration and "backup" issues with too little water intake.

REFERENCES CITED:

[1] Ashutosh, K, Methrotra, K, Fragale-Jackson, J. Effects of sustained weight loss and exercise on aerobic fitness in obese women. *J Sports Med Phys Fitness* 37.4 (1997): 252-257.

[2] Zachwieja, JJ et al. Short-term dietary energy restriction reduces lean body mass but not performance in physically active men and women. *Int J Sports Med* 22.4 (2001): 310-319.

[3] Niskanen, L et al. The effects of weight loss on insulin sensitivity, skeletal muscle compostion and capillary density in obese non-diabetic subjects. *Int J Obes Relat Metab Disord* 20.2 (1996):154-160.

[4] Mooney, JP, Burling, TA, Hartman, WM, Brenner-Liss, D. The abstinence violation effect and very low calorie diet success. *Addict Behav* 17.4 (1992): 319-324.

[5] Fawzy, FI, et al. comprehensive psychological approach to obesity. *Psychiatr Med* 1.3 (1983): 257-273.

[6] Fricker, J, Rozen, R, Melchoir, JC, Apfelbaum, M. Energy-metabolism adaptation in obese adults on a very-low-calorie diet. *Am J Clin Nutr* 53.4 (1991): 826-830.

[7] Lim, K, Murakami, E, Lee, S, Shimomura, Y, Suzuki, M. Effects of intermittent food restriction and refeeding on energy efficiency and body fat deposition in sedentary and exercised rats. *J Nutr Sci Vitaminol* 42.5 (1996): 449-468, 1996.

[8] Fricker, J, Rozen, R, Melchoir, JC, Apfelbaum, M. Energy-metabolism adaptation in obese adults on a very-low-calorie diet. *Am J Clin Nutr* 53.4 (1991): 826-830.

[9] Foster, GD et al. Controlled trial of the metabolic effects of a very-low-calorie diet: short and long-term effects. *Am J Clin Nutr* 51.2 (1990): 167-172.

10 Groff, J, Gropper, S, Hunt, S. *Advanced Nutrition and Human Metabolism* (Second Edition) (West Publishing, 1990) pgs. 204-205.

11 Chacon F, et al. Chronobiological features of the immune system. Effect of calorie restriction. *Eur J Clin Nutr* 56 Suppl 3 (2002): S69-72.

12 Groff, J, Gropper, S, Hunt, S. *Advanced Nutrition and Human Metabolism* (Second Edition) (West Publishing, 1990) pg. 184.

13 Baile CA, Della-Fera, MA, Martin, RJ. Regulation of metabolism and body fat mass by leptin. *Annu Rev Nutr* 20 (2000): 105-127.

14 McMinn, JE, Sindelar, DK, Havel, PJ, Schwartz, MW. Leptin deficiency induced by fasting impairs the satiety responses to cholecystokinin. *Endocrinology* 141.12 (2000): 4442-4448.

15 Frayn, KN, Karpe, F, Fielding, BA, Macdonald, IA, Coppack, SW. Integrative physiology of human adipose tissue. *Int J Obes Relat Metab Disord* 27.8 (2003):875-888.

16 Bates, SH, Myers, MG. The role of leptin receptor signaling in feeding and neuroendocrine function. Trends *Endocrinol Metab* 14.10 (2003): 447-452.

17 Tena-Sempere, M, Barreiro, ML. Leptin in male reproduction: the testis paradigm. *Mol Cell Endocrinol* 188.1-2 (2002): 9-13.

18 Harris, RBS. Leptin – much more than a satiety signal. *Annu Rev Nutr* 20 (2000): 45-75.

19 Jequier, E. Leptin signaling, adiposity, and energy balance. *Ann N Y Acad Sci* 967 (2002): 379-388.

20 Fried, SK, Ricci, MR, Russell, CD, Laferrere, B. Regulation of leptin production in humans. In Symposium: Adipocyte Function, Differentiation and Metabolism. San Diego, California: *Experimental Biology Meeting 2000*, ISBN: 0022-3166-00, (2000): 3127S-3131S.

21 Heymsfield, SB, et al. McCamish. Recombinant leptin for weight loss in obese and lean adults. *JAMA* 282.16 (1999): 1568-1575.

22 Menozzi, R., et al. Resting metabolic rate, fat-free mass and catecholamine excretion during weight loss in female obese patients. *Br J Nutr* 84.4 (2000): 515-520.

23 Parkin, JA, Carey, MF, Martin, IK, Stojanovska, L, Febbraio, MA. Muscle glycogen storage following prolonged exercise: effect of timing of ingestion of high Glycemic index food. *Med Sci Sportsd Exerc* 29.2 (1997): 220-224.

24 Murray, R, Paul, GL, Seilert, JG, Eddy, DE. Responses to varying rates of carbohydrate ingestion during exercise. *Med Sci Sports Exerc* 23.6 (1991): 713-718.

25 Mueller, WM et al. Evidence that glucose metabolism regulates leptin secretion from cultured rat adipocytes. *Endocrinology* 139.2 (1998): 551-558.

26 Kolaczynski, JW, Ohannesian, JP, Considine, RV, Marco, CC, Caro, JF. Response of leptin to short-term and prolonged overfeeding in humans. *J Clin Endocrinol Metab.* 81.11 (1996): 4162-4165.

27 Phillips, B. *Sports Supplement Review* (Third Edition) (Mile High Publishing, 1997) pg. 158.

28 Phillips, B. *Sports Supplement Review* (Third Edition) (Mile High Publishing, 1997) pg. 82.

29 Walberg, JL, et al. Macronutrient content of a hypoenergy diet affects nitrogen retention and muscle function in weight lifters. *Int J Sports Med* 9.4 (1988): 261-266.

30 Nutritional Biochemistry and Metabolism (Second Edition). (Elsevier Science Publishing Company, Inc., 1991) p. 283.

31 Westerterp-Plantenga, MS, Rolland, V, Wilson, SA, Westerterp, KR. Satiety related to 24 h diet-induced Thermogenesis during high protein/carbohydrate vs. high fat diets measured in a respiration chamber. *Eur J Clin Nutr* 53.6 (1999): 495-502.

32 Layman, DK, et al. A reduced ratio of dietary carbohydrate to protein improves body composition and blood lipid profiles durinig weight loss in adult women. *J Nutr* 133.2 (2003) : 411-417.

33 Tataranni, PA, Ravussin, E. Effect of fat intake on energy balance. *Ann N Y Acad Sci* 819 (1997): 37-43.

34 Phillips, B. *Sports Supplement Review* (Third Edition) (Mile High Publishing, 1997) pg. 229.

35 Dray F, Kouznetzova, B, Harris, D, Brazeau, P. Tole of prostaglandins on growth hormone secretion: PGE2 a physiological stimulator. *Adv Prostaglandin Thromboxane* Res 8 (1980):1321-1328.

36 Borkman, M, et al. The relation between insulin sensitivity and the fatty-acid composition of skeletal-muscle phospholipids. *N Engl J Med* 328.4 (1993): 238-244.

37 Pelikanova T, Kohout, M, Valek, J, Base, J, Kazdova, L. Insulin secretion and insulin action related to the serum phospholipids fatty acid pattern in healthy men. *Metabolism* 38.2 (1989): 188-192.

38 Miner, JL, et al. Conjugated Linoleic acid (CLA), body fat and apoptosis. *Obes Res* 9.2 (2001): 129-134.

39 Hargrave, KM, et al. Adipose depletion and apoptosis induced by trans-10, cis-12 conjugated Linoleic acid in mice. *Obes Res* 10.12 (2002):1284-1290, 2002.

40 Kanabrocki, EL, et al. Circadian variation of serum leptin in healthy and diabetic men. *Chronobiol Int* 18.2 (2001): 273-283.

41 Tipton, KD. "Timing of amino acid—Carbohydrate ingestion alters anabolic response of muscle to resistance exercise." *AmJ* Physiol 281 (2001):E197-E206.

42 Hulver, MW, Houmard, JA. Plasma leptin and exercise: recent findings. *Sports Med* 33.7 (2003): 473-482.

43 Garrow, JS, et al. The effect of meal frequency and protein concentration on the composition of the weight lost by obese subjects. *Br J Nutr* 45.1 (1981): 5-15.

44 Antoine JM, et al. Feeding frequency and nitrogen balance in weight reducing obese women. *Hum Nutr Clin Nutr* 38.1 (1984): 31-18.

45 Iwao S, Mori, K, Sato, Y. Effects of meal frequency on body composition during weight control in boxers. *Scand J Med Sci Sports* 6.5 (1996): 265-272.

46 Bertelsen JC, et al. Effect of meal frequency on blood glucose, insulin, and free fatty acids in NIDDM subjects. *Diabetes Care* 16.1 (1993): 4-7.

47 Fletchner-Mors, M, Ditschuneit, HH, Johnson, TD, Suchard, MA, Adler, G. Metabolic and weight loss effects of long-term dietary interventions in obese patients: four-year results. *Obes Res* 8.5 (2000): 399-402.

48 Howarth, NC, Saltzman, E, Roberts, SB. Dietary fiber and weight regulation. *Nutr Rev* 59.5 (2001): 129-139.

49 Yao, M, Roberts, SB. Dietary energy density and weight reduction. *Nutr Rev* 59.8 part 1 (2001): 247-258.

50 Pasman, WJ, Saris, WH, Wauters, MA, Westerterp-Plantenga, MS. Effect of one week of fiber supplementation on hunger and satiety ratings and energy intake. *Appetite* 29.1 (1997): 77-87.

51 Fuse K, Bamba, T, Hooda, S. Effects of pectin on fatty acid and glucose absorption on thickness of unstirred water layer in rat and human intestine. *Dig Dis Sci* 34.7 (1989): 1109-1116.

52 Raben, A, Jensen, ND, Marckman, P, Sandstrom, B, Astrup, A. Spontaneous weight loss during 11 weeks ad libitum intake of a low fat/high fiber diet in young, normal weight subjects. *Int J Obese Relat Metab Disord* 19.12 (1995): 916-923.

7 SUPPLEMENTS FOR FAT LOSS

What Works, What Doesn't and What To Look for

By Brett Hall, R D

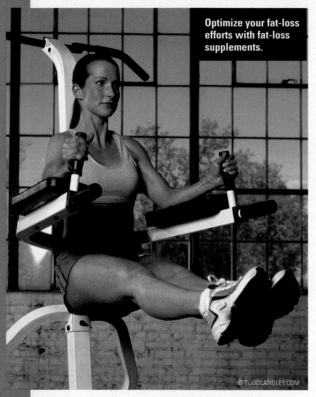

Optimize your fat-loss efforts with fat-loss supplements.

© TODDLANGLEY.COM

Fat-loss supplements may help burn fat, block fat storage, control caloric intake and suppress hunger, among other things. But what they can't do is transform your body from fat to fit all by themselves. They need your help. The use of fat-loss supplements must be combined with an effective fat-loss nutrition plan and consistent exercise in order to help you attain the lasting fat loss you desire. Think of fat-loss supplements as an "octane booster." You know that adding an octane booster to the gas in your car will make it go faster and perform more efficiently. But what good is it without the car? And what good is the car without gas? Only when you first have the car, and gas in the car, does the octane booster optimize your car's performance. And by starting out with a solid nutrition plan and exercise regimen, fat-loss supplements can, and will, help optimize your fat-loss performance.

But not every fat-loss supplement works. Even those touted as "miracle fat-loss cures" (especially those) can either lend no help to your fat-loss endeavors, or may hinder them or worse yet, pose some sort of health risk. This chapter examines the good, the bad and the equivocal ugly fat-loss supplements out there, giving you guidance on what to take, what to avoid and what to keep an eye on.

How Fat-Loss Supplements Work

In order to understand how the good fat-loss supplements actually do work, it's necessary to first get a feel for the basic metabolic mechanisms of fat loss. Now, don't panic; this isn't going to be all that complicated. As a matter of fact, it starts out so simple it's almost insulting. **To lose fat you have to burn more fat than you store.** But now let's ask the obvious question. How can you influence your metabolism in a way that leads to less fat storage and more fat burning?

First let's look at how to decrease fat storage. There are three main mechanisms by which fat storage can be reduced:

- **Absorb fewer calories than you burn each day.** This puts you in a negative calorie balance. Meaning there are simply no extra calories available to be stored as fat.
- **Keep your blood sugar level low to moderate, avoiding large spikes.** Consistently high, or regularly spiking, blood sugar levels induce your body to convert blood sugar to fat and store it in fat cells.
- **Block the entry of new fat into fat cells at the cellular level,** thereby decreasing the amount of fat deposited, even though there may be a surplus of fat or carbs floating around in your blood stream.

There are a variety of ways to help achieve each of these goals. Some are dietary (as mentioned in the last chapter) and some are through the use of supplements. We'll discuss these in detail shortly.

Next, how can you increase the amount of fat you burn each day? There are two main mechanisms here:

- **Increase the overall number of calories you burn each day.** Fat stores will naturally be used to fuel a portion of this increase in caloric expenditure–thus increasing the total amount of fat you burn each day.
- **Increase the ratio of fat fuel used to meet your overall daily caloric expenditure.** By increasing the proportion of fat (versus carbohydrates and proteins) used to supply your daily calorie needs, even if your overall caloric expenditure doesn't increase, the amount of fat burned each day will.

It's important to note that exercise is really the best way to achieve both of these goals; however, the use of specific supplements in conjunction with exercise can help catapult you more efficiently into a fat-burning zone. So let's take a look at which supplements those are and how they work.

Supplements That Work

Caffeine

- **What it is:**

It's the "buzz" in your morning cup of Joe. More technically it is a pharmacologically active compound that belongs to a group of nutrients called methylxanthines. It is found in abundance in coffee, tea, cocoa seed and kola nut. A typical cup of coffee contains about 100 milligrams of caffeine per cup, while tea contains about 50 milligrams and a soda has about 35 milligrams.

How it works:

Caffeine has a number of physiological effects when it comes to fat loss. Two of these effects appear to be the driving force behind caffeine's ability to help you lose fat. First of all, caffeine has the ability to increase resting energy expenditure (REE).[1,4,5,10] This is the number of calories you burn each day just sitting on the couch. A typical increase in REE from caffeine consumption is about 7 percent to 15 percent; however, different people do respond differently. For instance, as unfair as this is going to sound, lean people seem to experience a greater increase than overweight people.[1,10] People who are quite fit and exercise regularly appear to get the greatest benefit in terms of calorie burning enhancement.[32] The cool thing about this is that caffeine can be a potent weapon in your fat loss arsenal as you work to lose those last (and hardest) 5 to 10 pounds. Next, caffeine stimulates the breakdown and release of fat from fat cells.[2,6,41] This is known as lipolysis. By releasing fat from fat cells, caffeine helps to tip the scales of fuel utilization in your body away from carbs and protein and toward fat.

Both of these physiological effects are mediated by caffeine's ability to bind to a specific receptor site in your body that stimulates the release of a hormone called norepinephrine. Norepinephrine belongs to a class of compounds called catecholamines. These catecholamines orchestrate dozens of vital metabolic functions. Norepinephrine specifically acts directly upon the central nervous system (CNS)—causing the increase in REE—and upon the fat cell itself, stimulating lipolysis. And it is the combination of this dual effect of norepinephrine that makes caffeine such a potent fat-fighting compound.

What to look for:

The form you choose to consume your caffeine in isn't really all that important. Many of the studies performed have used pure caffeine in capsule or tablet form; however, one study used a highly caffeinated beverage, equivalent to about three cups of coffee. Researchers found that the beverage induced about a 12 percent increase in REE, as well as a significant increase in fat burning.[1] Interestingly, researchers used both lean and obese subjects in this study, and found that both increased their energy expenditure to a similar degree, but the lean folks burned more fat.

So feel free to use whatever form of caffeine you find convenient—they'll all work.

> **tip**
>
> Caffeine may help you lose those last 5 to 10 pounds.

Recommended use:

It takes a pretty hefty dose of caffeine to create the metabolic effects mentioned above—200 to 300 milligrams seem to be the threshold. If you're not used to consuming caffeine, this level could be a bit tough on the nerves. Try starting with 100 milligrams, two times per day and working your way up to 200 milligrams. If you are a current user, start with 200 milligrams and work your way up to 300 milligrams.

Timing of your caffeine intake is actually quite important. You want to take advantage of its fat-releasing effects by immediately burning the fat it releases. If you don't, all that fat floating around in your blood stream will more than likely find its way back to your love handles or thighs. So, the best time to take your two doses is the very first thing in the morning, at least 30 minutes before eating any food, and 30 to 45 minutes prior to your workouts. By doing so, you can burn up the released fat as fuel, avoiding the problem of re-deposition.

Another advantage of pre-exercise caffeination is that it has been proven to enhance endurance and overall athletic performance.[13,21,22,23] By shifting your fuel usage to fat, it spares valuable glycogen stores, allowing for more intense aerobic performance over a longer period of time.

Please consult your doctor before supplementing with caffeine if you have health issues such as high blood pressure or heart problems.

Calcium and Dairy Products

How they work:

As unlikely as it may seem, dairy products rich in calcium seem to help reduce body fat. Recent research has linked a greater consumption of dairy products with reduced weight gain and increased fat loss.[8,14,37,62,63] Most of the research thus far has been epidemiological, meaning that they are not "controlled" studies, but studies have looked at the correlation between overall dairy intake in a population as it relates to the level of body fat in members of that population. For instance, in adult women, calcium intake (mostly in the form of dairy) greater than 1,000 milligrams per day is associated with about a 30 percent lower level of body fat than in women who consume less than 600 milligrams per day.[26] And in 2- to 5-year-old kids, greater intakes of calcium were strongly correlated with a significantly lower body fat mass by the time they were 6 years old.[11]

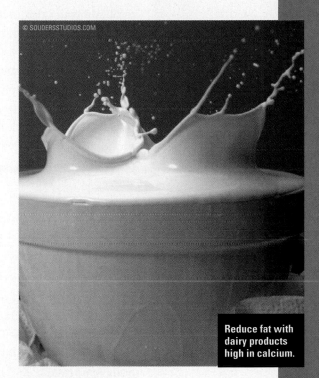

© SOUDERSSTUDIOS.COM

Reduce fat with dairy products high in calcium.

To help confirm these epidemiological findings, in 2002 researchers performed a controlled study in which they placed obese subjects on a reduced-calorie diet; however, one-third of the subjects received 800 milligrams of calcium per day as a supplement, one-third consumed 1,300 milligrams of calcium from low-fat dairy sources and one-third received a placebo. The results were really quite astounding. Over the course of the study, subjects in the placebo group lost an average of 6.4 percent of their body weight, while those in the supplement group lost 26 percent and the dairy group lost substantially more body weight.[64] And in the supplement and dairy groups 50 percent and 66 percent respectively of the fat was lost from the abdominal area. Good news for those of you looking for six pack abs.

It appears that calcium affects fat loss by influencing certain hormones involved in fat metabolism. Diets low in calcium tend to increase the level of hormones that create fat storage. By supplementing with calcium these hormones can be suppressed, thus decreasing fat deposition. One of the researchers in the study mentioned above summed up calcium's effects on fat loss as follows: "High-calcium diets attenuate adipocyte lipid (fat) accretion and weight gain during periods of over-consumption of an energy-dense diet, and to increase lipolysis and preserve thermogenesis during caloric restriction, thereby markedly accelerating weight loss."

So calcium actually seems to help you avoid weight gain during over-indulgence and accelerate fat loss when on a diet.

Recommended use: Shoot for an intake of 1,000 to 1,300 milligrams per day, taken in two to three doses. If using a calcium supplement, it is best to take it with food.

⊖ What to look for:

Even though most of the studies performed have used dairy sources of calcium, as you can see from the study above, supplemental calcium seems to work well—albeit maybe not quite as well. This may be due to the presence of other bioactive compounds in dairy products that support the effects of calcium. If you choose to use dairy foods to obtain your calcium intake, make sure to use non-fat or low-fat sources. That means that cheese is out, and skim milk is your best bet, with 302 milligrams of calcium per cup.

If you choose to use a supplement, be cognizant of the type of calcium used in the supplement. The most common form of calcium found in supplements is calcium carbonate. This is a very low-quality form and is poorly absorbed. Look for milk calcium, calcium citrate or calcium malate instead. They are all well absorbed. Also, look for a product that includes vitamin D. This helps further enhance absorption and utilization of the calcium.

Green Tea

⊖ What it is:

Green tea is pretty much exactly that—tea that is green. It's the stuff they serve you in the little porcelain pot in fine Chinese restaurants. It's green both due to the type of tea plant it comes from and because it is harvested early, before it matures completely. Green tea has been used for centuries by the Chinese and other Eastern cultures and has been assigned the ability to increase mental awareness, improve digestion and regulate body temperature. And more recently its been touted for its antioxidant and anti-carcinogenic properties, as well as its fat-fighting tendencies.

⊖ How it works:

Green tea contains a multitude of bioactive compounds called phytochemicals. The specific category of phytochemicals that have to do with fat loss are called catechin flavonoids. And it's one of these flavonoids in particular, called epigallocatechin gallate (EGCG), that has received the most attention from researchers. It has recently been discovered that EGCG has the unique ability to enhance thermogenesis (the burning of calories in the body) by inhibiting the enzyme that breaks down catecholamines.

Remember from above that caffeine affects fat burning by stimulating catecholamine (norepinephrine) release. EGCG works the same way, just from a different angle. While caffeine increases norepinephrine levels by stimulating their production, EGCG increases blood levels of norepinephrine and other active catecholamines by slowing their breakdown and clearance from the body.

Research has shown that on its own, EGCG increases calorie and fat burning to a very modest degree.[17] But when combined with caffeine, the thermogenic effect is about 200 percent greater.[17]

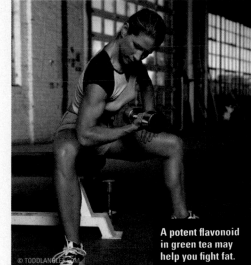

A potent flavonoid in green tea may help you fight fat.

Another recent study investigated the effect of green tea extract on energy expenditure and fat oxidation in three groups of overweight young men.[15] Group 1 consumed a green tea extract containing caffeine and EGCG; Group 2 consumed just caffeine; and Group 3 consumed a placebo. The researchers reported that the green tea extract increased 24-hour energy expenditure by 4 percent and fat burning was 10 percent higher compared to the placebo group. While this may not sound like a huge increase, every little bit helps in the fight against fat.

⊖ **What to look for:**

All green teas are not created equal. Simply drinking a few cups of brewed green tea is great, but the level of EGCG in different teas will vary widely and you would have to drink a lot of tea to get the dose of EGCG used in most studies. Look for a supplement containing an extract of green tea standardized for EGCG content.

Recommended use:
The dose found in the research to increase energy expenditure is 270 milligrams of EGCG taken three times per day. Try a supplement containing at least 500 milligrams of a green tea extract, standardized for EGCG, taken two to three times per day. Shoot for a total of 750 milligrams of EGCG per day.

Conjugated Linoleic Acid (CLA)

⊖ **What it is:**

CLA is a very specific fatty acid from the essential omega-6 family of fats. It is found in fairly large concentrations in beef and fatty dairy products. And because many of us tend to avoid consistent consumption of these foods, our dietary intake of CLA is usually quite low. While a specific required intake level has not yet been established, CLA is one of the essential fatty acids and has been shown to have numerous positive biological effects. These include the reduction of body fat storage, an increase in lean mass and protection against cardiovascular disease and many types of cancer. In fact, in 1996, the National Academy of Sciences stated that CLA is the only fatty acid shown unequivocally to inhibit cancer growth in experimental animals. So it is clear that CLA is essential for optimal health and a fit physique.

How it works:

As mentioned above, CLA has been shown to help increase lean mass and reduce body fat storage. Both of these effects will ultimately help you lose body fat—the increase in lean mass is caused by stimulating greater calorie and fat burning—and the

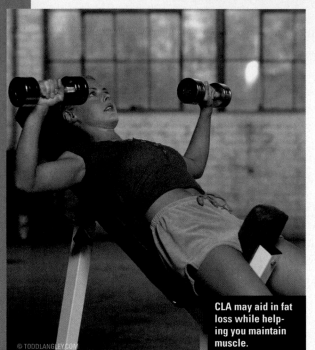

CLA may aid in fat loss while helping you maintain muscle.

© TODDLANGLEY.COM

reduction of fat storage by tipping the scales toward lipolysis. The mechanism by which CLA helps increase lean mass isn't well understood. But it appears to reduce fat storage by regulating several enzymes involved in fat metabolism. There are about a dozen studies investigating CLA's effect on body composition in humans.[9,29,31,38,47] And many of them have produced some impressive results. One study for example tested four different levels of CLA supplementation— 1.7grams, 3.4 grams, 5.1 grams and 6.8 grams per day. The study was 12 weeks long and included no exercise component or dietary controls. Results showed that the groups taking 3.4 grams and 6.8 grams of CLA experienced a significant reduction in body fat compared to the placebo group.[9] Interestingly there was no greater fat loss with 6.8 grams versus 3.4 grams. In another study, subjects consuming just 1.4 grams of CLA per day for 12 weeks reported a 4 percent decrease in body fat.[56] That's 1.6 pounds of pure fat loss in a 200-pound person with 20 percent body fat. Not bad for just popping a few grams of essential fats.

What to look for:

There are two forms of CLA. Their technical names are *cis-9,trans-11* and *trans-10,cis-12*. Suffice it to say, they are significantly distinct enough to posses different biological actions. And research suggests that optimally you want to use a product that contains both 9-11 and 10-12, with the ratio fairly heavily weighted toward the 9-11. The reason is that a couple of studies suggest that the pure 10-12 form may not be very effective and may even result in the development of insulin resistance. While taking a mixture of the two has been proven effective and produced no insulin resistance issues.[44,45]

Recommended use:
Most researchers have used dosage levels in the range of 1.5 to 6 grams per day. You may want to divide this into two to three servings per day. Try 1.5 grams of CLA two to three times per day.

Cayenne Pepper (capsaicin)

● What it is:

You all have heard of cayenne pepper, right? Well, this very same common spice is proving to be a hot little number in fat-loss supplementation. This particular pepper contains a compound called capsaicin. This is the stuff that makes this hot pepper hot. It is concentrated mainly in the seeds and membrane of the pepper. And besides its fat-loss effects, it has been studied for and used widely as a topical pain reliever.

● How it works:

There are two mechanisms by which researchers believe capsaicin helps to fight fat: First, an abundance of animal research has demonstrated that it has the ability to stimulate fat breakdown (lipolysis) from fat cells and to increase fat oxidation (the actual burning of the released fat).[28,30,40,46,61] Secondly, capsaicin appears to cause a feeling of fullness by stimulating appetite control centers in the brain. By creating a feeling of fullness, capsaicin decreases the sensations of hunger, consequently decreasing caloric intake.

A series of studies performed recently in humans tested the effects of capsaicin on appetite, energy intake, energy expenditure and fat oxidation. In these studies, subjects consumed appetizers with or without hot red peppers. Depending on the study, the subjects consumed 3 grams to 10 grams of hot red pepper in the appetizers, which were consumed with breakfast or right before lunch or dinner. The researchers then let them eat whatever they wanted to but measured the amount of food they consumed. The researchers found that when people had hot red pepper in their appetizers, they ate considerably less food at the next meal; furthermore, they experienced an increase in energy metabolism and fat oxidation.

● What to look for:

Try to find a supplement containing a cayenne pepper extract that is standardized for either capsaicin or for Scoville Heat Units (SHU). SHU is a measure of the amount of heat producing nutrients found in the product. This is basically capsaicin. Find a product that contains about 50 milligrams of capsaicin or 100,000 SHU per serving.

Recommended use:
Because capsaicin affects appetite, it is best to take your doses before your two largest meals of the day. And it is best to take 30 to 60 minutes prior to your meal, as some research suggests that taking it directly with your meal is ineffective.[34] So, take one dose of 50 milligrams of capsaicin, 30 to 60 minutes prior to your two largest meals of the day.

Banaba Leaf

⊖ **What it is:**

Banaba is a native plant of the Philippines. It is used as a folk medicine there among diabetics to help them control their blood sugar levels. The extract of the banaba leaf contains a variety of active compounds. The one researchers have become most interested in is called corosolic acid. This chemical appears to have insulin-like properties.

⊖ **How it works:**

As mentioned earlier, one of the main objectives of any fat-loss plan is to maintain a consistently low to moderate blood sugar level. By doing so, you can avoid forcing your body to convert blood sugar into fat for storage—and at the same time allow your body to draw on fat stores for use as fuel. Well, corosolic acid from the banaba leaf helps you do just that.

Animal research shows that it helps to improve the entry of blood sugar into cells in the body,[65,66] thereby helping to keep blood sugar levels low and consistent. One study even measured the effects of this blood sugar modulation on body fat loss. It was found that 12 weeks of supplementation lowered both body weight and body fat significantly.[66] And it did this without affecting the amount of food the animal actually consumed.

One human study measured the effects of an extract of banaba standardized for 1 percent corosolic acid on blood glucose levels in diabetics. It was found that a daily dosage of both 32 milligrams and 48 milligrams for two weeks significantly lowered blood glucose levels in all subjects.[67]

⊖ **What to look for:**

Definitely look for an extract of banaba standardized for 1 percent corosolic acid. "Glucosol™" or "GlucoTrim®" are the trade names of the ingredient upon which the actual research has been performed. Also, the research shows that the product is 50 percent more effective in a soft-gel capsule form rather than as an encapsulated powder.

> **Recommended use:**
> Research data suggest that while both 32 milligrams and 48 milligrams of corosolic acid per day are effective, 48 milligrams is significantly more so. So, if you know that you have trouble controlling your blood sugar levels, shoot for a daily dose of 48 milligrams in soft-gel form, divided into two to three servings per day.

Supplements That Might Work (Stay Tuned for More Research)

Phaseolamin

⊖ **What it is:**

Phaseolamin is an extract from white kidney beans. Scientists have known that phaseolamin inhibits alpha-amylase (the enzyme that breaks down starches in your stomach) for some time, but until recently commercial products containing phaseolamin were too weak to work in the body. The new phaseolamin products are 30 to 40 times more concentrated than previous commercial preparations.

⊖ **How it works:**

Phaseolamin partially inhibits the body's production of alpha-amylase, a starch-digesting enzyme found in the gut.[68,69] In doing so it decreases the efficiency with which your body can break down complex starches into simple sugars, namely glucose. And in order for starches to be absorbed into your system, they must first be reduced to glucose; thus, if you take a dose of phaseolamin before a starchy meal, a portion of the starch eaten simply passes through the digestive system without being digested or absorbed. Some research supports the concept that up to 66 percent of starch absorption can be blocked.

In theory this makes great sense. Lowering your absorption of carbs and calories could help you cut calories and control blood sugar. And there is some research to suggest that it might work to help reduce body fat. In one study, 40 obese volunteers were given daily doses of phaseolamin for 12 weeks. Body weight, body composition and blood pressure were recorded at baseline and every month during the study. The results show a significant difference in weight reduction in favor of the active group (3.5 kilograms versus 1.2 kilograms). Body composition measurements showed that about 85 percent of the reduction in the active group was fat loss.[70]

And in unpublished research, scientists at Northridge Hospital Medical Center performed a study with 50 obese patients randomly given either the supplement or a placebo. Those taking phaseolamin with meals dropped an average of 0.5 pounds a week, compared with 0.21 pounds in the placebo group. While it is not yet fully proven to be effective, stay tuned for more research.

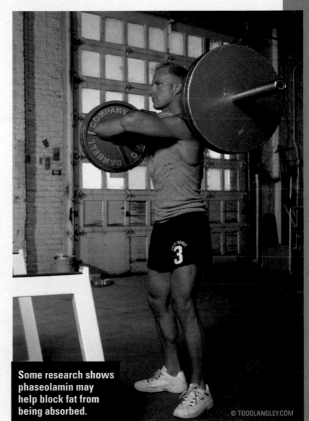

Some research shows phaseolamin may help block fat from being absorbed.

© TODDLANGLEY.COM

Octopamine

⊖ **What it is:**

This newly introduced compound is a neurochemical found in the brain tissue of various insects. It has a protein-like structure and seems to have differing activity in different species of animals, including being involved in the learning behavior of bumble bees.

⊖ **How it works:**

As mentioned earlier, catecholamines bind to various receptors in the body having a multitude of effects. Norepinephrine, for example, binds to three different receptors called adrenoceptors—namely alpha-1, alpha-2 and alpha-3 adrenoceptors. These three receptors have differing activities. Alpha-1 and alpha-2 tend to stimulate the central nervous system and cause the "buzz" you get from the stimulation of norepinephrine by caffeine. Alpha-3 is more focused on lipolytic (fat-burning) actions. This is why caffeine gives you a buzz and helps burn fat.

But octopamine is a bit different. Research shows that octopamine really only binds to the number 3 receptor.[71,72] In theory, this would mean that octopamine has the ability to stimulate lipolysis without the caffeine-like buzz; however, no human studies have been done to test this effect on actual fat loss. More research is needed.

Chitosan

⊖ **What it is:**

Chitin is a non-soluble, naturally occurring polysaccharide found in the shell of various shellfish like crabs and shrimp. Chitosan is produced by hydrolyzing (adding water molecules) to chitin. By doing so, chitosan takes on a weak positive electrical charge and becomes soluble in an acid environment. It is considered a soluble form of fiber.

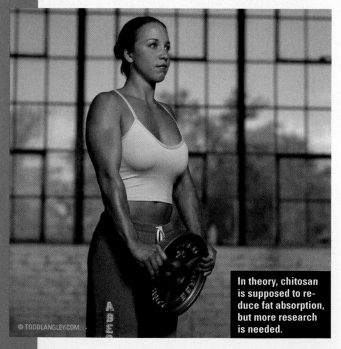

In theory, chitosan is supposed to reduce fat absorption, but more research is needed.

© TODDLANGLEY.COM

⊖ **How it works:**

Chitosan is known as a "fat binder." The idea is that, taken right before or with a high-fat meal, it will irreversibly bind to some of the dietary fat, thus rendering it unabsorbable. The mechanism by which it does this is quite interesting: As chitosan solublizes in the stomach acid, it takes on a weak positive electrical charge. This charge allows chitosan to emulsify (break down) the dietary fats in your stomach. Then as this mass of emulsified fat and chitosan moves into the intestine, the change in pH creates an insoluble gel. This gel of fat and chitosan then passes, unabsorbed, through the intestine and out of the body.

There have been a variety of animal studies showing that chitosan is indeed very effective at reducing fat absorption; however, the initial human studies were not quite as positive. The first study performed to measure the effects of chitosan on fat loss showed no effect after four weeks of treatment.[42] Two other studies, actually measuring the amount of fat in the feces of subjects using chitosan also found no effect (i.e., no increase in fat in the feces versus placebo).[19,20]

But quite recently a new, more rapidly soluble form of chitosan has been introduced to the market and tested in a controlled study. In this study, 59 overweight subjects were given a dose of chitosan before their two largest meals of the day over an eight-week period. They did not alter their diet or any other lifestyle parameter. The results showed that the chitosan group lost 2.2 pounds over the study period, while the placebo group gained 3.3 pounds.[73]

It appears that this more soluble form of chitosan may be more effective than the old stuff. But one interesting thing seems to take place with chitosan usage. Subjects appear to eat fatty foods more freely when they believe they are protected from absorbing the fat. Hence the weight gain in the placebo group. So, if you choose to try this product, keep in mind it's not a license to eat whatever you want, but a possible tool to help you cut the amount of fat you absorb from the fatty foods you are already eating. Keep your eyes out for more research on this newer form of chitosan as well.

Chromium

Chromium is found in many nutritional supplements.

⊝ **What it is:**

Chromium is an essential trace mineral required for normal carbohydrate and fat metabolism and is necessary for optimal insulin activity and maintenance of normal blood glucose levels.

⊝ **How it works:**

The idea behind the use of chromium for weight loss has to do with blood sugar control. As mentioned above, controlling blood sugar levels is key to controlling fat storage and promoting fat loss. And because chromium is a vital cofactor in the function of insulin, carbohydrate metabolism and blood sugar control, folks figured supplementing with chromium would optimize these processes, thereby promoting fat loss. This theory was tested in a now famous study and (surprisingly enough) found to be correct. Supplementing subjects with chromium did indeed appear to enhance fat loss. Since then, this study has been challenged by a number of researchers.[12,18,30,33] Although this nutrient holds promise, more research is needed. First of all, the original theory behind chromium's fat-loss action is not quite correct. You need chromium to properly metabolize carbs and control blood sugar—but you only need so much. Most Americans consume plenty of chromium every day to meet their needs.[3] One study found that excessive chromium supplementation resulted in damage to chromosomes in hamsters. Additional studies have confirmed this finding and added damage to mitochondria and early cell death to the list. Keep in mind that the dosages used in these studies were very high; much higher than what is found in dietary supplements. But there is still some concern that chromium may accumulate in cells, and long-term use may result in cellular levels that could cause problems. As stated previously, this interesting nutrient needs more research. Many nutritional supplements already contain chromium, and at this point, research indicates you don't need to supplement your diet with any more than that.

Medium-Chain Triglycerides (MCT)

What they are:

MCTs are what you might call a "designer oil." Unlike long-chain triglycerides (LCT), which are found in abundance in our food supply, MCTs are not. As a matter of fact they are very rare, but they can be made. They are created by connecting three medium-chain fatty acids to a glycerol molecule backbone.

How they work:

MCTs are metabolized more rapidly than other fats and thus are poorly stored.[7] Because of this, some researchers and individuals in the supplement industry refer to MCTs as "light fats" or "fatless fats." Because MCTs are oxidized more quickly and stored less efficiently than other fats, it has been hypothesized that MCTs may aid in the control of body fat in humans.

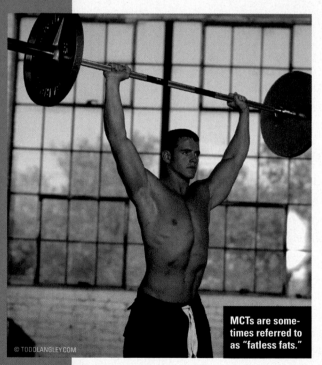

MCTs are sometimes referred to as "fatless fats."

© TODDLANGLEY.COM

A number of research studies have investigated the use of MCTs in the control of food intake, energy expenditure and body weight/composition of humans.[16,25,48,49,57,58] In regard to food intake, when MCTs were consumed during breakfast, the amount of food consumed at lunch was significantly less.[58] Also, the insulin responses to the meals were lower.

Energy expenditure is also greater following the consumption of a meal with MCTs. In one study, the thermic response to food was 12 percent greater with the consumption of MCTs compared to long-chain triglycerides.[25] Furthermore, resting energy expenditure is elevated for 24 hours when MCTs are consumed with breakfast, lunch and dinner,[16] and when MCTs are consumed consistently for four weeks.[48,49] During a 12-week study, people lost significantly more body fat when they consumed MCTs on a daily basis,[57] and very few side effects were reported in all of these studies.[16]

The only drawback is that MCTs are really only effective when they are used in place of other fats, not when they are added on top of your current fat intake.

Pyruvate

⊖ **What it is:**

Pyruvate is an intermediary compound created in your body during the process of converting blood sugar into functional energy. It sits at a pivotal point in the energy production process. During anaerobic exercise it is converted into lactic acid, and during aerobic exercise it's converted into ATP, the final energy source that drives muscular contraction.

⊖ **How it's supposed to work:**

The supposed fat-fighting effects of pyruvate were stumbled upon when researchers were assessing its effects on alcohol consumption in mice. They found that mice supplemented with pyruvate (plus another nutrient called dihydroxyacetone [DHAP]) with their daily dousing of alcohol accumulated less fat in their liver.[51] This finding eventually lead to human research that found that pyruvate, both in combination with DHAP and by itself, was able to enhance weight loss or prevent weight gain in humans.[27,50,53,54] However, the effect was small, only amounting to about 2 pounds of weight loss over a month. And researchers have never fully been able to explain why pyruvate has this effect.

⊖ **Why it doesn't work:**

Granted, even though the effect of pyruvate is small, and the mechanism of action is not really understood, there is research showing it has an effect in humans. But here's the kicker: the dosage of pyruvate used in each of these studies varied between 20 and 53 grams per day.[50,52,53] However, if you take a look at any of the pyruvate products on the market today, the recommended daily dose is 2 to 3 grams per day. And there is absolutely no evidence to suggest that this dose has any effect on fat loss whatsoever.

Marketers of pyruvate pull this smoke and mirrors game with the dosage because pyruvate is expensive stuff. They know they could never sell a product suggesting an effective dose, as it would end up costing you about $20 per day.

Food Sources of Calcium

The following is a list of easy to consume foods and drinks that contain moderate to high amounts of calcium.[6,7]

1 8 ounces of skim milk (302 milligrams)
2 8 ounces low-fat plain yogurt (274 milligrams)
3 Half cup of part-skim ricotta cheese (337 milligrams)
4 Half cup of low-fat cottage cheese (69 milligrams)
5 Orange juice, calcium-fortified (300 milligrams)
6 Boiled artichoke (135 milligrams)
7 Half cup of broccoli (47 milligrams)
8 Navy beans (61 milligrams)
9 Sesame seeds (88 milligrams)
10 Sardines, with bones (242 milligrams)
11 8 ounces spinach (244 milligrams)

Hydroxycitric Acid (HCA)

⊖ **Why it doesn't work:**

Hydroxycitric acid (HCA) is a compound extracted from the skin of a native Indian fruit called Garcinia cambogia.

⊖ **How it's supposed to work:**

HCA has the ability to inhibit the action of an enzyme called ATP-citrate-lyase, the key enzyme for the synthesis of fat from carbohydrates.[36] By doing so, it is thought that HCA can decrease the production and storage of new fat in fat cells, even if blood sugar levels get too high.

HCA has also been reported to suppress food intake[35,55] and decrease weight gain[43] in rats. The mechanism for the suppression of food intake is not really understood.

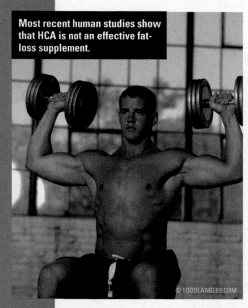
Most recent human studies show that HCA is not an effective fat-loss supplement.

⊖ **Why it doesn't work:**

It's simple. Most recent human research says it doesn't work. The few human studies that have been performed all show negative results. In one study, 135 people were divided into two groups who both followed a 1,200-calorie diet.[23] One group received 1,500 milligrams of HCA, the other group received a placebo. At the end of the 12 weeks, the placebo group lost 9 pounds and 2.2 percent body fat while the HCA group lost 7 pounds and 1.4 percent body fat. Not a happy outcome for the marketers of HCA.

In another study, 500 milligrams of HCA or a placebo were consumed three times per day for two weeks. Both groups lost the same amount of weight, about 2.2 pounds, and HCA did not affect food intake or appetite.[39] Again, the results in these studies are not supportive of HCA being an effective fat-loss supplement.

To be fair it should be pointed out that both of these studies required people to follow low-calorie diets. And when food and carbohydrate intakes are low, it's unlikely that carbohydrates are being converted to fat. It would be interesting to see a high-carb study with HCA.

Carnitine

● **What it is:**

Carnitine is a non-essential amino acid. It can be synthesized from the essential amino acid lysine, and therefore deficiencies are rare.

● **How it's supposed to work:**

There is a special structure within each of our cells called the mitochondria. These little organelles are the "power plants" for our cells. They are responsible for converting fat into useable energy. But before that can happen, the fat has to get into the mitochondria. It does so through what is known as an "active transport" mechanism, meaning the fat has to enter through a specific "door" with the help of a specific co-factor. And in this case, the co-factor is carnitine.

Knowing this, scientists theorized that supplementing with carnitine—thus increasing the levels of available carnitine in muscle cells—would enhance the uptake and burning of fat in mitochondria. It seems to make sense, but the science proves otherwise.

⊖ Why it doesn't work:

In order for carnitine supplementation to actually increase fat uptake and oxidation in muscle cells, it would have to effectively increase the amount of carnitine in the muscle cells; unfortunately, this doesn't appear to be the case. Research shows that carnitine supplementation of 6 grams per day for 14 days failed to increase muscle carnitine content at all.[60]

Even though this research seemed pretty conclusive, researchers decided to try carnitine again in an eight-week study with overweight women, thinking that maybe there would be other mechanisms by which carnitine would help with fat loss. After consuming 4 grams of carnitine per day for eight weeks and exercising for 30 minutes, four days per week, results showed that there were no differences in the amount of fat lost between the carnitine and the placebo group.[59]

While it's clear that this carnitine doesn't work for fat loss, some studies indicate it may have other benefits when it comes to muscle growth and recovery, as discussed in Chapter 9 and Chapter 11.

The Straight Skinny on Ephedra

By now everyone has heard of this infamous herb. Touted for decades as the magic bullet for fat loss, it has recently fallen into disfavor with the powers that be and is not long for this world (at least in the United States). With all of the hype and press surrounding ephedra, it can be hard to decipher the truth about this herbal supplement. Here is the straight scoop on this potent herb and its infamous history:

The use of ephedra dates back some 5,000 years in China. It was (and still is) used there to treat respiratory ailments due to its bronchodilating effects. As a matter of fact, derivatives of ephedra, such as pseudo-ephedrine, are used today in over-the-counter cold and asthma medications here in the United States.

There are a variety of different strains of the ephedra herb. Each strain contains different levels of the active compound, ephedrine, which is responsible for ephedra's biological effects. Ephedra sinica is the most commonly used form. This raw herb, which contains about 2 percent ephedrine, is concentrated until a final extract is produced containing anywhere from 8 percent to 25 percent ephedrine. This is the stuff that is used in modern-day supplements.

Ephedrine is known as a beta-andrenergic agonist, meaning that it stimulates an overall increase in central nervous system and fuel utilization activity in the body. It does so by promoting the release of norepinephrine from a gland in the brain. Norepinephrine then binds to a variety of receptors in the body, causing a multitude of physiological effects, including—an increase in metabolic rate, increase in body temperature, increase in release of fat from fat cells, increased fat oxidation and accelerated heart rate, etc. It is the combination of enhanced fat oxidation and the general increase in metabolic rate that lend to ephedrine's fat-loss effects.

Dozens of studies have been performed using ephedrine, either in combination with caffeine or by itself, as an aid to weight loss. The great majority of these studies have shown that ephedrine, taken in the proper dose over an extended period of time, is a very effective fat-loss aid.[74,75,76,77,78]

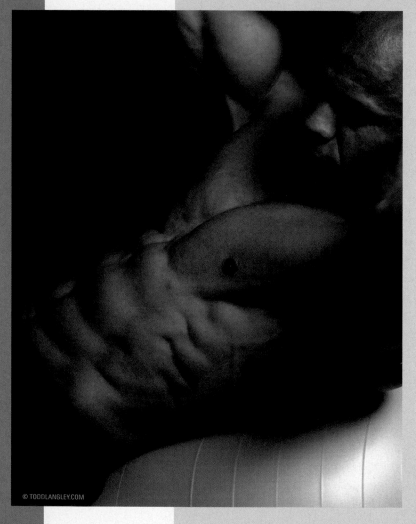

© TODDLANGLEY.COM

However, ephedrine has been the subject of scrutiny. First and foremost, it may cause nervousness, sleeplessness and anxiety, along with a variety of other excitatory responses—namely an increase in heart rate and a transient increase in blood pressure. These side effects have not demonstrated any adverse reactions in research subjects, outside of mild discomfort.

The issue is this: For healthy people, it appears that ephedrine can be a safe product to use. However, for people already suffering from high blood pressure, heart conditions or other metabolic disorders, it may exacerbate those issues.

In light of this issue, and in response to a variety of complaints from consumers about adverse reactions to ephedrine intake, the FDA has made the landmark decision to classify ephedrine as a "controlled substance" and pull it from the supplement market. Soon it will only be available as a prescription medication.

Putting the Supplements That Work To Work for You

What	How Much	When	What Form
Caffeine	200 to 300 mg per serving	Take one serving first thing in the morning, at least 30 minutes before breakfast, and/or one serving 30 to 45 minutes before your daily workout.	You can use coffee, a pure caffeine like caffeine HCL or an herbal caffeine extract like from Guarana.
Calcium	1,000 to 1,300 mg per day	Split your daily intake up into 2 to 3 servings per day. It is best to take with meals to aid in absorption.	Calcium as a component of dairy products seems to be best. Or one of these types of supplements is fine as well: milk calcium, calcium citrate, calcium malate. Avoid calcium carbonate as it is not well absorbed.
Green Tea	270 mg of EGCG per serving	Take 2 to 3 servings per day. Optimally two of these doses should be taken with your caffeine supplement.	Use a green tea extract standardized for EGCG and/or total catechins, so you know exactly what level of EGCG you're getting.
CLA	1.5 g per serving	Take 2 to 3 servings per day, with or without food; it doesn't matter.	Only use CLA that is composed of a mixture of the cis-9,trans-11 and trans-10, cis-12 forms, with the greatest portion being cis-9, trans-11.
Capsaicin	50 mg per serving	Take 2 servings per day 30 to 60 minutes before your two largest meals of the day.	Most likely you will find capsaicin as an extract of cayenne pepper. Make sure it provides at least 100,000 SHU per dose.
Banaba Leaf	32 to 48 mg per day	Split this daily dose up into 2 servings, taken between meals is best.	It's important to find a product standardized to 1% corosolic acid. Look for the trade names "Glucosol" or "GlucoTrim" to know you are getting a pure product.

To simplify things there are a few quality products that combine some of these ingredients for easier use:

- **EAS® Thermo DynamX®**—contains the proper forms and effective doses of green tea extract, calcium and caffeine.
- **EAS® Carb DynamX™**—contains the proper form and effective dose of banaba leaf extract.
- **EAS® CLA**—possesses the desired blend of cis-9, trans-ll and trans-10, cis-12 isomers.

REFERENCES CITED:

[1] Acheson, KJ, Zahorska-Markieqicz, B, Pittet, Ph, Anantharaman, K and Jequier, E. Caffeine and coffee: their influence on metabolic rate and substrate utilization in normal weight and obese individuals. *Am J Clin Nutr* 33 (1980): 989-997.

[2] Anderson, DE and Hickey, MS. Effects of caffeine on the metabolic and catecholamine reponse toexercise in 5 and 28 degrees C. *Med Sci Sports Exerc* 26 (1994): 453-458.

[3] Anderson, RA and Kozlovsky, AS. Chromium intake, absorption and excretion of subjects consuming self-selected diets. *Am J Clin Nutr* 41 (1985): 1177-1183.

[4] Arciero, PJ, Bougopooulos, CL, Nindl, BC and Benowitz, NL. Influence of age on the thermic response to caffeine in women. *Metabolism* 49 (2000): 101-107.

[5] Arciero, PJ, Gardner, AW, Benowitz, NL and Poehlman, ET. Relationship of blood pressure, heart rate and behavioral mood state to norepinepherine kinetics in younger and older men following caffeine ingestion. *Eur J Clin Nutr* 52 (1998): 802-812.

[6] Astrup, A, Toubro, S, Cannon, S, Hein, P, Breum, L and Madsen, J. Caffeine: a double-blind, placebo-controlled study of its thermogenic, metabolic, and cardiovascular effects in healthy volunteers. *Am J Clin Nutr* 51 (1990): 759-767.

[7] Bach, AC, Ingenbleek, Y and Frey, A. The usefulness of dietary medium-chain triglycerides in body weight control: fact or fancy? *J Lipid Res* 37 (1996): 708-726.

[8] Barr, SI. Increased dairy product or calcium intake: is body weight or composition affected in humans? *J Nutr* 133 (2003): 245S-248S.

[9] Blankson, H, Stakkestad, JA, Fagertun, H, Thom, E, Wadstein, J and Gudmundsen, O. Conjugated linoleic acid reduces body fat mass in overweight and obese humans. *J Nutr* 130 (2000): 2943-2948.

[10] Bracco, D, Ferrarra, JM, Arnaud, MJ, Jequier, E and Schutz, Y. Effects of caffeine on energy metabolism, heart rate, and methylxanthine metabolism in lean and obese women. *Am J Physiol* 269 (1995): E671-678.

[11] Carruth, BR and Skinner, JD. The role of dietary calcium and other nutrients in moderating body fat in preschool children. *Int J Obes* 25 (2001): 559-566.

[12] Clarkson, PM. Effects of exercise on chromium levels: is supplementation required? *Sports Med* 23 (1997): 341-349.

[13] Costill, DL, Dalsky, GP and Fink, WJ. Effects of caffeine ingestion on metabolism and exercise performance. *Med Sci Sports* 10 (1978): 155-158.

[14] Davies, KM et al. Calcium intake and body weight. *J Clin Endocrinol Metab* 85 (2000): 4635-4638.

[15] Dulloo, AG et al. Efficacy of a green tea extract rich in catechin polyphenols and caffeine in increasing 24-h energy expenditure and fat oxidation in humans. *Am J Clin Nutr* 70 (1999): 1040-1045.

[16] Dulloo, AG, Fath,i M, Mensi, N and Girardier, L. Twenty-four-hour energy expenditure and urinary catecholamines of humans consuming low-to-moderate amounts of medium-chain triglycerides: a dose-response study in a human respiratory chamber. *Eur J Clin Nutr* 50 (1996): 713-715.

[17] Dulloo, AG, Seydoux, J, Girardier, L, Chantre, P and Vandermander, J. Green tea and thermogenesis: interactions between catechin-polyphenols, caffeine and sympathetic activity. *Int J Obes* 24 (2000): 252-258.

[18] Evans, GW. The effect of chromium picolinate on insulin controlled parameters in humans. *Int J Biosocial Med Research* 11 (1989): 163-180.

[19] Gades, MD and Stern, JS. Chitosan supplementation does not affect fat absorption in healthy males fed a high-fat diet, a pilot study. *Int J Obes* 26 (2002): 119-122.

[20] Gades, MD and Stern, JS. Chitosan supplementation and fecal fat excretion. *Obes Res* 11 (2003): 683-688.

[21] Graham, TE. Caffeine and exercise: metabolism, endurance and performance. *Sports Med* 31 (2001): 767-807.

[22] Graham, TE, Hibbert, E and Sathasivam, P. Metabolic and exercise endurance effects of coffee and caffeine ingestion. *J Appl Physiol* 85 (1998): 883-889.

[23] Heymsfield, SB et al. Garcinia cambogia (hydroxycitric acid) as a potential antiobesity agent. *JAMA* 280 (1998): 1596-1600.

[24] Graham, TE and Spriet, LL. Metabolic, catecholamine, and exercise performance responses to various doses of caffeine. *J Appl Physiol* 78 (1995): 867-874.

[25] Hill, JO, Peters, JC, Yang, D, Sharp, T, Kaler, M, Abumrad, NN and Greene, HJ. Thermogenesis in humans during overfeeding with medium-chain triglycerides. *Metabolism* 38 (1989): 641-648.

[26] Jacqmain, M, Doucet, E, Despres, JP, Bouchard, C and Tremblay, A. Calcium intake, body composition, and lipoprotein-lipid concentrations in adults. *Am J Clin Nutr* 77 (2003): 1448-1452.

[27] Kalman, D, Colker, CM, Stark, R, Minsch, A, Wilets, I and Antonio, J. Effect of pyruvate supplementation on body composition and mood. *Curr Therap Res* 59 (1998): 793-802.

[28] Kawada, T, Hagihara, KI and Iwai, K. Effects of capsaicin on lipid metabolism in rats fed a high fat diet. *J Nutr* 116 (1986): 1272-1278.

[29] Kelley, DS and Erickson, KL. Modulation of body composition and immune cell functions by conjugated linoleic acid in humans and animal models: benefits vs. risks. *Lipids* 38 (2003): 377-386.

[30] Kobayashi, A et al. Capsaicin activates heat loss and heat production simultaneously and independently in rats. *Am J Physiol* 275 (1998): R92-R98.

[31] Kreider, RB, Ferreira, MP, Greenwood, M, Wilson, M and Almada, AL. Effects of conjugated linoleic acid supplementation during resistance training on body composition, bone density, strength, and selected hematological markers. *J Strength Cond Res* 16 (2002): 325-334.

[32] LeBlanc, J, Jobin, M, Cote, J, Samson, P and Labrie, A. Enhanced metabolic response to caffeine in exercise-trained human subjects. *J Appl Physiol* 59 (1985): 832-837.

[33] Lefavi, RG et al. Efficacy of chromium supplementation in athletes: emphasis on anabolism. *Int J Sports Nutr* 2 (1992): 111-122.

[34] Lejeune, MPGM, Kovacs, EMR and Westerterp-Plantenga, MS. Effect of capsaicin on substrate oxidation and weight maintenance after modest body-weight loss in human subjects. *Br J Nutr* 90 (2003): 651-659.

[35] Leonhardt, M and Langhans, W. Hydroxycitrate has long-term effects on feeding behavior, body weight regain and metabolism after body weight loss in male rats. *J Nutr* 132 (2002): 1977-1982.

[36] Lowenstein, JM. Effect of (-)-hydroxycitrate on fatty acid synthesis by rat liver in vivo. *J Biol Chem* 246: 629-632, 1971.

[37] Melanson, EL, Sharpt, TA, Schneider, J, Donahoo, WT, Grunwald, GK and Hill, JO. Relation between calcium intake and fat oxidation in adult humans. *Int J Obes* 27 (2003): 196-293.

[38] Mougios, V et al. Effect of supplementation with conjugated linoleic acid on human serum lipids and body fat. *J Nutr Biochem* 12 (2001): 585-594.

[39] Ntambi, JM, Choi, Y, Park, Y, Peters, JM and Pariza, MW. Effects of conjugated linoleic acid (CLA) on immune responses, body composition and stearoyl-CoA desaturase. *Can J Appl Physiol* 27 (2002): 617-627.

[40] Ohnuki, K, Haramizu, S, Oki, K, Watanabe, T, Yazawa, S and Fushiki, T. Administration of capsaite, a non-pungent capsaicin analog, promotes energy metabolism and suppresses body fat accumulation in mice. *Biosci Biotechnol Biochem* 65 (2001): 2735-2740.

[41] Patwardhan, RV et al. Effects of caffeine on plasma free fatty acids, urinary catecholamines, and drug binding. *Clin Pharmacol Ther* 28 (1980): 398-403.

[42] Pittler, MH, Abbot, NC, Harkness, EF and Ernst, E. Randomized, double-blind trial of chitosan for body weight reduction. *Eur J Clin Nutr* 53 (1999): 379-381.

[43] Rao, RN and Sakariah, KK. Lipid-lowering and antiobesity effect of (-)hydroxycitric acid. *Nutr Resesarch* 8 (1988): 209-212.

[44] Riserus, U, Basu, S, Jovinge, S, Fredrickson GN, Arnlov J and Vessby B. Supplementation with conjugated linoleic acid causes isomer-dependent oxidative stress and elevated C-reactive protein: a potential link to fatty acid-induced insulin resistance. *Circulation* 106 (2002): 1925-1929.

[45] Riserus, U, Brismar, K, Arner, P and Vessby, B. Treatment with dietary trans 10 cis 12 conjugated linoleic acid causes isomer-specific insulin resistance in obese men with the metabolic syndrome. *Diabetes Care* 25 (2002): 1516-1521.

[46] Salimath, BP and Satyanarayana, MN. Inhibition of calcium and calmodulin-dependent phosphodiesterase activity in rats by capsaicin. *Biochem Biophys Res Comm* 148 (1987): 292-299.

[47] Smedman, A and Vessby, B. Conjugated linoleic acid supplementation in humans - metabolic effects. *Lipids* 36 (2001): 773-781.

[48] St-Onge, MP, Bourque, C, Jones, PJH, Ross, R and Parsons, WE. Medium- versus long-chain triglycerides for 27 days increases fat oxidation and energy expenditure without resulting in changes in body composition in overweight women. *Int J Obes* 27 (2003): 95-102.

[49] St-Onge, MP, Ross, R, Parsons, WD and Jones, PJH. Medium-chain triglycerides increase energy expenditure and decrease adiposity in overweight men. *Obes Res* 11: 395-402, 2003.

[50] Stanko, RT and Arch, JE. Inhibition of regain in body weight and fat with addition of 3-carbon compounds to the diet with hyperenergetic refeeding after weight reduction. *Int J Obes Relat Metab Disord* 20 (1996): 925-930.

[51] Stanko, RT, Mendelow, H, Shinozuka, H and Adibi, SA. Prevention of alcohol-induced fatty liver by natural metabolites and riboflavin. *J Lab Clin Med* 91 (1978): 228-235.

[52] Stanko, RT, Reynolds, HR, Lonchar, KD and Arch, JE. Plasma lipid concentrations in hyperlipidemic patients consuming a high-fat diet supplemented with pyruvate for 6 wk. *Am J Clin Nutr* 56 (1992): 950-954.

[53] Stanko, RT, Tietze, DL and Arch, JE. Body composition, energy utilization, and nitrogen metabolism with a severely restricted diet supplemented with dihydroxyacetone and pyruvate. *Am J Clin Nutr* 55 (1992): 771-776.

[54] Stanko, RT, Tietze, DL and Arch, JE. Body composition, energy utilization, and nitrogen metabolism with a 4.25 MJ/d low-energy diet supplemented with pyruvate. *Am J Clin Nutr* 56 (1992): 635.

[55] Sullivan, AC, Triscari, J, Hamilton, JG and Miller, ON. Effect of (-)-hydroxycitrate upon the accumulation of lipid in the rat: II. Appetite. *Lipids* 9: 129-134, 1973.

[56] Thom, E, Wadstein, J and Gudmundsen, O. Conjugated linoleic acid reduces body fat in healthy exercising humans. *J Int Med Res* 29 (2001): 392-396.

[57] Tsuji, H et al. Dietary medium-chain triacylglycerols suppress accumulation of body fat in a double-blind, controlled trial in healthy men and women. *J Nutr* 131 (2001): 2853-2859.

[58] Van Wymelbeke, V, Himaya, A, Louis-Sylvestre, J and Fantino, M. Influence of medium-chain and long-chain triacylglycerols on the control food intake in men. *Am J Clin Nutr* 68 (1998): 226-234.

[59] Villani, RG, Gannon, J, Self, M and Rich, PA. L-carnitine supplementation combined with aerobic training does not promote weight loss in moderately obese women. *Int J Sports Nutr Exerc Metab* 10 (2000): 199-207.

[60] Vukovich, MD, Costill, DL and Fink, WJ. Carnitine supplementation: effect on muscle carnitine and glycogen content during exercise. *Med Sci Sports Exerc* 26 (1994): 1122-1129.

[61] Yoshica, T, Yoshioka, K, Wakabayashi, Y, Nishioka, H and Kondo, M. Effects of capsaicin and isothiocyanate on thermogenesis of interscapular brown adipose tissue in rats. *J Nutr Sci Vitaminol* 34 (1988): 587-594.

[62] Zemel, M. Calcium modulation of adiposity. *Obes Res* 11 (2003): 375-376.

[63] Zemel, MB, Shi, H, Greer, B, Dirienzo, D and Zemel, PC. Regulation of adiposity by dietary calcium. *FASEB J* 14 (2000): 1132-1138.

[64] Zemel, MB, et al. Dietary calcium and dairy products accelerate weight and fat loss during energy restriction in obese adults. *Am J Clin Nutr* 75(suppl 2) (2002): 342S.

[65] Kakuda, T et al. Hypoglycemic effect of extracts from Lagerstroemia speciosa L. leaves in genetically diabetic KK-AY mice. *Biosci Biotechnol Biochem* 60.2 (1996): 204-8.

[66] Suzuki, Y et al. Antiobesity activity of extracts from Lagerstroemia speciosa L. leaves on female KK-Ay mice. *J Nutr Sci Vitaminol* (Tokyo) 45.6 (1999): 791-5.

[67] Judy, WV et al. Antidiabetic activity of a standardized extract (Glucosol) from Lagerstroemia speciosa leaves in Type II diabetics. A dose-dependence study. *J Ethnopharmacol* 87.1 (2003): 115-7.

[68] Yoshikawa, H et al. Characterization of kintoki bean (Phaseolus vulgaris) alpha-amylase inhibitor: inhibitory activities against human salivary and porcine pancreatic alpha-amylases and activity changes by proteolytic digestion. *J Nutr Sci Vitaminol* (Tokyo) 45.6 (1999): 797-802.

[69] Nakaguchi, T et al. Structural characterization of an alpha-amylase inhibitor from a wild common bean (Phaseolus vulgaris): insight into the common structural features of leguminous alpha-amylase inhibitors. *J Biochem* (Tokyo) 121.2 (1997): 350-4.

[70] Thom, E. A Randomized, Double-blind, Placebo-controlled Trial of a New Weight-reducing Agent of Natural Origin. *J Int Med Res* 28 (2000): 229-233.

[71] Carpene, CJ et al. Selective activation of beta3-androceptors by octopamine: comparative studies in mammalian fat cells. *Naunyn Schmiedebergs Arch Pharmacol* 359.4 (1999): 310-321.

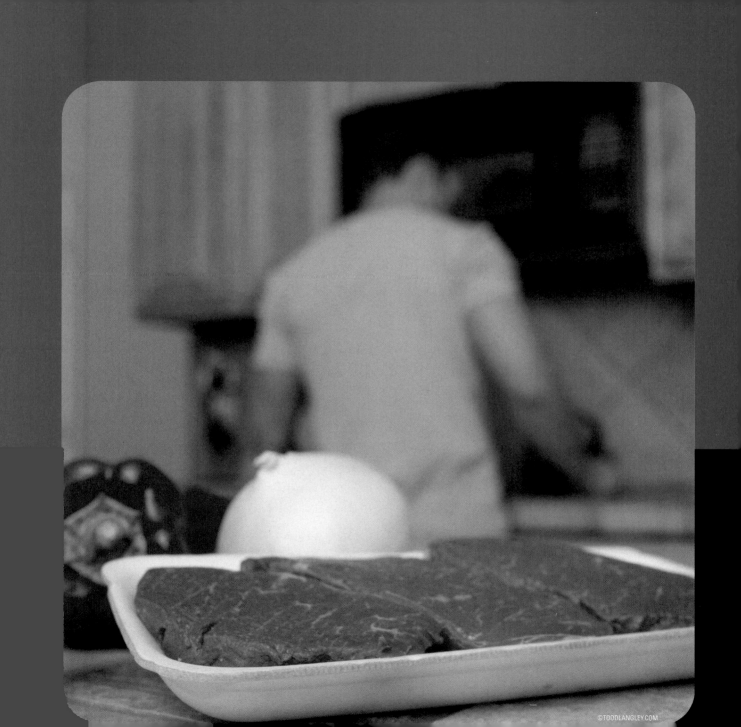

LEAN MASS
& STRENGTH ⊕

part three

8 NUTRITION FOR LEAN BODY MASS AND STRENGTH

A Balanced Nutrition Plan for Muscle Growth

By Jose Antonio, Ph.D., C.S.C.S., FACSM

If your goal is to build a well-muscled, lean physique, you need to use the right building blocks. In other words: You need to eat the right foods at the right time. If you do that, you've won half the battle in your quest for the perfect body, or at least you'll have the physique and the fitness to keep up with your kids as they run you ragged through Disney World. Or you can partake in that pick-up basketball game at the local park knowing that you'll be fine the next day. Achieving a certain level of lean body mass will not only make you look good, it's good for you.

The focus of this chapter will be on nutrition for gaining lean body mass—muscle. Strength, though it is a nice "side effect," is really more of a secondary issue. Unless you're training for a powerlifting or weight lifting competition, gaining muscle is perhaps where your emphasis should be.

Why Can't We Be Like the Black Bear?

Before bears go into winter hibernation, they pig out and gain lots of weight. Then they go to sleep during the winter months. Think of what would happen to you if you slept for several months straight. If you answered, "I'd lose a lot of weight," you're wrong; you'd be dead (of starvation). But the bear can literally sleep for months, wake up, shake the cobwebs from his thick skull and be absolutely fine. Bears have an uncanny ability to burn fat while they hibernate without losing any muscle. In fact, some scientists actually took muscle biopsies from black bears before and after they hibernated and found that they had no change in muscle fiber number or size after hibernation.[1]

So bears have somehow adapted to hibernation by preserving lean body mass and using their body fat stores for energy. Imagine if humans had it so easy. Unfortunately, we don't; however, unlike the bear, we have access to an unlimited number, amount and type of foods, foods that can promote lean body mass gain. So before you go into hibernation, let's see how the body regulates lean body mass.

Common terms you should know

- **Anabolism**—building up of tissue mass
- **Catabolism**—breaking down of tissue mass
- **Synthesis**—same as anabolism
- **Degradation**—same as catabolism
- **Proteolysis**—breakdown of protein
- **Lipolysis**—breakdown of fat
- **Glycolysis**—breakdown of carbohydrates

Making More Muscle—The Sum of Anabolism and Catabolism

What are the mechanisms behind gaining muscle? It's actually quite simple: Your body's metabolism is the sum total of all anabolic and catabolic events. If your body weight hasn't changed in years, then you could rightly assume that the rate of tissue anabolism is equal to the rate of catabolism. If your goal is to gain muscle, the rate of muscle protein synthesis or anabolism must exceed that of proteolysis or catabolism. Think of the "water in the bucket" analogy.

Let's say your body is represented by a bucket of water (150 pounds) that has small holes in the bottom of the bucket. Each day you pour water in the bucket and that water represents calories (protein, carbs, fat and maybe a little alcohol). But since there are holes in the bucket, some of that proverbial water (i.e., energy and macronutrients) is burned for fuel and utilized.

To gain weight, you need to pour more water (i.e., calories and macronutrients) in the bucket than leaves the bucket. To lose weight, the opposite is true.

Muscle-Building Nutritional Guidelines

Before delving into the type of foods essential for building muscle, let's talk about the nutrition guidelines you'll be following. In Chapter 6, you learned how to keep a seven-day food diary to establish your maintenance calorie level, and then you *decreased* your daily calorie intake by about 15 percent in order to lose fat. In this case, since you're interested in gaining muscle, you'll need to *add* about 10 percent to 15 percent to your maintenance calorie level, divided among six small daily meals (to learn more about establishing your maintenance calorie level, go to Chapter 6).

If you have access to the Internet, there are also some calculators that are available for predicting calorie needs, such as the Harris-Benedict formula. It's quite simple; just plug in your age, sex, activity level, height and weight. If you go to the following Web site, it makes it as easy as a point and few clicks: www.annecollins.com/calories/calorie-needs-men.htm. Once again, when the site calculates your calorie needs, you'll need to add approximately 10 percent to 15 percent to ensure you're getting the calories necessary for gaining muscle.

As recommended throughout this book, a macronutrient ratio of 40 percent protein, 40 percent carbohydrates and 20 percent fat is recommended. Please turn to Chapter 4 to learn how to calculate a 40/40/20 ratio.

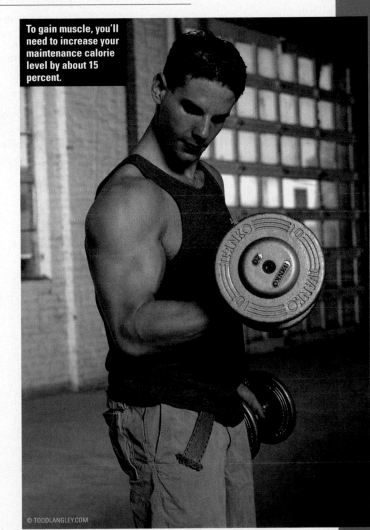

To gain muscle, you'll need to increase your maintenance calorie level by about 15 percent.

© TODDLANGLEY.COM

Muscular Macronutrients

As you learned in Chapter 1, the macronutrients are carbohydrates, fat and protein. Both carbohydrates and protein contain four calories per gram, whereas fat has nine; however, not all calories are created equal. Furthermore, within each subset of the macronutrients, you have "good" and "bad" carbs, protein and fat.

Now don't think this is merely calories in versus calories out. That's part of the equation. But keep in mind that the kind of food you eat affects the kind of weight gain and weight loss that result. For instance, if you pour "protein" into your proverbial "bucket," you are less apt to gain fat weight because your body burns more energy digesting the protein. This is called the thermic effect of feeding. Thus, pouring protein in your bucket is not the same as pouring table sugar. In short, the type of macronutrient that you pour into your bucket will directly affect the nature of your body weight alterations.

Carbohydrates: Fuel for Muscle-Building Exercise

Because carbohydrates serve as the primary fuel source for intense exercise, you can't do a low-carb diet without expecting a compromise in your exercise abilities. Though some might suggest that if you do a low-carb diet, eventually your body adapts to this by oxidizing or burning fat more efficiently; however, keep in mind that intramuscular carbohydrates (i.e., glycogen stored in your muscle cells) are the main fuel source during intense exercise, including lifting weights and intense cardio. Though strength athletes do not need the amount of carbohydrates (for a given body weight) that an endurance athlete would, it would be unwise for you to restrict carbohydrate consumption if you want to gain lean body mass. Half the battle is making sure you eat nutrient-dense carbohydrates (i.e., brown rice, whole-grain bread, oats, etc.) in a regular fashion and limit the high-glycemic, nutrient-sparse carbs.

Which of the Three Major Macronutrients Are Essential?

In the *American Journal of Clinical Nutrition*[2], Dr. Eric C. Westman of Duke University Medical Center says that the currently established essential nutrients are "water, energy, amino acids, essential fatty acids, vitamin E, vitamin K, thiamine, riboflavin, niacin, vitamin B_6, pantothenic acid, folic acid, biotin and vitamin B_{12}, minerals, trace minerals, electrolytes and ultratrace minerals."[3] (Note the absence of specific carbohydrates from the list.)

From this list, you must be thinking, if carbohydrates are not "essential" per se, then why is everyone telling me to eat them? First of all, don't confuse "essential" with "important." It may be true that as long as you're eating plenty of essential amino acids (protein) and essential fatty acids, you'll be alive and healthy. But you "need" to eat carbs, not to sustain life, but to sustain your ability to exercise and to expedite your recovery. So don't go super low in the carbs, or you may end up with super low energy.

Why Low Is the Way To Go

Think "low," as in Glycemic Index, that is. As you know, the Glycemic Index (GI) is how much your blood glucose (sugar) rises after eating a specific kind of carbohydrate. Interestingly, simple sugars or carbohydrates do not always have a higher glycemic index than complex carbohydrates; for example, fruit sugar or fructose barely causes a rise in blood glucose. Table sugar is higher. But in general, the low-glycemic items also tend to be the healthiest. Here's why:

- ⊕ If you consume a low-glycemic carbohydrate roughly 60 to 90 minutes before training, this may help your exercise performance.
- ⊕ Because high-glycemic foods cause a surge in blood glucose, and then insulin, you'll end up getting hungrier sooner. Thus, you'll be more apt to overeat.
- ⊕ High-glycemic foods may increase your risk of coronary artery disease.

Carb Facts for Muscle Growth

Carbs are essential to a solid muscle growth nutrition plan. Here are a few tips to keep in mind:

- ⊕ Carbs should make up roughly 40 percent of your daily calories.
- ⊕ Eat natural, unprocessed carbohydrates.
- ⊕ The right types of high-glycemic carbs have their place; they're usually best consumed immediately after a weight-training workout (see sidebar).

What About Carb Loading?

Unless you're an ultra-endurance athlete, there's no need to carb load, simple as that. Here's a fun fact for you: For every gram of muscle glycogen stored, you will also store 2.7 grams of water.[4] That might be why you feel bloated after a carb-eating binge.

Is There a Good Time to Eat High-Glycemic Carbs?

Absolutely! Immediately before, during and after exercise, it is best for you to consume high-glycemic carbohydrates. For more detail on this strategy called nutrient timing, go to Chapter 10.

Sample Guidelines for Gaining Muscle Mass

EXAMPLE #1:
A 200-pound male, 20 years old, 5 feet 10 inches tall, with "heavy" activity levels would need 3,561 calories.

Macronutrient breakdown (based on 40% protein, 40% carbs, 20% fat):
Protein—1,424 calories or 356 grams
Carbs—1,424 calories or 356 grams
Fat—713 calories or 79 grams of fat
Meal frequency—6 meals per day
Average calories per meal—593.5 calories
Average grams per meal (protein/carbs/fat)—59/59/13

EXAMPLE #2:
A 150-pound male, 40 years of age, 5 feet 8 inches tall, with a "moderate" activity level would need 2,467 calories.

Macronutrient breakdown (based on 40% protein, 40% carbs, 20% fat):
Protein—987 calories or 247 grams
Carbs—987 calories or 247 grams
Fat—493 calories or 55 grams
Meal frequency—6 meals per day
Average calories per meal—411 calories
Average grams per meal (protein/carbs/fat)—41/41/9

Fat: The Good, The Bad, The Ugly

Besides protein (i.e., essential amino acids), fat is the other essential macronutrient, meaning you need to eat fat because your body doesn't normally make certain essential fatty acids (i.e., linoleic and linolenic acid). It's best that you consume 20 percent (give or take) of your calories as fat. Take a close look at someone on a very low-fat diet. They look unhealthy. Their skin is dry, their hair brittle and their mood resembles a shark that missed its last feeding. Despite the plethora of low-fat and fat-free foods, don't let the marketers fool you. You need a certain amount of healthy dietary fat. Without the proper fat, you'll compromise your health and well-being. Fat is needed for energy, insulation, hormone production, cell membrane structure and function and a slew of other things.

Dietary Fats 101

The confusing thing about fat is that there are so many kinds. You have healthy fats and lethal fats. Some fats impact blood lipids favorably and improve health outcomes. And some fats might even help you lose body fat. So let's go over some of the major categories of fat. This summary will give you the rudiments of fat physiology. With these tools, you can make more sensible dietary choices.

Good Fats: The MUFAs and PUFAs

MUFAs are monounsaturated fats and PUFAs are polyunsaturated fats. On a more palatable level, MUFAs are healthy fats found in nuts, avocados and oils. Olive oil is perhaps the best known of the MUFAs; however, don't forget canola. According to sports nutritionist Cassandra Forsythe, "canola oil is 60 percent MUFA, second only to olive oil, which contains 75 percent. And more importantly, canola oil contains the least saturated fat and no trans fats."

DHA and EPA—Fabulous Fats

DHA and EPA are unsaturated omega-3 fats and deserve special mention. They may be the most important PUFAs you should consume. Joseph Chromiak, Ph.D., concurs: "The EPA and DHA found in fish fat is an excellent and healthy fat; so combined with fish protein, you really do have one of the highest quality foods." There is laundry list of wonderful things these fats do. For instance, research has shown that treatment with EPA improved blood vessel function in individuals with heart disease.[6] Fish, in and of itself, is a solid source of muscle-building protein, but the valuable fats found in fish have other benefits as well:

➕ EPA and DHA may reduce risk of death from heart disease.[7]
➕ EPA may reduce injury to the heart.[8]
➕ EPA and DHA may lower blood fat (triglycerides).[9,10]

MUFA consumption may decrease your risk of heart disease and may even help you lose body fat; for example, a 30-week study in which subjects consumed lots of peanuts—which are high in MUFAs—they lowered their serum or blood levels of fat (specifically triglycerides) and reduced their cardiovascular disease risk.[5]

PUFAs are sort of a mixed bag. Most Americans get plenty of linoleic acid (an omega-6 PUFA) but usually not enough of linolenic acid (an omega-3 PUFA). Linoleic acid is found in corn, cottonseed and soybean oils, whereas linolenic acid is found in high concentrations in walnuts and flax, along with some in soybean oil. Thus, some PUFAs are more beneficial than others; for example, the omega-3 fats found in fish oil or fat (i.e., eicosapentanoic acid or EPA, docosahexanoic acid or DHA) are great for you, yet most Americans get very little in their diets. On the other hand, we tend to eat too much of the omega-6 fats found in vegetable oils at the expense of not enough omega-3s. Some research recommends a 1:4 ratio of omega 3s to 6s; however, most Americans probably eat closer to a 1:20 ratio; that is, they consume 20 times more omega 6s than 3s. This could increase the risk of the number of inflammatory-related diseases.

Another Good Fat—Conjugated Linoleic Acid (CLA)

Conjugated linoleic acid (CLA) has received a bit more press, probably because it's a good fat-loss supplement. According to a recent study, besides having a dramatic effect on weight loss in mice (this is true), CLA may help you regain lean body mass after going off a diet.

Scientists took 26 men and 28 women and put them on a very-low calorie diet for three weeks. How low? About one cheeseburger's worth of calories per day (~500 calories). After these three weeks of famine, they had them take either 1.8 grams of CLA, 3.6 grams of CLA or a placebo daily for 13 weeks. The very-low calorie diet lowered body weight, fat mass and fat-free mass significantly. Obviously with any diet, losing fat-free mass—which is mainly muscle—is not a good thing. But after the 13 weeks of intervention and going back on a normal diet, they found that the CLA groups regained fat-free mass better than the placebo. Interestingly, the low-dose CLA produced a better fat-free mass gain than the higher dose (6.2 percent versus 4.6 percent); the placebo gained roughly 3 percent in fat-free mass. This means that if you've lost weight, it might be a good idea to supplement with about 1.5 grams of CLA daily if you want to regain some of the fat-free mass you may have lost.

Fat Affects Testosterone Levels

If you're thinking low-fat diets are the way to go, think again. If you're a guy, eating too little fat will turn you from a burly man into a girlie man. OK, maybe you won't turn into high-heel wearing chick, but it may affect levels of the omnipresent hormone, testosterone—the crème de la crème of muscle-building hormones. Researchers at Penn State University examined how diet fits into the anabolic puzzle.[12] They had 12 men perform a variety of weight-training exercises and measured their testosterone levels. They found that the men who ate more fat, whether it be the monounsaturated or saturated variety, tended to have higher levels of resting testosterone. Although diet and exercise affect steroid hormones, scientists don't yet know all the pieces to this wacky puzzle; until then, however, your best bet is to consume plenty of healthy fats.

Bad Fats—Trans and Saturated Fats

These two fats are a deadly duo. If you enjoy living, limit your consumption of these fats. Unlike the MUFAs or PUFAs, saturated fats have no carbon double bonds. That is, all of their carbons are "saturated" with as many hydrogen molecules as possible (hence the name!). Saturated fats are solid at room temperature. So that delicious morsel of fat from that grilled steak is probably high in saturated fat. *Trans* fat (also known as *trans* fatty acids) are made when food manufacturers turn liquid oils into solid fats; however, a small amount of *trans* fat occurs naturally in animal-based foods. Just like saturated fats, trans fats are not your best friend.[11] They can elevate the "bad" cholesterol (LDL) and thus increase your risk of heart disease. Next time, read a food label. If it says "partially hydrogenated" or "hydrogenated," then there's trans fats in it. You'll find trans fats in foods such as margarines, cookies, snacks, fried foods and even peanut butter.

Fat Facts for Muscle Growth

If you're like most normal people, you don't necessarily care what the structural or biochemical differences are between different types of fat. So here is the message that you need to take home:

- Fat should make up roughly 20 percent of your calories.
- Limit intake of saturated and trans fats (basically avoid processed foods).
- Eat fish fat once a week; they have lots of the healthy PUFAs (omega 3s).
- Use olive oil-based salad dressing.
- Eat nuts; they have lots of healthy MUFAs.
- If you exercise a lot, getting needed calories from fat may be required.

Protein: The King of Muscle Growth

According to Lonnie Lowery, Ph.D., an exercise physiologist at Kent State University, "To gain lean body mass, you need to consume more protein than the RDA; whole-protein sources such as milk, eggs, whey and meats are great." In terms of what your body is made up of, protein is second only to water. You are probably well aware of the importance of protein for gaining lean body mass. Keep in mind, protein, fat and carbs form a trio that you can't just haphazardly consume in the hopes that it'll all end up where you want it to. Systematic eating produces systematic results. Don't forget that!

How Much Protein Can I Consume?

To be honest, nobody knows the answer to this question. But at the same time, it would be headstrong and foolish to think that your 85-year-old grandma and the 315-pound offensive tackle for a football team both have the same limitations when it comes to digesting and absorbing protein. There are studies in which levels of 30 grams of protein are fed to subjects, and this amount produces a tremendous rise in blood amino acid levels. A good starting point may be 30 grams of protein per meal. Assuming you eat 30 grams a sitting and you eat six times daily, that's about 180 grams of protein. That's good if you weigh 180 pounds or less; if you're a sumo wrestler, football player or bodybuilder, you'll need to up the protein dose per meal or increase meal frequency.

How Much Protein Should I Eat?

This issue has been the subject of debate by every expert ranging from registered dieticians and exercise physiologists to scientists and doctors. Part of this food fight revolves around the misguided notion that eating more protein than the Recommended Dietary Allowance (RDA) will cause your kidneys to quit, but there is no scientific evidence that consuming two or even three times the RDA for protein (if you're a normal, healthy individual) is harmful; unless, of course, your kidneys don't already work.

According to noted exercise physiologist, Darryn Willoughby, Ph.D., "The hazards of eating a high-protein diet are overstated. If you're healthy, eating more than the RDA is fine. If you have kidney problems, see your physician." Current research suggests that 1.5 grams to 2.0 grams per kilogram per day are needed for those interested in packing on some muscle.[13] In other words, try to eat about 1 gram of protein daily per pound of body weight.

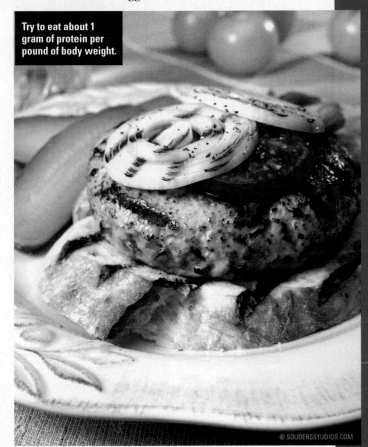

Try to eat about 1 gram of protein per pound of body weight.

© SOUDERSSTUDIOS.COM

So Many Proteins, So Little Time

Basically, the protein you eat should have the entire complement of essential amino acids. Incomplete proteins, such as peanuts, do not contain all essential amino acids.

One way scientists compare the quality of protein sources is through something called the biological value or BV. The BV measures the amount of protein retained per gram of protein absorbed. If a given protein provides all the essential amino acids in the correct proportions and is readily absorbed, the BV score will approach 100. On the other hand, if the protein is deficient in one essential amino acid, then its BV score will be much lower. Foods with excellent BV are milk, whey, casein, egg, meats and fish. Plant sources tend to be inferior.

In addition, scientists have discovered that the manner in which your body digests protein (i.e., slow proteins [casein] versus fast proteins [whey]) also affects how your body responds. More on that later.

When Should I Eat Protein?

According to strength and conditioning specialist David Sandler, C.S.C.S., of Florida International University, "Anyone who is trying to gain lean body mass via the participation in high-volume, heavy-resistance exercises needs to eat small frequent meals that contain protein. This will enhance muscle protein anabolism and expedite the adaptive response."

In one study, six resistance-trained men performed a "typical" bodybuilding workout, and researchers found that muscle protein synthesis was increased at four and 24 hours after exercise but returned to pre-exercise levels after 36 hours post-exercise.[14]

As a general rule, it probably takes about two days for muscle protein synthesis to drop back to baseline. What does this mean? Your muscles "grow" when you're not exercising, especially when you're sleeping. Hence, it is critical that you feed your muscles nutrients throughout the day. Thus, eat frequent, small meals daily. (You can see more on this in Chapter 6.)

Top Muscle-Building Protein Picks

Fish—The Champion of Proteins

As you learned earlier, fish (or the healthy fat in fish) may have a number of benefits, including increased cardiovascular health and protection against strokes.[16,17]

Also, eating fish improves your insulin sensitivity.[18] Some investigators believe it's related to the amino acid arginine. Others have theorized that the high lysine content of fish may also confer benefits. Ultimately, the increased insulin sensitivity means that you need less insulin to transport glucose and amino acids into your cells. By preventing drastic increases in insulin, you can limit the amount of fat you gain and is key when you're trying to gain muscle. Try to eat fish once or twice a week.

Whey Works

It is the second most abundant protein derived from milk. (Casein is the most abundant milk protein.) It's found mainly in meal-replacement powders, protein powders and ready-to-drinks and contains all of the essential amino acids and is particularly high in the branched-chain amino acids. Whey is considered a "fast" acting protein.[19] For example, if you consume a 30-gram serving of whey on an empty stomach, levels of blood amino acids peak about one hour afterward and return to pre-meal levels by three to four hours. This absorption profile makes whey a very anabolic protein; in fact, a whey protein meal produces a 68 percent increase in protein synthesis; however, it doesn't blunt protein breakdown (Casein protein does. More on that later).[20]

FINAL SCORE: Meat Protein May Be Superior to Plant Protein for Muscle Growth

Scientists have found that eating a meat-containing diet is superior to a lacto-ovovegetarian diet with regard to gaining skeletal muscle mass.[15] Nineteen overweight men participated in this 12-week study. Nine men consumed a diet that derived 50 percent of their protein calories from meat (beef, chicken, fish, etc.), while the other 10 men consumed a lacto-ovovegetarian diet. That is, they could not consume meats; however, they could eat egg and dairy products. All test subjects lifted weights for the 12-week duration. Subjects in both groups improved their strength by up to 38 percent with no real differences between meat-eaters and non-meat eaters. But when they measured body composition, there was a definite difference. The lacto-ovo group had no change in fat mass and a slight decrease (-1.2 percent) in lean body mass. On the other hand, the meat-eaters experienced a 4.6 percent decrease in fat mass coupled with a 2.7 percent increase in lean body mass.

The bottom line is this: Consuming meats as part of your overall eating program is better than a vegetarian-based diet, at least when it comes to putting on muscle.

One study found that supplementing with whey protein during a six-week resistance training program increased strength and muscle mass more than just training alone.[21] Clearly, supplementing with whey is a better alternative than no supplementation at all.

Not only will whey protein help you put on muscle, but this stuff has potent effects on the immune system.[22] One study found that whey protein helped stabilize or reverse tumor growth in patients with metastatic carcinoma.[23] Of course, whey can give you tremendous recovery benefits as well. According to exercise scientist Ron Mendel, Ph.D., "Immediately after exercise, drink a protein shake that combines a fast-acting protein like whey with a high-glycemic index carb."

Casein—The "Slow" Protein

Casein is the main protein in milk. Besides drinking milk, you can obtain casein in various meal-replacement powders, protein powders, cottage cheese and ready-to-drinks. Casein "clots" in your stomach, making its absorption a bit slower than whey, hence, it's designated a "slow-acting" protein. Casein has a strong anti-catabolic effect, and you could describe casein as the "opposite" of whey. They're both great proteins but they act in quite the opposite manner. Casein has a lower anabolic effect (31 percent versus 68 percent) when compared to whey; however, casein has a very profound anti-catabolic effect, meaning that this protein inhibits protein breakdown.[24] This has profound implications for the proper use of casein. Because casein is digested slowly, it produces a slow but steady rise in amino acids. Blood levels peak about one to two hours after consuming casein and remain elevated for up to seven hours. In head-to-head comparisons of casein versus whey, casein seems to promote a better net gain in muscle protein. Nevertheless, if you were to compare one feeding of casein (30 grams) versus repeated small servings of whey (equaling 30 grams) the net anabolic effect would be similar.

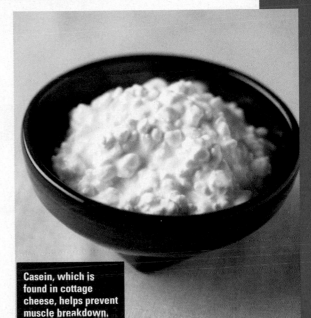

Casein, which is found in cottage cheese, helps prevent muscle breakdown.

In a 12-week study comparing the changes in body composition in three different groups following reduced-calorie diets—a diet-only group, a second group that strength-trained and supplemented with casein and a third group that strength-trained and supplemented with whey[25]—researchers found that body fat loss and lean body mass gains were greatest in the casein group followed by the whey group (and then the control group). According to the study's authors, casein supplementation improved nitrogen retention; also, they felt that casein provided a good anti-catabolic effect.

In other words, casein is an excellent protein that improves lean body mass gain when taken as part of a reduced-calorie diet. According to noted sports nutritionist Jeffrey Stout, Ph.D., author of *Supplements for Strength-Power Athletes*, "Casein is a great protein to take before going to bed. Because it's absorbed slowly, you'll get a nice stream of amino acids into your body. This will help you recover as well as assist you in gaining lean body mass."

Milk—Not Just for Kids

Ancient Middle Easterners first domesticated animals for their meat roughly 10,000 years ago. Oddly, it wasn't until 3,000 years later (or 7,000 years ago) that animals were first used for their milk.[26] And milk isn't just for kids. Adults could meet their protein and calcium requirements via a few glasses of the white stuff. Besides, there are other reasons to drink milk; for example, milk contains all of the essential amino acids.[27] According to the *Journal of Dairy Science*, "Bioactive peptides [in milk] may function as health care products, providing therapeutic value for either treatment of infection or prevention of disease."[28]

Keep in mind that if you're trying to get lean stay away from whole milk and stick to skim. Skim milk is an excellent food source that's perfect as an evening protein supplement. Because the majority of the protein in milk is casein (a "slow" protein), you'll get a slow and sustained elevation of amino acids throughout the night while you sleep. This will insure that your body has the amino acids it needs to facilitate muscle recovery … and build muscle. According to coach and personal trainer, Juan Carlos Santana, C.S.C.S., "Milk, especially skim milk, is a great way to get protein; and it's inexpensive as well. I highly recommend skim milk or non-fat milk powder for many of the athletes I train."

EGGcellent Tidbits[31]

OSTRICH EGGS

If you're an egg lover, then you'd love the ostrich egg. The ostrich is the largest bird in the world. One ostrich egg contains roughly 1,600 calories, 137 grams of protein, 110 grams of fat and roughly 10 grams of carbs! That's equal to about two dozen chicken eggs. Talk about a muscle-gaining omelet.

ORGANIC EGGS

Organic eggs come from hens who weren't exposed to commercial fertilizers, pesticides or herbicides. Thus, the egg is a bit more expensive than regular eggs. As far as nutrition is concerned, organic eggs are no different than non-organic eggs.

FREE-RANGE EGGS

Free-range eggs are from hens that have been raised outdoors; however, because of weather constraints, this doesn't mean these hens are running around like wild animals in Yellowstone. Let's just say they let them out for a daily jog. The nutrient content is the same for free-range eggs as it is with regular eggs. And they cost more, too.

Eggs—A Cost-effective Protein

Eggs are a rich source of thiamine, riboflavin, pantothenic acid, folic acids, vitamin B_{12}, biotin, vitamin D, vitamin E and phosphorus.[29] Seems like a complete food, right? In one large study of 27,000 people,[30] it was discovered that "the daily nutrient intake of egg consumers was significantly greater than that of non-consumers." For instance, vitamins B_{12}, C, E and A were consumed in greater quantities in the egg consumers. And get this: Those who reported eating four or more eggs daily had lower blood cholesterol levels than those who ate one egg or less daily. Not only is egg protein great, but it's very affordable. According to Chris Mohr, R.D., "Where else can you get 80+ grams of protein, like what is found in a dozen eggs, for under a dollar?" And don't be so quick to throw out the yolks. While egg white omelets (three to five egg whites with one whole egg) are an excellent food, the evidence for whole eggs being harmful is just not supported by the evidence. But if you're trying to cut back on calories, egg whites will suffice as a protein source.

The Meat of the Matter—Beef, Chicken and Pork
Beef

Beef has gotten a bad rap, but it does have a place in your muscle-building arsenal. In one study, 11 men consumed a beef-containing diet while 10 men ate a vegetarian diet for 12 weeks.[32] During this time all subjects participated in weight training three days per week. The beef-eating group experienced an increased hemoglobin concentration and hematocrit compared with the vegetarian group. This would mean they'd have a greater capacity to carry oxygen in their blood—definitely a plus if you exercise.

Beef contains all of the essential amino acids; moreover, beef is an excellent protein source and is loaded with zinc and iron as well. Also, beef isn't as bad as its reputation. For example, a study published in *Nutrition* found that overweight women—who exercised and consumed a restricted-calorie diet with either lean beef or chicken as the main protein source—demonstrated weight loss, as well as decreases in body fat percentage, total cholesterol and LDL cholesterol.[33] The key is that you need to consume *lean* beef. The fat content between different kinds of beef can be quite variable.[34]

Weight Loss With Chicken or Beef

Losing weight doesn't mean you have to give up your favorite cut of steak or chicken; in fact, complete proteins like beef and chicken play a critical part in your diet, especially if you're trying to lose weight and preserve or gain muscle. One study looked at changes in body weight and lipid profiles in a 12-week, randomized, controlled trial in which overweight women followed a lower-calorie diet with lean beef or chicken as the primary protein source. In addition, they took part in a fitness walking program.[36] Both groups lost body fat and had a drop in LDL cholesterol levels (the "bad" cholesterol). According to the study's authors, "weight loss and improved lipid profile can be accomplished through diet and exercise, whether the dietary protein source is lean beef or chicken."

- 70 percent lean, 30 percent fat (ground beef)
- 80 percent lean, 20 percent fat (ground chuck)
- 85 percent lean, 15 percent fat (ground round)
- 90 percent lean, 10 percent fat (ground sirloin)

An easy way to remember which beef source has the least fat content is to remember that those at the beginning of the alphabet (ground **B**eef) have the most fat and those near the end of the alphabet (ground **S**irloin) have the least.

Keep in mind that if dietary fat is a concern, it should be noted that beef fat may not entirely deserve its bad rep. According to Lonnie Lowery, Ph.D., a sports nutrition scientist and former amateur bodybuilder, "It is controversial whether components of beef fat (stearic acid) actually increase cardiovascular risk like other saturated fats. And a little fat, along with the solid nature of beef, provides a dieter with superior satiety (fullness and satisfaction) compared to liquids. Beef cuts like eye of round and 90 percent lean (or leaner) hamburger add dietary variety and are a richer source of nutrients than many foods. For the many athletes who get too few calories (hypoenergetic), even the extra fat could be advantageous if consumed in moderation. And another thing that many athletes forget is that beef contains creatine. And we all know how effective creatine is for promoting gains in muscle size!" For muscle growth, your best bet is to consume lean cuts of beef at least once or twice per week.

Chicken

Chicken is a great protein source and is perhaps the single most consumed dietary protein. Like beef, the fat content of chicken can vary dramatically especially if you eat the skin. For instance, a 100-gram serving of light meat chicken with skin contains 222 calories and 10.85 grams of fat compared to 173 calories and 4.51 grams of fat if you remove the skin. That's 141 percent more fat (with skin)! Chicken contains all of the essential amino acids, and because of its complete amino acid profile and the universally loved taste of chicken, it's a favorite amongst fitness enthusiasts. Similar to lean beef, chicken consumption as part of a well-rounded diet can help decrease total cholesterol and LDL cholesterol.[35] As part of a muscle-growth plan, chicken may very well be a staple. Just be sure to eliminate the skin.

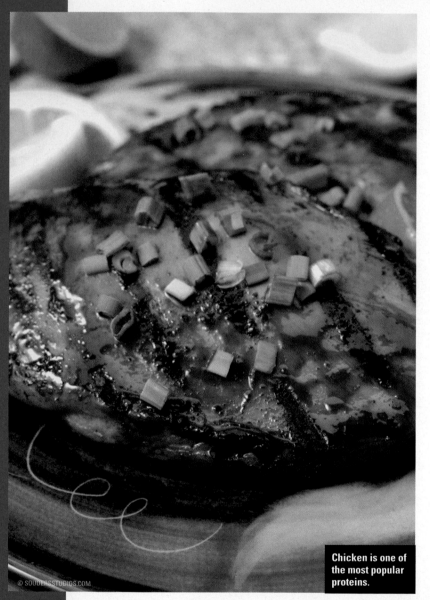

Chicken is one of the most popular proteins.

© SOUDERSSTUDIOS.COM

Pork

Pork protein has some interesting effects.[37] Danish scientists examined the effects of three macronutrient diets: pork-meat protein, soy protein and carbohydrate on 24-hour energy expenditure. They took 12 young, slightly overweight, non-smoking men and had them consume one of the three diets for four days followed by a one- to 10-week "washout" period. Thus, all subjects went through all three treatments and therefore served as their own controls. For the two higher protein diets, protein made up approximately 30 percent of the total calories, while on the lower protein diet, protein made up only 11 percent of total calories. Fat intake was the same for all three treatments.

LEAN BODY MASS & STRENGTH

So what happened? With regard to 24-hour energy expenditure, the pork-consuming group burned 3.9 percent more calories than the carb group and 1.9 percent more calories than the soy group. In addition, when the investigators looked at sleeping energy expenditure, basal metabolic rate and diet-induced thermogenesis, they found that pork was highest, followed by soy and then carbohydrates. There is plenty of evidence to show that protein in general has a greater thermogenic effect than carbohydrates.[38] But it is clear that there are differences between proteins.

For instance, the consumption of a well-balanced mixture of amino acids produces a greater thermogenic response than one with a lower biological value.[39] And we know that pork protein has higher levels of histidine, methionine and leucine than soy protein. This might promote greater thermogenesis and protein synthesis.[40] Certainly, this study, as well as others, makes it crystal clear that meat is an important source of protein. As a way to enhance metabolic rate, meat is an excellent source; furthermore, it is a superior way to acquire the building blocks of protein, amino acids are all necessary for serious muscle growth.

Pork is an excellent source of amino acids.

© SOUDERSTUDIOS.COM

Last But Not Least …

Soy—A Solid Plant Source of Protein

Soy is the best non-animal source of protein and is often accused of being inferior to animal-source protein because it can be limiting in the amino acid methionine. However, methionine supplementation in an adult's diet is usually not necessary because at levels normally consumed, soy protein provides sufficient amounts. It's been shown that soy protein is comparable in digestibility to other high-quality protein sources such as meat, milk, fish and egg. According to Darryn Willoughby, Ph.D., an associate professor of exercise physiology at Texas Christian University, "Soy protein's powerful antioxidant capabilities provide significant health and anti-cancer benefits. This is probably due to the presence of isoflavones, saponins, phytic acid and protease inhibitors." In fact, a recent study found that a soy-based meal replacement formula was "effective at lowering body weight, fat mass and reducing LDL cholesterol."[41]

This means that soy, similar to casein, may have a significant anti-catabolic effect—it helps decrease muscle breakdown. Chinese scientists from Nanjing Agricultural University examined the effects of daidzein, an isoflavone in soy protein, on various hormonal parameters in rats.[42] In the male rats, body weight, as well as muscle weight, increased more in the daidzein-fed rats than the control rats. Blood urea nitrogen decreased, whereas blood testosterone levels increased. In female rats, body weight gain per day actually decreased by 19 percent. Also, a study from the same university in China found that total isoflavones extracted from red clover improved body weight gain and increased serum testosterone levels (by 36 percent) in males.[43] In addition, a study from the Applied Research Institute in Japan found that soy protein may reduce body fat in obese animals.[44]

Thus, if you're one who shies away from eating our vertebrate pals, then chowing down on tofu, soy milk and assorted other soy products may be a good alternative for getting the essential amino acids you need to build muscle.

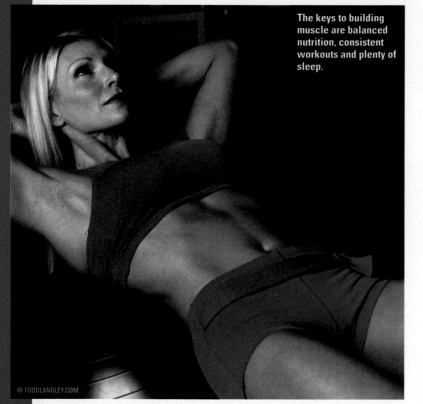

The keys to building muscle are balanced nutrition, consistent workouts and plenty of sleep.

© TODDLANGLEY.COM

Putting It All Together

So you want to build muscle? No problem. Let's assume you're hitting the weights and you're getting plenty of sleep. The last part of this mass-building trio is nutrition. With nutrition, pick those foods that are best for your health and for promoting gains in muscle protein. We've just given you a variety to choose from and a plan to follow.

A Sample Grocery List for One Week

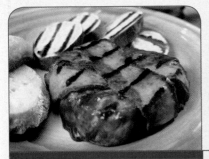

PROTEIN

20 ounces fish
(salmon, tuna, etc)

2 dozen eggs
(mostly egg whites; but three to four whole eggs/week is fine)

6 pieces skinless chicken breast

1 can tuna (in water)

Half gallon skim milk

24 ounces lean cuts of beef

2 cartons low-fat cottage cheese

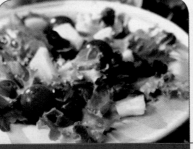

CARBOHYDRATES

Vegetables (preferably fresh; canned is second choice):

Spinach
Bok choy
Tomatoes
Cucumbers
Cabbage
Green beans
Broccoli

Whole-grain, slow-cook oatmeal
Brown rice
Sweet potatoes

Fruits:
Strawberries
Blueberries
Bananas
Pears
Plums
Peaches
Mangoes

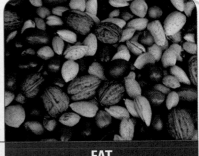

FAT

1 jar all-natural peanut butter

1 can nuts

Fish oil (if you don't eat fish)

Flax seed oil

NUTRITIONAL SUPPLEMENTS

Essential fatty acid blend

EAS CLA

EAS Phosphagen HP™

Individual meal-replacement packets (EAS Myoplex® Original)

1 jug protein powder (EAS Precision Protein™ or MyoPro Whey™)

Nutrition bars
(EAS Myoplex® Deluxe bars, EAS Myoplex® Carb Sense® bars)

EAS products can be found online at www.eas.com, by calling 1-800-297-9776 or by going to an authorized specialty retailer.

The Take-Home Message
on Nutrition for Muscle Growth

1. Choosing the correct macronutrients is key to building a lean physique.
2. To gain lean body mass, rates of anabolism must exceed rates of catabolism.
3. The three major macronutrients are carbohydrate, protein and fat.
4. Carbohydrates, also known as starches and sugars, contain 4 calories per gram.
5. Stored carbohydrates are the main fuel source for intense exercise.
6. Your daily carbohydrate fare should consist mainly of high-fiber, low-glycemic, unprocessed carbohydrates.
7. Low-glycemic carbohydrates provide sustained energy and may decrease your risk of cardiovascular disease.
8. The best time to eat a high-glycemic carbohydrate is pre-, during and post-exercise.
9. Carbohydrate loading is not necessary for gaining muscle.
10. Fat is an essential macronutrient.
11. Fat contains 9 calories per gram.
12. The MUFAs and PUFAs are healthy fats.
13. Fish fat contains DHA and EPA, two very healthful fats.
14. CLA may assist you in gaining muscle while losing body fat.
15. Trans and saturated fat consumption should be limited; these may increase your risk of cardiovascular disease.
16. Eating too little fat might decrease levels of testosterone.
17. Protein is an essential macronutrient; its building blocks are amino acids.
18. Protein contains 4 calories per gram.
19. Eat approximately 1 gram of protein per pound of body weight daily.
20. Eat high-quality protein, usually from animal sources.
21. Science has not yet determined how much protein is ideal for each meal.
22. Meat protein is better than plant protein for gaining lean body mass.
23. Fish is the single best protein source.
24. Whey is a fast protein that is highly anabolic.
25. Casein is a slow protein that is highly anti-catabolic.
26. Milk is a great protein; it is 80 percent casein and 20 percent whey.
27. Whole eggs are an excellent protein with lots of vitamins and minerals.
28. Beef is an excellent source of protein, iron and zinc.
29. Skinless chicken is a great low-fat source of protein.
30. Soy is the best non-animal source of protein.
31. There is no evidence that eating high-protein diets (two to three times the RDA) is harmful to your health.
32. Gaining lean body mass requires dedication and work.

REAL WORLD MUSCLE-BUILDING STRATEGIES

By now, you are well aware that eating to gain lean body mass is a chess match of sorts. You've got to know when to move your pawn, the bishop, the queen, the rook, the knight and then the big daddy of them all, the king. Suffice it to say that if you move the wrong pieces at the wrong time, then you'll be further from achieving your physique goals. Here are some scenarios you may very well deal with on a daily basis and nutrition strategies that should help:

1. Normal meals—You want to sit down and just enjoy a healthy, muscle-building meal. In this case, it is best you consume a high-fiber carbohydrate such as brown rice or sweet potatoes. Add to that fibrous vegetables (as much as you can stomach) and a lean protein source (i.e., skinless chicken). On occasion, eat beef for its high content of zinc and iron. In summary: a starchy high-fiber carb, lean protein source, fibrous vegetables. If you love salad, use a moderate amount of olive-oil based dressing. The MUFAs in the olive oil are good for your health.

2. Snacks—As an anabolic snack, stick to the various ready-to-drink protein shakes that contain roughly 20 to 25 grams of protein, preferably a combination of slow and fast proteins (i.e., whey and casein; a touch of soy for women).

3. On the run—To get your healthy fats, snack on peanuts and nuts such as almonds, walnuts, cashews, etc. This will give you plenty of the healthy MUFAs and PUFAs.

4. A once-a-week must—Go to the sushi bar and eat fish; especially the fatty kind, such as salmon. If you can't stomach the thought of fish, take a fish oil capsule that contains DHA and EPA.

5. No time to cook a regular meal—Consume a slow protein that is mainly casein or milk protein. Casein protein clots into the stomach and delays its emptying from your gut; this results in a slower release of amino acids into your blood. This is good for muscle gain. Look for milk or casein protein as the first protein ingredient on the protein powder label.

6. Before going to bed—Eat a meal composed primarily of casein or slow protein. This will help offset the long period (eight hours or so) of not eating. Alternatively, try cottage cheese. It's a great source of slow protein.

7. Immediately before a workout—Consume a high-glycemic carbohydrate with just a touch of protein; perhaps something like 10 grams of carbs and 5 grams of whey protein; that way, you won't get an upset stomach but you'll provide fuel for exercise and some amino acids to initiate the recovery process.

8. During your workout—Consume a sports drink if you are working out for an hour or more. Try adding 1 teaspoon of whey protein; the small amount of whey will assist with recovery, and the sugar in the sports drink will provide you with extra energy.

9. Immediately after a workout—Consume a fast-acting protein such as whey combined with a high-glycemic carbohydrate; there are various recovery powders that you can buy that do this job well. For some healthy fat, add a teaspoon of flax oil or peanut butter (blend it, of course). (See Chapter 10 for more details.)

10. If you have a flexible schedule—It may be best to consume whey protein frequently (every three to four hours) during the course of the day; even if it's a small dose (~10 grams). Because it is more easily digested (than casein), it will be easier for you to feed frequently and get your needed amino acids. On top of this, make sure you're eating your regular meals.

Sample Muscle-Building Nutrition Plan

Here is a sample meal plan for a 200-pound, 25-year-old active male who is 5'10". This should give you an idea of what you can do when building your own muscle-building nutrition plan.

	Meal	Nutritional Facts	
1	**BREAKFAST ** ** Omelet (5 egg whites, 1 whole egg) 1 cup of oatmeal 8 ounces skim milk	Calories: Protein: Carbohydrates: Ratio*:	450 46 grams 48.5 grams 41/43/16
2	**SNACK ** ** Meal-replacement bar— EAS Myoplex Deluxe	Calories: Protein: Carbohydrates: Ratio*:	340 24 grams 44 grams 28/52/20

3	**LUNCH ** **
	2 cups diced, cooked white meat
	  (no skin) chicken
	Salad with 2 tablespoons olive
	  oil dressing
	½ cup of steamed cooked brown rice
		Calories:
		Protein:
		Carbohydrates:
		Ratio*:
			545
			43 grams
			46 grams
			32/34/34

4	**1 HOUR POST-WORKOUT ** ** 8 ounce broiled Porterhouse steak 1 cup of steamed broccoli ½ cup steamed brown rice Water	Calories: Protein: Carbohydrates: Ratio*:	590 68 grams 31 grams 46/21/33
5	**DINNER ** ** 12 ounce baked cod with lemon and garlic ½ cup of corn Water	Calories: Protein: Carbohydrates: Fat: Ratio*:	496 60 grams 55 grams 4 grams 48/44/7
6	**SNACK ** ** 1 cup of low-fat cottage cheese 1 cup blueberries OR EAS Myoplex CarbSense nutrition shake blended with fruit	Calories: Protein: Carbohydrates: Fat: Ratio*:	247 29 grams 26 grams 3 grams 47/42/11

* (protein/carbohydrates/fat)

Daily Totals:
Calories:
~3,167 calories

Average Ratio (not including pre-, during and post-workout): ~40:40:20 (protein/carbohydrates/fat)

** Please see Chapter 9 and Chapter 10 for nutritional supplement recommendations.

REFERENCES CITED:

1. Tinker, DB et al. Protein use and muscle-fiber changes in free-ranging, hibernating black bears. *Physiol Zool* 71 (1998): 414-424.

2. Westman, EC. Is dietary carbohydrate essential for human nutrition? (letter to the editor). *Am J Clin Nutr* 75 (2002): 951-953.

3. Harper, AE. Defining the essentiality of nutrients. In: Shils MD, Olson JA, Shihe M, Ross AC, eds. *Modern nutrition in health and disease.* (Ninth edition). (William and Wilkins, 1999).

4. McArdle, WD et al. *Sports & Exercise Nutrition* (Baltimore, 1999).

5. Alper, CM and Mattes, RD. Peanut consumption improves indices of cardiovascular disease risk in healthy adults. *J Am Coll Nutr* 22 (2003): 133-41.

6. Tagawa, T et al. Long-term treatment with eicosapentanoic acid improves exercise-induced vasodilation in patients with coronary artery disease. *Hypertens Res* 25 (2002): 823-9.

7. Von Schacky, C. The role of omega-3 fatty acids in cardiovascular disease. *Curr Atheroscler Rep* 5 (2003): 139-45.

8. Chen, H et al. Eicosapentanoic acid inhibits hypoxia-reoxygenation-induced injury by attenuating upregulation of MMP-1 in adult rat myocytes. *Cardiovasc Res* 59 (2003):7-13.

9. Grimsgaard, S et al. Highly purified eicosapentanoic acid and docosahexanoic acid in humans have similar triacylglyerol-lowering effects but divergent effects on serum fatty acids. *Am J Clin Nutr* 66 (1997): 649-59.

10. Raastad, T et al. Omega -3 fatty acid supplementation does not improve maximal aerobic power, anaerobic threshold and running performance in well-trained soccer players. *Scand J Med Sci Sports* 7 (1997): 25-31.

11. Lichtenstein, AH. Dietary fat and cardiovascular disease risk: quantity or quality? *J Womens Health (Larchmt)* 12 (2003): 109-14.

12. Volek, JS et al. Testosterone and cortisol in relationship to dietary nutrients and resistance exercise. *Journal of Applied Physiology* 82.1 (1997): 49-54.

13. Lemon, PW. Is increased dietary protein necessary or beneficial for individuals with a physically active lifestyle? *Nutrition Reviews* 54 (1996): S169-S175.

14. MacDougall, JD et al. The time course for elevated muscle protein synthesis following heavy resistance exercise. *Canadian Journal of Applied Physiology* 20 (1995): 480-486.

15. Campbell, WW et al. Effects of an omnivorous diet compared with a lactoovovegetarian diet on resistance-training induced changes in body composition and skeletal muscle in older men. *American Journal of Clinical Nutrition* 70 (1999): 1032-9.

16. Erkkila, AT et al. n-3 Fatty acids and 5-y risks of death and cardiovascular disease events in patients with coronary artery disease. *Am J Clin Nutr* 78.1 (2003):1-2.

17. He, K et al. Fish consumption and risk of stroke in men. *JAMA* 288.24 (2002):3130-6.

18. Lavigne, C et al. Cod and soy proteins compared to casein improve glucose tolerance and insulin sensitivity in rats. *Am J Physiol Endocrinol Metab* 278 (2000): E491-E500.

19. Dangin, M et al. The digestion rate of protein is an independent regulating factor of postprandial protein retention. *Am J Physiol Endocrinol Metab* 280 (2001): E340-E348.

20. Boirie, Y et al. Slow and fast dietary proteins differently modulate postprandial protein accretion. *Proc Natl Acad Sci USA* 94 (1997):14930-14935.

21. Burke, DG et al. The effect of whey protein supplementation with and without creatine monohydrate combined with resistance training on lean tissue mass and muscle strength. *Int J Sport Nutr Exerc Metab* 11.3 (2001): 349-64

22. Bounous, G and Gold, P. The biological activity of undenatured dietary whey proteins: role of glutathione. *Clinical Investigative Medicine* 14 (1991): 296-309.

23. Kennedy, RS et al. The use of whey protein concentrate in the treatment of patients with metastatic carcinoma: a phase I-II clinical study. *Anticancer Research* 15.6B (1995): 2643-2649.

24. Boirie, Y et al. Slow and fast dietary proteins differently modulate postprandial protein accretion. *Proc Natl Acad Sci USA* 94 (1997): 14930-14935.

25. Demling, RH and DeSanti, L. Effect of a hypocaloric diet, increased protein intake and resistance training on lean mass gains and fat mass loss in overweight police officers. *Ann Nutr Metab* 44.1 (2000): 21-9.

26. http://www.newscientist.com/news/news.jsp?id=ns99993310 accessed from NewScientist.com on 10-20-03.

27. Berardi, J. (eds. Antonio J, Stout J). *Sports Supplement Encyclopedia.* (Nutricia, 2001). Pg 24.

28. Clare, DA and Swaisgood, HE. Bioactive milk peptides: a prospectus. *J Diary Sci* 83:1187-1195.

29. Van Niekerk, PJ et al. The nutritional composition of South African eggs. *South African Medical Journal* 83 (1993): 842-6.

30. Song, WO et al. Nutritional contribution of eggs to American Diets. *Journal of the American College of Nutrition* 19 (2000): 556S-562S.

31. http://www.hormel.com/cm/templates/kitchen/knowledge.asp?articleid=282&zoneid=54; Hormel foods website accessed 10-19-03.

32. Wells, AM et al. Comparisons of vegetarian and beef-containing diets on hematological indexes and iron stores during a period of resistive training in older men. *J Am Diet Assoc* 3.5 (2003): 594-601.

33. Melanson, K et al. Weight loss and total lipid profile changes in overweight women consuming beef or chicken as the primary protein source. *Nutrition* 19 (2003): 409-14.

34. http://www.dispatch.com/news/food/food00/food0517/282614.html

35. Scott, LW et al. Effects of beef and chicken consumption on plasma lipid levels in hypercholerolemic men. *Arch Intern Med* 154 (1994): 1261-7.

36. Melanson, K et al. Weight loss and total lipid profile changes in overweight women consuming beef or chicken as the primary protein source. *Nutrition* 19.5 (2003): 409-14.

37. Mikkelsen, PB et al. Effect of fat-reduced diets on 24-h energy expenditure: comparisons between animal protein, vegetable protein, and carbohydrate. *American Journal of Clinical Nutrition* 72 (2000): 1135-1141.

38. Whitehead, JM et al. The effect of protein intake on 24-h energy expenditure during energy restriction. *International Journal of Obesity and Related Metabolic Disorders* 20 (1996): 727-32.

39. Pitkanen, O et al. Branched-chain and mixed amino acid solutions and thermogenesis in postoperative patients. *Nutrition* 10 (1994): 132-7.

40. Tsujinaka, T et al. Modulation of thermogenic response to parenteral amino acid infusion in surgical stress. *Nutrition* 12 (1996): 36-9.

41. Allison, DB et al. A novel soy-based meal replacement formula for weight loss among obese individuals: a randomized controlled clinical trial. *Eur J Clin Nutr* 57 (2003): 514-22.

42. Wang, J and Han, ZK. Effects of daidzein on muscle growth and some endogenous hormone levels in rats. *American Journal of Clinical Nutrition* 68.6S (1998): 1539S.

43. Wang, J and Han, ZK. Effects of total isoflavones of red clover on male broiler growth and serum testosterone concentrations. *American Journal of Clinical Nutrition* 68.6S (1998): 1539S.

44. Yamamoto, T et al. Soy protein and its hydrolysate reduce body fat of dietary obese rats. *American Journal of Clinical Nutrition* 68.6S (1998): 1540S.

9 NUTRITIONAL SUPPLEMENTS FOR STRENGTH AND LEAN BODY MASS

How to Take Your Muscle Growth to the Next level

By Jeffrey R. Stout, Ph.D., and Ash Batheja, M.S., C.S.C.S.

In a landmark study printed in the *Journal of Applied Physiology*, researchers set out to determine which nutritional supplements actually promoted measurable lean mass and strength gains, and which could be safely cast aside as pretenders. [41] In this meta-analysis—where numerous studies are examined and analyzed, held up or dressed down, lauded or laughed at—only two supplements emerged unscathed. Just two supplements—in an evaluative process that encompassed a time period stretching from 1967 to 2001—could be recommended for adding muscle and strength.

AND THE WINNERS ARE ...

The two? Creatine and beta-hydroxy-beta-methylbutyrate, better known as HMB. Now, many supplements could not be included in the study simply because they did not meet a predetermined set of experimental criteria. More than likely, there are other supplements that are helpful in promoting lean mass and strength gains, but it's not likely that any are of the caliber of creatine and HMB. Meanwhile, in the stark reality known as the "other end of the spectrum," some supplements can now safely be described as hot air in a capsule.

And so it really boils down to two. With creatine, as the researchers discovered, you can expect net lean mass gains of 0.36 percent per week. For someone with 150 pounds of lean mass, that's a musculature gain of one half pound a week. Two pounds a month. Six pounds in three months. With HMB, the gains are a nearly identical 0.28 percent per week.

The expected strength gains obtained from these two supplements are even more impressive. Creatine delivers a 1.09 percent weekly boost in strength, with HMB superior at 1.40 percent per week. To put this in perspective, if your maximum bench press is 250 pounds, a compounded 1 percent weekly gain would push your max to 260 pounds in just one month. Use both supplements, train hard and eat right, and you might surpass that figure significantly.

Perhaps it's not surprising that these two supplements are superior to all others. Creatine, especially, has experienced an unprecedented amount of fanfare, from hardcore bodybuilders to casual gym-goers, underground publications to mass media outlets. Its worth and value is unquestioned, and the latest research only adds to its legacy. It would be unfair to say that HMB is just as popular, but this paramount study certainly establishes that it, too, belongs.

Accordingly, this chapter will focus predominately on these two supplements. It will outline their history, their composition and their efficacy. You will learn why they work, how they work and how to make them work. The chapter will also examine other supplements, but without solid research it must be stated that none will ever reside in the same category as creatine and HMB. Some have promise, yes, but only time will bear out their fate. Quite naturally, however, the chapter will begin with the most successful sports supplement in history—creatine.

Creatine

One of the greatest discoveries in the history of sports supplementation was the revelation that muscle creatine stores could be elevated by oral ingestion of the dietary supplement creatine.[24] From there, the innumerable studies that would follow touched off a firestorm of interest in the supplement, and since then, no supplement has even remotely established the same scientific support as has creatine. Why has creatine

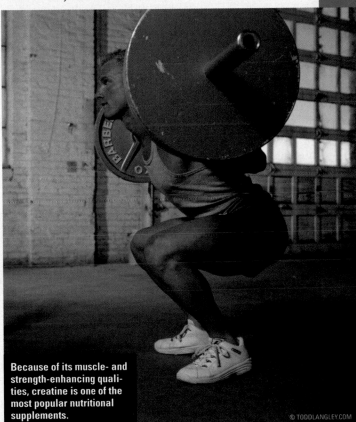

Because of its muscle- and strength-enhancing qualities, creatine is one of the most popular nutritional supplements.

become such a driving force in the sports supplement arena since it was first brought to the market in the early 1990s? Simple. It works!

Creatine supplementation can build muscle, improve strength and power, and may also help you improve aerobic performance, although researchers aren't entirely certain how this occurs. While the distinct methods by which creatine exerts its impressive effects still require further examination, it is a virtual certainty that creatine is highly effective for numerous athletic pursuits, making it one of the most popular supplements ever produced.

A Brief History of Creatine

Contrary to what you might read in popular bodybuilding and fitness magazines, the discovery of creatine was not made in the United States. While its use in this country was certainly popularized by the flood of studies performed by U.S. scientists, the scientific discovery of creatine itself was actually made in the 1800s. Some of the earliest research on creatine as an ergogenic aid was performed in the former Soviet Republic. In fact, it was research that was far superior to anything taking place in the United States at the time.[31]

The Russians essentially pioneered the use of creatine as a sports supplement. Evidence suggests that it was being used successfully by Russian athletes as early as the 1970s and 1980s, well before it gained overwhelming popularity here in the early

1990s. With the Russians' early discovery of creatine's effectiveness, combined with their superior training methods, they were placed in rarefied athletic company for much of the Cold War, when information was not shared freely with their Western counterparts.[31]

The Soviets attained a dominant athletic position in the Olympic Games shortly after World War II and much of their success could be attributed to their incredibly advanced research testing in exercise and muscle biochemistry. Of course, their secretive nature about such testing became a Russian trademark, and it wasn't the least bit surprising that they neglected to share any of their findings with the West, particularly the United States.

The Russians first established that oral creatine supplements could improve athletic performance in short, intense activities such as sprints and weight lifting. By comparison, this identical discovery wasn't made in the West until the 1990s. In addition, the Russians discovered that creatine is found in higher concentrations within fast-twitch muscle fibers (as opposed to slow-twitch), and that regular exercise increases levels of creatine within these fibers. They figured that higher levels of creatine would likely improve performance, and soon, they were confident that they could turn out superior athletes by boosting creatine stores within muscle. In developing what was likely the first oral creatine supplement ever produced, they did exactly that.[31]

Given the initial progress made by the Russians, it's evident that creatine isn't a new supplement. In fact, many of the critical questions surrounding creatine—proper dosing, the

On the Forefront: Creatine Plus Beta-Alanine

Beta-alanine is an amino acid produced naturally in the body and found in foods such as chicken. In and of itself, it is a fairly innocuous amino acid. But once it's plugged into the metabolic pathway in your body it produces another biochemical called carnosine, which is a powerful buffering agent. It has the ability to neutralize lactic acid buildup in your muscles, and it accounts for up to 60 percent of your body's natural lactic acid buffering action. The build-up of lactic acid in muscles is one of the main limiting factors in muscular performance. Therefore, the more carnosine your muscles hold, the longer you'll be able to delay the accumulation of lactic acid in your muscles during intense exercise, and the longer you'll be able to exercise at peak levels.

One recent study demonstrated this effect when scientists correlated the bicycle sprint performance of subjects with their naturally-occurring muscle carnosine levels. They found that there is a very strong relationship between the amount of carnosine in the muscle and the ability to perform at peak levels throughout the sprint. Those with high levels of carnosine significantly outpaced their lower-carnosine counterparts in the sprint—especially in the last 10 seconds of a 30-second sprint. This type of reserve power when you really need it is what every athlete looks for.

And it doesn't take much beta-alanine to substantially raise your carnosine levels. Research shows that just 3.2 grams of beta-alanine taken over a four-week period can increase muscle carnosine content by up to 42 percent. And that's enough to make a noticeable difference in the gym.

What's really interesting is that beta-alanine may actually help creatine work better in your body—not by getting more creatine into your muscle cells, but using the creatine that's there and making it act more effectively on your muscles.

Creatine only works within a very limited pH range. In other words, if your muscles become too acidic due to lactic acid buildup, creatine simply won't work like it's supposed to. So by effectively buffering lactic acid, carnosine (secondary to beta-alanine supplementation) supports optimal creatine effectiveness.

upper limit of stored creatine in the human body, time period of discontinuance necessary to restore baseline levels, and agents that improve creatine absorption—were addressed long before creatine was ever brought to the forefront of sports supplementation.

In roughly 1833, a French scientist named Chevreul first identified creatine, although it wasn't until approximately 1847 that a Dr. Liebig provided evidence linking creatine to muscle tissue. In 1922, human studies were reviewed dating back to 1910, in which subjects ingested 1 to 20 grams of creatine per day for six days.[28] Case study reports in 1926 also detail human subjects consuming 2.5 grams of creatine, four times per day for 10 days.[12] In the 1970s, researchers concluded that the increase in total creatine content in muscle may somehow be mediated by insulin.[14] It would take another 17 years before the Harris (1992) study ignited the creatine explosion and 21 years before scientists (again) shed light on the theory that uptake of creatine into muscle was mediated by insulin.[20,24]

How Creatine Works

Approximately 95 percent of all the creatine stored in the human body is found in skeletal muscle. Creatine is naturally produced in the body from the amino acids methionine, arginine and glycine[47] and is available through the diet from foods like fish and beef.[74] However, the powdered form is not only more convenient, it's also much more practical. For instance, you would have to ingest roughly 2 ½ pounds of raw meat to equal one 5-gram serving of supplemental creatine.

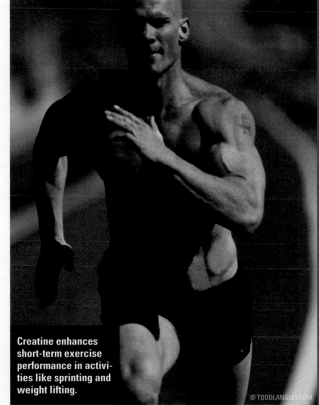

Creatine enhances short-term exercise performance in activities like sprinting and weight lifting.

© TODDLANGLEY.COM

Your body utilizes a few different methods for producing energy , but the ultimate source of that energy is always a chemical known as adenosine triphosphate, or ATP. For you to run, walk, lift weights and even breathe, your body must either derive energy from its immediate ATP stores or it must create it using stored glucose or fats. The problem is, your body only has enough immediate ATP to last for about three to five seconds of intense activity, which is typical of a weight-training set or an all-out sprint. This is one of the reasons why you can only sprint at full speed for a short time or why you fatigue quickly during your 5-rep max on the bench press—your ATP is depleted rapidly, and it takes a few minutes to regenerate.

That leaves us with glucose and fats. Either one can be used to create ATP, but it takes time. You can't go all-out on a lift or a sprint and expect a meaningful contribution from carbs or fats—they simply can't produce ATP quickly enough. These systems are very valuable, however, for providing sustained energy during longer term exercise bouts. These just aren't the kind of activities that are going to pack on mass. No one got big running marathons.

The key, then, is to enhance short-term exercise performance by increasing your immediate ATP stores. Knowing this, researchers, for years, focused on how to do just that, but it was futile since you couldn't really increase ATP beyond existing levels. In fact, taking ATP itself made no difference. Why? Simple. The limiting factor in this case was not ATP, but rather a chemical known as phosphocreatine (PCr).

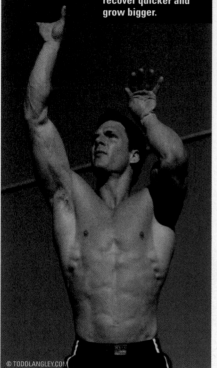

Creatine may help you run faster, jump higher, recover quicker and grow bigger.

© TODDLANGLEY.COM

Chemically speaking, once you utilize an ATP molecule for energy, it's reduced to ADP, or adenosine diphosphate. ADP, lacking one phosphate, is basically useless unless a companion chemical can donate the additional phosphate, allowing ADP to once again become an energy providing ATP molecule. That companion chemical is, of course, phosphocreatine.

Therefore, by increasing the levels of PCr within muscle, you could regenerate ATP like never before. You would be stronger. You would perform, say, 8 reps with a weight that was previously a 5-rep max. Your 3-rep max would be your 6-rep max. You could work out with greater poundages for longer periods of time. Run faster, jump higher, recover quicker. Grow bigger.

This is exactly what the ingestion of a creatine supplements allows. With the absorption of creatine into muscle, you've provided a greater pool of phosphocreatine, allowing faster and more prolific regeneration of ATP, the ultimate source of energy. This is why creatine has attracted the attention of the weight-training community, the athletic community, the scientific community and even the medical community. The research emphatically supports its use, and its mechanisms for enhancing strength and lean body mass are practical and purposeful, as outlined by the following:

➕ Increased ability to train at higher intensities and workloads, thus providing greater stimulus for training adaptations.[10]

➕ Increased protein synthesis secondary to increased muscle cell hydrations.[6, 25]

➕ An increase in myosin heavy-chain mRNA and protein expression, which basically stimulates the building of new muscle.[75, 76]

➕ Increase in satellite cell activity.[15] Satellite cells are cells that are attached to the muscle cell membrane. When activated, they are involved in repairing damaged muscle and aid in increasing muscle size and/or increasing muscle fiber number.

Creatine Enhances Strength

After numerous research studies validated the success of oral creatine in elevating the body's phosphocreatine stores, over 20 studies have reported that creatine supplementation enhances muscle strength and lean body mass responses to resistance training.[53,70] With a firm understanding of the mechanisms responsible for these enhancements, the following is a brief rundown of the most comprehensive studies and their results.

Dr. Earnest and colleagues were the first to investigate chronic creatine use on strength and power, and instead of using a traditional set of untrained individuals, they examined creatine's effects on resistance-trained men.[16] The subjects—men with 10 years of weight training experience—received a 28-day supply of creatine, and after just 14 days of supplementation, they demonstrated significantly greater sprint capacity. After receiving the full 28-day complement of creatine, both muscular strength and total lifting volume improved. Several other studies also showed creatine's positive effect on strength and power.[37,62,63]

Longer studies on creatine have also demonstrated similar positive results. One in particular involved untrained, sedentary women who supplemented four daily servings of creatine (5-gram doses), for four days, followed by a 70-day maintenance period of 2.5-gram, twice-daily servings.[67] During this latter "maintenance" period, the women underwent a resistance-training program. After five and 10 weeks of creatine supplementation, strength was significantly greater in the creatine group versus a group that trained without creatine. Furthermore, after stopping the resistance-training program, a smaller group continued to take 5 grams of creatine daily for an additional 10 weeks. The researchers discovered that, despite the fact that the women were no longer working out, the continued use of creatine delayed decreases in strength that occurred in subjects that ceased both training and creatine use. In other words, creatine maintained some of their strength gains even when they quit training!

Creatine Builds Muscle

During the initial explosion of interest surrounding creatine, the question of whether creatine was effective at building muscle mass was largely up for debate. Many of the studies focused on strength and athletic performance enhancement, and it was thought that much of the body weight gains could be attributed to excess water retention. However, researchers soon discovered that, in addition to the improvement of strength, creatine supplementation has a significant effect on body composition. In fact, there are now a multitude of studies that have demonstrated creatine's prowess in spurring lean body mass gains.

One of the better studies to date studied the effects of creatine supplementation on experienced weight-trained men.[69] The investigators began the subjects with 25 grams per day for seven days, followed by a maintenance dose of 5 grams per day for 77 days. Their training targeted all of the major muscle groups and spanned three or four days per week. After the 12-week training and supplementation period, the creatine-supplemented group gained an average of 9.5 pounds of lean body mass compared to only 4.6 pounds in placebo group. That represents a whopping 107 percent difference.

Figure 1 is an average of several studies that examined the effects of creatine supplementation on lean body mass. It is apparent that there is a wide range of responses—gains encompassed anywhere from 0 to 10 pounds—with the average gain being approximately 5 pounds. Factors such as training status, duration of the study, gender, dosage, training program and others affect your response to creatine supplementation. However, the fact remains that in every properly-designed training study reviewed, creatine supplementation enhanced the effect of training on lean body mass gains greater than training alone.

did you know?

Factors Affecting Creatine Supplementation Research
- training status
- duration of study
- gender
- dosage
- training program

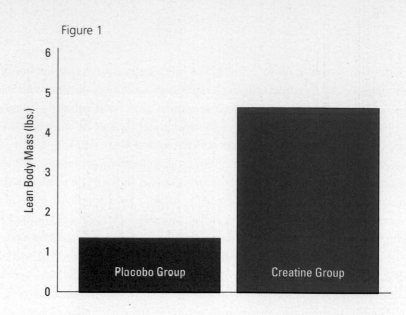

Figure 1

Average lean body mass change after creatine supplementation. Blue represents placebo group and purple is creatine group. Data averaged from various studies.[5,16,32,33,3 7,45,47,48,54,67,69]

Nutrients That Enhance the Effects of Creatine

Creatine Plus HMB

HMB is a metabolite of the amino acid leucine, a compound found in all dietary protein and an essential building block of protein in all tissues.[44]As outlined at the outset of this chapter, studies have shown that HMB supplementation alone may increase strength and lean body mass in exercising individuals. Other studies have also suggested that HMB may have protein-sparing or anti-catabolic action (more on HMB later). Thus, combining HMB and creatine may have a synergistic effect for strength athletes or anyone looking to pack on lean muscle mass.

A recent study, published in the journal *Nutrition*, may have proved that the combination of HMB and creatine is the most naturally potent method for gaining strength and lean mass.[30]After three weeks of training, the researchers found that the creatine plus HMB supplement group experienced a 28 percent greater strength increase over the HMB-only group and held a 25 percent advantage over the creatine-only group, thus validating the advantage of using both creatine and HMB.

Creatine Plus Carbohydrates

When it comes to nutrients that enhance the effect of creatine, some of the most solid research has been performed using the powerful combination of carbohydrates plus creatine.

The main benefit of adding carbohydrates to your creatine is that it increases creatine uptake within the body. Obviously, the more creatine you can absorb, the greater the corresponding effect. Carbohydrates, especially if they're the "fast-acting" kind—such as glucose—can indirectly aid creatine absorption by stimulating the release of insulin from the pancreas. Insulin is a powerful hormone that effectively "shuttles" protein, carbohydrates and, in this case, creatine, into muscle cells. Therefore, if you can enhance the release of insulin when taking creatine, you can send more of it to muscle cells, which may augment its already positive effects. Again, it's the presence of carbohydrates in the blood stream that allow this to happen.

So what does the research have to say? One study reported that ingesting 5 grams of creatine 30 minutes after consuming 93 grams of simple sugars resulted in a 60 percent increase in total muscle creatine concentration when compared to a group that consumed creatine alone.[20] That's quite an improvement, and it stands to reason that an enhancement such as this should also lead to elevated improvements in performance and physique-related measures. Countless other studies have supported the addition of carbohydrates to creatine for physique- and performance-enhancement,[37] and some studies show this is possible by adding fewer carbohydrates.[56,58,62]

Creatine Plus Phosphates

Phosphates are one of the most abundant minerals in the body, and are extremely important in human metabolism. Approximately 80 percent to 90 percent of the phosphates in the body combine to form calcium phosphate, which is used for the development of bones and teeth. Other phosphate salts, such as sodium phosphate, are involved in acid-base balance. The remainder of the body's phosphates is found in a variety of organic forms, including phospholipids, which help cell membranes and DNA. Furthermore, phosphates are essential to the normal function of most of the B vitamins involved in the energy processes within the cell.

To put it simply, phosphates may help exercise performance through their ability to buffer lactic acid, improve the body's ability to deliver oxygen to contracting muscles, and enhance the cardiovascular system's ability to deliver more nutrients to the muscle, which is important for muscle growth.[7]

Now, what about the theory of synergy between phosphates and creatine? First, you must understand that when creatine is ingested, it enters the blood stream as free creatine. It can only exert its powerful effects when it's "phosphorylated" within the muscle cell, which is a fancy way of saying that a phosphate is attached to it (the same goes for glucose to make glycogen). Here's the key: the amount of creatine that is phosphorylated, and thus the amount that is effective may be dependent on how much phosphate is available, and the human body can only supply a limited amount. Thus, if you have inadequate phosphates available, lower muscle creatine levels may result, despite the fact that you may be supplementing with creatine.

Why is this important? Obviously, if more creatine is phosphorylated, then more of it is effective, and you will likely experience greater gains. We know that the

The Potential Medicinal Uses of Creatine

As a result of case studies and the mechanisms by which it can improve strength and prevent muscle losses, creatine has launched itself into a new category of sport supplement—an ergogenic aid that can positively influence the realm of medicine and disease.

Creatine may play a vital role in the treatment of many common diseases and rehabilitation. In 1928, Dr. Hunter first stated that patients with muscular diseases retained less creatine than healthy subjects.[29] Creatine has since been discovered to play a role in such diseases as gyrate atrophy (muscular atrophy of the retina), muscular dystrophy, rheumatoid arthritis, firbromyalgia, congestive heart failure, neuromuscular disease, stroke/ neurodegenerative disese and postoperative surgical recovery.[4,64] Whether or not creatine supplementation can effectively treat these diseases is inconclusive, but recent work is very promising.

Creatine Case Study

When a nutritional supplement advances beyond the confines of barbells and sporting arenas and into the forefront of medicine, you've found a product that can profoundly affect a person's entire way of life. The latest advancements concerning the medicinal effects of creatine suggest that it is in fact one of those supplements—and likely the only one—that can make significant improvements in the lives of the physically challenged.

Take, for example, a case study published in *Medicine and Science in Sports and Exercise* involving the use of creatine in the treatment of neurologic disorders.[61] It tracks the difficult life of an individual we'll call E.M., a 27-year-old medical student who suffers from myasthenia gravis, a neurological condition that results in muscle wasting, fatigue and weakness. E.M. was an avid weight lifter that, three months prior to his diagnosis of myasthenia gravis in 1995, had noticed sharp drops in his strength and visible muscle atrophy. At one point, E.M. had bench pressed 300 pounds, but at the time of his diagnosis he could no longer perform even a single push-up. And, despite use of medications and surgery on his thymus, none of his previous strength or musculature had even remotely returned.

In 1999, he had an exacerbation of his disease and underwent a repeat thymectomy as treatment in April. Following his sternotomy and thymic tissue removal, and three months of restricted exercise, he started a training program that included the use of supplemental creatine.

Since the use of creatine was part of an organized research study, his body mass index (BMI) was calculated, and body part measurements were taken in order to record baseline diameter values. He kept a detailed workout log from the beginning of July until early December 1999. Again, previous to his trial of creatine supplementation, he was unable to gain appreciable muscle mass or make even minimal gains in strength, no matter how diligently he trained. His weight had dropped to 170 pounds, roughly a 15- to 20-pound decline from his normal weight. However, as a result of his 15-week trial with creatine, he was able to gain approximately 11 pounds of muscle mass while maintaining the same body fat percentage, and his strength also returned. Prior to the study, he could only bench press 30-pound dumbbells for three sets of 10. After training and using supplemental creatine, he was soon able to press 60- to 65-pound dumbbells for three sets of 10, an astounding increase in strength for any individual, let alone one suffering from a neurologic disorder.

regeneration of ATP (needed for muscle contraction) is crucial for allowing repeated reps and sets in the gym, and this process relies heavily on creatine phosphate and glycolysis. So, taking phosphates with creatine may be a one-two punch at improving performance by increasing creatine phosphate levels (more energy for training) in the muscle, which also delays fatigue by increasing oxygen to working muscles and buffering lactic acid.

The research proves it. In one study, researchers investigated the effect of supplemental creatine alone versus creatine plus phosphates on muscle power.[73] Male and female subjects were given either 5 grams of creatine four times daily, or 5 grams of creatine plus 1 gram of sodium phosphate four times per day, for five days. The results showed that the combination of creatine plus phosphate resulted in a significantly higher muscle power output.

A more recent study examined the effects of creatine versus creatine plus phosphate on anaerobic working capacity.[18] At the end of the experiment, the subjects who took creatine plus phospate scored 104 percent greater than the placebo group, and 67 percent better than the creatine group. Pretty impressive, and precisely why many creatine products now also contain phosphates.

Creatine Plus Protein

We know that carbohydrates can enhance the positive performance effects of creatine, but what about protein? If it does, in fact, work synergistically with creatine, it would likely be accomplished through different mechanisms, since carbohydrates are primarily a fuel source, while much of protein's contribution to exercise includes repair of damaged muscle fibers through the provision of amino acids needed for muscle protein gain (i.e., hypertrophy).

Like weight training itself, creatine has been shown to enhance muscle protein synthesis. Therefore, it would seem to make sense that combining protein with creatine would be a powerful combo for gaining strength and lean body mass. In a study examining the effects of resistance training and whey protein supplementation— with and without creatine—on lean body mass and muscle

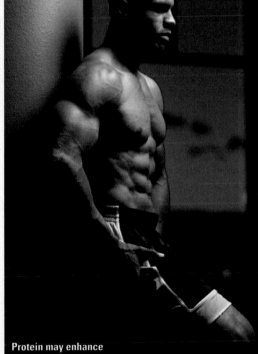

Protein may enhance creatine's effects.

strength, 36 men supplemented with either whey protein, whey protein and creatine or a placebo over the course of a six-week resistance-training program. The results? Significantly greater strength and lean body mass for the group taking the combination of whey protein and creatine. And, quite naturally, this supports the theory that protein enhances the already potent effects of creatine.[9]

Creatine Plus Glutamine

For starters, we know that the building blocks of proteins are amino acids, and that the best sources of proteins contain the highest percentage of essential amino acids. Essential amino acids, of course, are those that you must obtain from your diet. In the case of glutamine, however, it's considered a "conditionally essential amino acid."

Interestingly, glutamine (not carbohydrates or fat) is the preferred fuel source for rapidly dividing cells such as intestinal cells and your immune system cells. Glutamine also has a role in acid-base balance, as a nitrogen carrier and as a precursor for important macromolecules (i.e., proteins, nucleic acids). Furthermore, under certain stressful catabolic conditions, glutamine may be needed as part of your diet; hence the term "conditionally essential." Can you think of activities that foster a stressful catabolic condition? That's right, exercise, and more specifically, weight training. Since weight training is catabolic (rest and recovery is anabolic), pumping iron puts a strain on glutamine reserves. And because glutamine makes up roughly 61 percent of the amino acid pool in skeletal muscle, the loss of muscle glutamine may be a signal of muscle breakdown. So, it now becomes "essential" that intramuscular glutamine stores are maintained,[1] and quite conceivable that adding glutamine to your creatine supplementation program may be a good idea.

In a recent study, 29 male and female college track athletes were randomly divided into three groups: a creatine-only group, a creatine plus glutamine group and a placebo group.[38] During the seven weeks of supplementation, all treatment groups went through an identical resistance-training program, but the creatine-only and the creatine plus glutamine groups were the only ones that demonstrated significant increases in lean body mass.

But was the creatine plus glutamine group any better? Actually, not statistically. What should be pointed out is that the creatine plus glutamine group did show 26 percent greater lean body mass gains than the creatine-only group, only this was not deemed significant enough, as permitted by the study design. Therefore, future investigations should repeat this study with more subjects and for a longer period of time.

The Future of Creatine

While creatine has definitely left its mark on the athletic and fitness worlds, the coming years may find creatine launching itself into arenas far more important than those that reward strength and speed. Whether it's the training table or hospital bed, creatine is rapidly becoming a safe, effective supplement for an incredible array of applications. Without question, athletes will continue to use creatine to improve advanced function. However, it is now possible to visualize creatine as instrumental in simply promoting function in people with delicate health. Weakness and poor endurance are hallmarks of many disease processes, and to date few medicinal choices exist for improving these conditions. Since creatine has already proven itself superior in these areas athletically, it will only be fitting to find it as a preeminent topic of future medical research.

Creatine: Recommendations For Use

Whether your goal is to gain muscle, become stronger or improve athletic performance, the manner in which you use creatine is virtually the same. The only real decision you have to make is whether to "load" or not. The loading phase, as its termed, refers to the first five to seven days of dosing, in which roughly 20 to 30 grams are ingested daily (in divided 5-gram doses) to fully saturate the muscles with creatine.

tip

Optimize Your Creatine Intake:

• Take a 5-gram dose after your workout
• Take with at least 30 grams of a fast-acting carbohydrates (EAS Phosphagen HP)
• Drink plenty of water

Research has confirmed that this method is, in fact, effective at substantially increasing creatine levels.[21] It's also important to mention that once you've achieved this level of saturation, you only need to maintain it with a once-daily 5-gram dose. Excess intake will not increase muscle creatine levels further.

The loading method is also effective at achieving a rapid weight gain, most of which is likely water weight, and which may or may not be a desirable effect. If, for instance, you want to avoid a rapid weight gain, research has demonstrated that you don't have to load. One study confirmed that you could achieve the same level of muscle creatine saturation by using just 3 grams per day, although it would take a month to attain it, whereas you could do it in six days of daily 20- to 30-gram doses.[27] It all depends on how fast you want to get there, and if you're trying to avoid a rapid water weight gain (in which case you would not load).

But how much should you take? Does everybody need the same dose? Simply put, the answer lies in your body weight. Specifically, the more you weigh, the more you need. A proper loading dose is usually an amount equal to your body weight multiplied by 0.1364 grams of creatine daily. For a 200-pound person, that's roughly 27 grams of creatine daily, split into dosages of 4 to 5 grams each. And for the maintenance phase, interestingly enough, the researchers discovered that you could maintain your elevated

The Creatine Controversy—How Safe Is It?

Creatine Safety—People Under 18

Currently, there is no published scientific evidence which suggests that regular creatine supplementation causes harm to people under 18. Despite any unfounded claims made to the contrary, this statement is fact. Perhaps any negativity addressed at creatine could be countered by the following—an intriguing series of studies involving the role of creatine in guanidinoacetate methyltransferase deficiency, a novel inborn error of metabolism.[59] In this and other investigations, creatine supplementation has been used as replacement therapy to treat infants with congenital defects in which they fail to produce normal amounts of bodily creatine.[60] Interestingly, they have found long-term (22 months) oral administration of creatine monohydrate (4 to 8 grams per day) normalizes brain and total body levels of creatine and also improves motor function, and this occurred with absolutely no harmful effects. Furthermore, the dose given would be the equivalent of approximately 100 grams daily (for an average size individual) for nearly two years. As a comparison, the current recommended daily dose is 3 to 5 grams, an intake that is twenty fold less. Keep in mind that for the most part, creatine supplementation is not necessary for anyone under 18.

Creatine Safety—Healthy Adults

Creatine has reportedly been linked to a myriad of health problems, ranging from the mild (e.g., muscle cramps) to the critical (e.g., renal failure). It should be clear that in normal healthy individuals, these purported ill effects have no factual basis. The published scientific evidence clearly shows that creatine supplementation in normal healthy adults poses little to no risk. To make things a bit more concise and thorough, we've included the following table, which lists the anecdotal side effects and safety concerns and allays them with what has actually been found in controlled studies.

In a retrospective study on the safety and side effects of creatine, investigators concluded "there were no differences in the reported incidence of muscle injury, cramps or other side effects" as compared to control groups not receiving creatine. [57] Another study also reported on the safety of creatine and concluded "there is no evidence for deleterious effects in healthy individuals." [50]

Recently, another study concluded that long-term (21 months) creatine supplementation while training does not significantly affect clinical markers of health in athletes. [34] Again, this basically supports what others have concluded— that creatine is not harmful to the body.

	Anecdotal Reports and Concerns	Actually Shown in Controlled Research Studies
Nausea	X	
Vomiting	X	
Diarrhea	X	
Renal Failure/Kidney Disease	X	
Liver Failure	X	
Cardiovascular Stress	X	
Heat Exhaustion	X	
Cramping	X	
Muscle Strains/Tears	X	
Cancer	X	
GI Distress	X	X
Weight Gain	X	X

Table 2. Anecdotal reports versus actual data

An additional study concluded that creatine supplementation while training does not increase the incidence of cramping or injury and, perhaps surprisingly, they also reported that creatine supplementation may actually reduce the incidence of dehydration, cramping and/or injury during intense training. [22,23] This suggests that the anecdotal claims of cramping and muscle strains supposedly caused by creatine are likely related to poor hydration habits or over-exertion during exercise, rather than by some physiological effect of creatine.

And what of the ongoing claims that creatine poses a negative stress on renal and kidney function, as raised in both the general population and scientific communities? Well, to date, no study has shown a link between creatine use and renal failure, aside from creatine use in subjects with existing renal dysfunction.[17] Neither short-, medium- or long-term creatine use has been shown to negatively impact kidney function.[49,51,55]

One potential side effect, if you can consider it one, is that the use of creatine has consistently resulted in weight gain. Of course, this depends upon whom you ask, as weight gain may be a welcome offshoot for some. If you're a competitive jockey or swimmer, then weight gain is probably unwanted, but an offensive lineman in football or competitive bodybuilder likely wouldn't mind it. GI (gastrointestinal) distress is one undesirable effect that has also been noted in the literature, but it's only been found to occur when creatine is consumed just prior to or during exercise.[68] The high amount of simple sugars that often accompanies carbohydrate intake may also be, in part, to blame for stomach upset since sugar slows gastric emptying in the gut.

Thus, a reasonable interpretation of the scientific literature would lead a reasonable person to the following conclusion: regular creatine supplementation in normal healthy adult individuals "does not cause serious adverse health effects, including kidney damage."

levels of muscle creatine by taking just 2 grams per day. However, they discovered that this amount was not sufficient to maintain levels of performance. So, a 5-gram maintenance dose appears to be ideal.[69]

As for improving its effectiveness, creatine should be ingested with at least 30 grams of a fast-acting carbohydrate, such as glucose, to improve absorption. This was discussed in previous sections, as was the effectiveness of adding compounds such as phosphates. And when it comes to timing, post-workout is an ideal time to take your 5-gram maintenance dose, since your muscle creatine levels drop somewhat following intense exercise.

HMB (beta-hydroxy-beta-methylbutyrate)

As we discussed at the outset of the chapter, only two supplements can justifiably and consistently claim that they are powerful enough to improve lean body mass and strength. In creatine, we've covered one, with its relatively simple mechanisms and volumes of successful research. In HMB, we have a supplement with similarly compelling research, but nevertheless it remains research that is, at times, quite complex.

HMB is a metabolite of the amino acid leucine, an essential building block of protein in all tissues that is found in all dietary protein. [43] Among the amino acids, leucine holds a special place. In addition to being an essential amino acid, it's also one of the three branched chain amino acids (the other two are isoleucine and valine), a trio of compounds that together possess unique performance-enhancing effects. But what ultimately separates leucine from the other two, and from all other amino acids for that matter, is its role in regulating protein synthesis and protein breakdown.

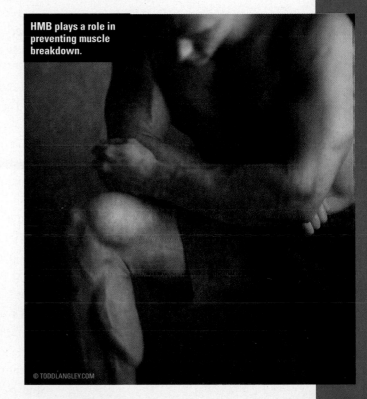

HMB plays a role in preventing muscle breakdown.

© TODDLANGLEY.COM

Before we delve into the connection between HMB and leucine, we must first set the stage with a little history of leucine and its first metabolite, a compound called ketoisocaproate, better known as KIC. Early research on KIC demonstrated that it could duplicate most, if not all, of the effects of leucine in tissues. These effects included decreased protein breakdown and increased protein synthesis, two prerequisites for recovery and lean muscle gain.[13,40] Additional studies also supported these effects.[8,11,39]

Here's where it gets interesting. Scientists speculated that there was a "mystery" compound behind all these protein-sparing effects. The data with KIC indicated that the leucine effect was, in fact, not due to leucine but instead due to a downstream product. Thus, the same question remained: Was the effect due to KIC itself or some further breakdown product in the pathway (of which, by the way, there are about eight additional biochemicals)? In the early 1980s, scientists suggested an alternative metabolic pathway of leucine metabolism, one which indicated that KIC's effects were being executed by an enzyme distinct to, you guessed it, HMB.

Scientists at Iowa State University were the first to test the hypothesis that this HMB metabolite was responsible for the potent effects of leucine and KIC on protein metabolism. This led them first to a series of successful animal experiments and, in research spanning the last 10 years, to humans. These extensive studies suggest that HMB may be the bioactive component of leucine metabolism that plays a regulator role in protein metabolism.[43,44] In other words, it was the key that unlocked the complex door of protein synthesis and anti-catabolism (prevents protein breakdown).

Research in animals suggests HMB plays some role in protein metabolism, especially in stressful situations. Although no one is certain of the mechanism(s) behind HMB, scientists have been working on two hypotheses:[43]

Hypothesis 1: HMB may regulate enzymes responsible for muscle tissue breakdown. This theory is supported by the evidence found in several studies where biochemical indicators of muscle damage (CPK and 3-MH) decreased in the blood.

Hypothesis 2: HMB may be an essential component of the cell membrane. Scientists propose that under stressful situations, the body may not make enough HMB to satisfy the increased needs of tissues. It could also be that stress may alter enzymes or concentration of certain biochemicals that decrease normal HMB production. Either scenario requires dietary supplementation of HMB for skeletal muscle system to function maximally.

Take 1 gram of HMB three times a day with meals for best results.

© TODDLANGLEY.COM

Evidence That HMB Enhances Strength and Lean Body Mass

The first human study with HMB showed that after just one week of training and supplementation, muscle protein breakdown in a group given 3 grams of HMB decreased 44 percent (compared with the placebo group).[43] Also, muscle breakdown muscle damage continued to be lower in the HMB group for the entire three-week study.

OK, so there were some encouraging results in the level of biochemical indicators of muscle damage, but what about real-life, tangible progress? Well, the research also focused on that, and found that strength increased in both of the HMB-supplemented groups: 23 percent for a group taking 1.5 grams per day, and 29 percent for the 3-gram group. So, we have an initial study on HMB indicating that it may reduce the damaging effects of resistance exercise on muscle, with the pleasant consequence of increasing maximal strength in response to exercise. Several other studies have shown positive gains in strength in both men and women from supplementing with 3 grams of HMB a day and engaging in a weight-training program.[19,42,46,72]

The effects of HMB on lean body mass are also promising, even if the research may not be as comprehensive as the literature on strength augmentation. Like studies on creatine, most investigations will emphasize its strength- and performance-enhancing effects while viewing the influence on lean body mass as secondary. That's just reality within the research community, since gaining strength or improving performance is simply deemed more important than packing on muscle.

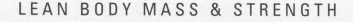

Nevertheless, one study recently reported that HMB supplementation tended to increase lean body mass in 70-year-old adults participating in a strength-training program.[71] And, in an extensive study more specific to the traditional weight-training demographic,[46] the HMB group had greater gains in strength and lean body mass and, according to the investigators, "This study showed, regardless of gender or training status, HMB may increase upper body strength and minimize muscle damage when combined with an exercise program."

HMB—Recommendations For Use

As complex as HMB's mechanisms are, it has been shown to increase muscle strength and enhance recovery and muscle breakdown. Take 1 gram, three times a day with meals.

Miscellaneous Mass- and Strength-Enhancing Nutrients

⊕ Essential Amino Acids

Amino acids are the building blocks of protein in the body, and are essential for making structural proteins, enzymes and certain hormones and neurotransmitters. Amino acids are also involved in the metabolic pathways that affect exercise metabolism.[36] Further, it's been suggested that additional protein (amino acids) may enhance muscle tissue growth and even serve as a potential energy source during exercise.[35] All amino acids are termed either essential or non-essential, with essential amino acids (EAAs) being those that are not made by the body and must be obtained through the diet. EAAs include the following: isoleucine, leucine, valine, lysine, methionine, phenylalanine, threonine and tryptophan. High amounts of EAAs can be found in animal-based protein (e.g., beef, pork, chicken, milk proteins such as whey and casein and eggs) and most nutrition shakes.

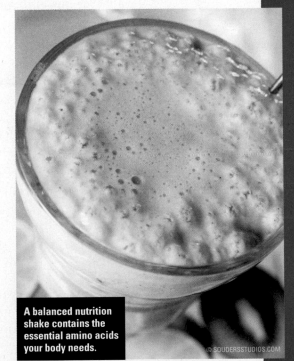

A balanced nutrition shake contains the essential amino acids your body needs.

© SOUDERSSTUDIOS.COM

So, if you ingested additional EAAs, could it lead to strength and mass gains? Well, scientists recently demonstrated that the consumption of EAAs can, in fact, augment muscle protein synthesis in healthy human subjects.[52,65] For example, one study examined the effects of EAAs in six healthy adults (three men, three women). The study was simple—the researchers placed the subjects on a resistance-training program and followed it with the consumption of either 40 grams of EAAs or a placebo. Investigators found that EAAs were very effective at stimulating muscle growth. This was followed up with the same protocol (but with only 6 grams of EAA and 36 grams of sugar), which showed a significantly greater muscle growth with the EAA supplement (when given after resistance exercise versus the placebo supplement).

More recently, a study researched whether the timing of EAA supplementation had an effect on muscle protein metabolism. Specifically, the study examined whether taking 6 grams of EAA plus 35 grams of sucrose immediately before training or immediately after training, had a different impact on muscle protein metabolism.[66] Interestingly, they discovered that if you consumed this mixture immediately before weight training, net muscle protein accretion or gain was more than double than if you consumed it immediately after weight training. An examination of the data shows that EAA consumed with sugar before exercise produces a 158 percent greater anabolic effect than consuming after training.

The available evidence from short-term studies using 6 grams to 40 grams of EAA suggests that it may enhance the anabolic stimulus of weight training. However, more evidence is needed to determine the long-term benefits of EAA supplementation on strength and lean body mass.

✚ Vitamin C

Vitamin C, also known as ascorbic acid, is a water-soluble vitamin found in many fruits and vegetables, and is one of the more important antioxidants present in the human body. But the body can't make it by itself, so you must obtain it through the diet. Vitamin C has many functions in the body, many of which are vital to the athlete or active person. Its primary role is the synthesis of collagen, which is important for the strengthening of cartilage, tendons and bones. It also plays a critical role in the formation of neurotransmitters and hormones, both of which are released during exercise for the purpose of stimulating muscle growth and breaking down carbohydrates and fat for energy. In addition, vitamin C is involved in the synthesis of red blood cells—which are vital to delivering oxygen to the muscle—and is a powerful antioxidant that prevents the buildup of free radicals in the body. Free radicals, we know, can lead to muscle and tendon damage, as well as a host of other unwanted effects.

Past studies show that supplementing vitamin C at doses between 500 milligrams and 3,000 milligrams per day may improve strength, power

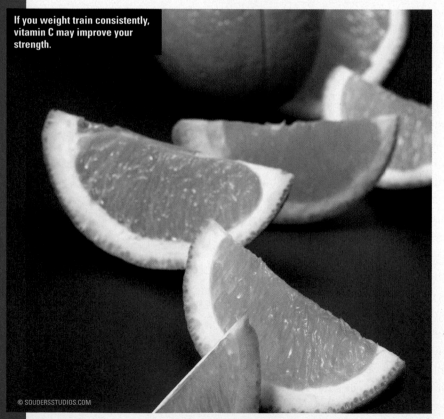

If you weight train consistently, vitamin C may improve your strength.

© SOUDERSSTUDIOS.COM

and endurance.[3,26] More recently, scientists examined the effects of vitamin C on the development of strength during eight weeks of weight training, and sure enough, vitamin C supplementation provides an advantage and results in a measurable strength improvement in conjunction with weight training.[2]

As usual, more research is always needed, but so far, it would appear that 500 milligrams to 1,000 milligrams per day of vitamin C would benefit the strength athlete. Naturally, it would behoove all athletes (and non-athletes as well) to consume a plethora of fruits and vegetables to get adequate vitamin C. However, it may be necessary to take supplemental vitamin C to reach the desired daily allotment of 500 milligrams to 1,000 milligrams.

Past, Present and Future

The past has taught us the importance of an increased protein intake for recovery and lean mass/strength gains, it has taught us of the remarkable influence of supplements such as creatine and HMB, and it has taught us the relative differences and benefits of the varied types of carbohydrates, protein and fat. From high- and low-glycemic carbohydrates, to whey and casein protein, to omega-3 and omega-6 fatty acids, the past and current sports nutrition climate has signaled the next advancement in a strikingly rapid evolution—nutrient timing (more on this in Chapter 10). Among the more promising areas is most certainly the influence of nutrients on the neural systems of recovery, as preliminary research on the subject can attest. Continued advancements in nutrient combinations and their timings is also an exciting development.

The future, or evolution, of sports nutrition is a continual process, building

A Nutritional Supplement Plan for Gaining Lean Mass and Strength

7 A.M. BREAKFAST
1 gram HMB (EAS HMB)
Antioxidant/multivitamin blend
1 teaspoon flax seed oil

10 A.M. MID-MORNING SNACK

12 P.M. LUNCH
1 gram HMB (EAS HMB)
6 grams EAAs**
1 teaspoon flax seed oil

1 P.M. STRENGTH-TRAINING WORKOUT

2 P.M. POST-WORKOUT MEAL*
5 grams mixed creatine blend***
(EAS Phosphagen HP)
1 gram HMB (EAS HMB)
3 grams EAAs**
1 teaspoon flax seed oil

5 P.M. DINNER

8 P.M. PRE-BED SNACK*

* See Chapter 8 for nutrition recommendations for gaining lean mass and strength

** Most nutrition shakes or protein powders contain the amount of essential amino acids (EAAs) that you need. You can also find EAA supplements at any specialty nutrition store or health food store.

*** If you choose to "load" your creatine, take 20 to 30 grams of creatine in divided doses of 5 grams for five to seven days before maintaining with 5 grams a day, taken after workouts.

upon past and current research to navigate the delicate maze that leads to performance and physique enhancement. With remarkable strides made in the last decade, we should expect the next 10 years to be marked by similar progress. Regardless of what the next great frontier may be its impact will most certainly be felt in athletic arenas, gyms and physiques across the globe.

REFERENCES CITED:

[1] Antonio, J and Street, C. Glutamine: A potentially useful supplement for athletes. *Can J Applied Phys* 24 (1999): 1-14.

[2] Beam, WC et al. The effect of chronic ascorbic acid supplementation on strength following istonic strength training. *Med Sci Sports Exer* 30 (1998): S219.

[3] Bramich, K et al. The effects of two levels of ascorbic acid on muscular endurance, muscular strength and on VO2 max. *Int Clin Nutr Rev* 7 (1987): 5.

[4] Balsom, PD et al. Creatine in humans with special reference to creatine supplementation. *Sports Medicine* 18 (1994): 268-280.

[5] Becque, MD et al. Effects of oral creatine supplementation on muscular strength and body composition. *Med Sci Sports Exer* 32 (2000): 654-658.

[6] Bemben, MG et al. Creatine supplementation during resistance training in college football athletes. *Med Sci Sports Exerc* 33 (2001): 1667-1673.

[7] Bucci, L. *Nutrients as ergogenic aids for sports and exercise* (CRC Press, 1993).

[8] Buckspan, R et al. Alpha-Ketoisocarpoate is superior to leucine in sparing glucose utilization in man. *Am J Phys* 251 (1986): E648-E653.

[9] Burke, DG et al. The effect of whey protein supplementation with and without creatine monohydrate combined with resistance training on lean tissue mass and muscle strength. *Int J Sport Nutr Exerc Metab* 11 (2001): 349-364.

[10] Casey, AD et al. Creatine ingestion favorably affects performance and muscle metabolism during maximal exercise in humans. Part 1. *Am J Phys* 271 (1996): E31-E37.

[11] Cerosimo, E et al. alpha-Ketoisocaproate, not leucine, is responsible for nitrogen sparing during progressive fasting in normal male volunteers. *Surgical Forum* 34 (1983): 96-98.

[12] Chanutin, A. The fate of creatine when administered to man. *J Bio Chem* 67 (1926): 29-41.

[13] Chua, B et al. Effect of leucine and metabolites of branched chain amino acids on protein turnover in heart. *J Bio Chem* 254 (1979): 8358-8362.

[14] Crim, MC et al. Creatine metabolism in men: urinary creatine and creatinine excretion with creatine feeding. *J Nutr* 105 (1974): 428-438.

[15] Dangott, B et al. Dietary creatine monohydrate supplementation increases satellite cell mitotic activity during compensatory hypertrophy. *Int J Sports Med* 21 (2000):13-16.

[16] Earnest, CP et al. The effect of creatine monohydrate ingestion on anaerobic power indices, muscular strength and body composition. *Acta Physiol Scand* 153 (1995): 207-209.

[17] Edmunds, JW et al. Creatine supplementation increases renal disease progression in Han :SPRD-cy rats. *Am J Kidney Dis* 37 (2001): 73-78.

[18] Eckerson, J et al. The effect of creatine phosphate supplementation on anaerobic working capacity following 2 and 6 days of loading in men. *J Str Cond Res* 15 (2001): 392.

[19] Gallagher, PM et al. B-hydroxy-B-methylbutyrate ingestion, part I: Effects on strength and fat free mass. *Med Sci in Sports and Exer* 32 (2000): 2109-2115.

[20] Green, AL et al. Carbohydrate ingestion augments skeletal muscle creatine accumulation during creatine supplementation in humans. *Am J Physiol* 271 (1996): E821-826.

[21] Greenhaff, PL et al. Influence of oral creatine supplementation of muscle torque during repeated bouts of maximal voluntary exercise in man. *Clin Sci* 84 (1993): 565-571.

[22] Greenwood, M et al. Cramping and injury incidence in collegiate football payers are reduced by creatine supplementation. *J Athl Train* 38 (2003): 216-219.

[23] Greenwood, M et al. Creatine supplementation during college football training does not increase the incidence of cramping or injury. *Mol Cell Biochem* 244 (2003): 83-88.

[24] Harris, RC et al. Elevation of creatine in resting and exercised muscle of normal subjects by creatine supplementation. *Clin Sci* 83 (1992): 367-374.

[25] Haussinger, D et al. Cellular hydration state: an important determination of protein catabolism in health and disease. *Lancet* 341 (1993): 1330.

[26] Howald, H et al. Ascorbic acid and athletic performance. *Annals of the New Your Academy of Sciences* 258 (1975): 458-464.

[27] Hultman, E et al. Muscle creatine loading in men. *J Appl Physiol* 81 (1996): 232-237.

[28] Hunter, A. The physiology of creatine and creatinine. *Physiol Rev* 2 (1922): 580-626.

[29] Hunter, A. *Monographs on Biochemistry: Creatine and Creatinine* (Logman, Green and Co. Ltd., 1928).

[30] Jowko, W et al. Creatine and beta-hydroxy-beta-methylbutyrate (HMB) additively increase lean body mass and muscle strength during a weight-training program. *Nutrition* 17 (2001): 558-566.

[31] Kalinski, MI. State-sponsored research on creatine supplements and blood doping in elite soviet sport. *Perspectives in Biology and Medicine* 46 (2003): 445-451.

[32] Kelly, VG and Jenkins, DG. Effect of oral creatine supplementation on near maximal strength and repeated sets of high-intensity bench press exercise. *J Stength Cond Res* 12 (1998): 109-115.

[33] Kirksey, KB et al. The effects of 6 weeks of creatine monohydrate supplementation on performance measures and body composition in collegiate track and field athletes. *J Str Cond Res* 13 (1999): 148-156.

[34] Kreider, RB et al. Long-term creatine supplementation does not significantly affect clinical markers of health in athletes. *Mol Cell Biochem* 244 (2003): 95-104.

[35] Kreider, R et al. Amino acid supplementation and exercise

performance. *Sports Medicine* 16 (1993): 190-209.

[36] Kreider, R et al. Effects of protein and amino acid supplementation on athletic performance. Sportscience. [Online]. Available: sportsci.org/jour/9901/rbk.html. (1999).

[37] Kreider, R et al. Effects of creatine supplementation on body composition, strength, and sprint performance. *Med Sci Sports Exer* 30 (1998): 73-82.

[38] Lehmkuhl, M. The effects of 8 weeks of creatine monohydrate and glutamine supplementation on body composition and performance measures. *J Strength Cond Res* 17 (2003): 425-438.

[39] Mitch, W et al. Nitrogen sparing induced by leucine compared with that induced by its keto-analogue, alpha-Ketoisocaproic in fasting, obese man. *J Clin Inves* 67 (1981): 553-562.

[40] Mortimore, GE et al. Multiphasic control of hepatic protein degradation by regulatory amino acids, general features and hormonal modulation. *J Bio Chem* 262 (1987): 16322-16327.

[41] Nissen, SL and Sharp, RL. Effect of dietary supplements on lean mass and strength gains with resistance exercise: a meta-analysis. *J Appl Physiol* 94 (2003): 651-659.

[42] Nissen, S et al. Effects of feeding beta-hydroxy-beta-methylbutyrate (HMB) on body composition and strength in women. *Federation of American Societies for Experimental Biology Journal* 11 (1997): A150.

[43] Nissen, S et al. Effect of beta-hydroxy-beta-methylbutyrate (HMB) supplementation on strength and body composition of trained and untrained males undergoing intense resistance training. *Federation of American Societies for Experimental Biology Journal*. 10 (1996): A287.

[44] Nissen, S et al. Effec of leucine metabolite beta-hydroxy-beta-methylbutyrate on muscle metabolism during resistance-exercise training. *J Appl Physol* 81 (1996): 2095-2104.

[45] Noonan, D et al. Effects of varying dosages of oral creatine relative to fat free body mass on strength and body composition. *J Strength Cond Res* 12 (1998): 104-108.

[46] Panton, LB et al. Nutritional supplementation of leucine metabolite beta-hydroxy-beta-methylbutyrate (HMB) during resitance training. *Nutrition* 16 (2000): 734-739.

[47] Pearson, D et al. Long-term effects of creatine monohydrate on strength and power. *J. Str Cond Res* 13 (1999):187-192.

[48] Peeters, BM et al. Effect of oral creatine monohydrate and creatine phosphate supplementation on maximal strength indices, body composition, and blood pressure. *J. Strength Cond Res* 13:3-9, 1999.

[49] Portmans, JR et al. Effect of short term creatine supplementation on renal responses in men. *Eur J Appl Physiol* 76(1997): 566-567.

[50] Portmans, JR et al. Adverse effects of creatine supplementation: fact or fiction ? *Sports Medicine* 30 (2000):155-170.

[51] Portmans, JR et al. Long-term oral creatine supplementation does not impair renal function in healthy athletes. *Med. Sci. Sports Exerc* 32 (1999): 1108-1110.

[52] Rasmussen, BB et al. An oral essential amino acid-carbohydrate supplement enhances muscle protein anabolism after resistance exercise. *J Appl Physiol* 88 (2000): 386-392.

[53] Rawson, ES et al. Effects of creatine supplementation and resistance training on muscle strength and weightlifting performance. *J Strength Cond Res* 17 (2003): 822-31.

[54] Rawson, ES et al. Effects of 30 days of creatine ingestion in older men. *Eur J Appl Physiol* 80 (1999): 139-144.

[55] Robinson, TM et al. Dietary creatine supplementation does not affect some haematological indices, or indices of muscle damage and hepatic and renal function. *Brit J Sports Med* 34 (2000): 284-288.

[56] Robinson, TM et al. Role of submaximal exercise in promoting creatine and glycogen accumulation in human skeletal muscle. *J Appl Physiol* 87 (1999): 598-604.

[57] Schilling, BK et al. Creatine supplementation and health variables: a retrospective study. *Med Sci Sports Exerc* 33 (2001): 183-188.

[58] Steenge, GR et al. Protein and carbohydrate induced augmentation of whole body creatine retention in humans. *J Appl Physiol* 89 (2000): 1165-1171.

[59] Stockler, S et al. Creatine replacement therapy in guanidinoacetate methyltransferase deficiency, a novel error of metabolism. *Lancet* 348 (1996): 789-790.

[60] Stockler, S et al. Guanidino compounds in guanidinoacetate methyltransferase deficiency, a new inborn error of creatine synthesis. *Metabolism* 46 (1997):1189-1193.

[61] Stout, JR et al. Effects of resistance exercise and creatine supplementation on myasthenia gravis: a case study. *Med Sci Sports Exerc* 33 (2001): 869-872.

[62] Stout, JR et al. The effects of creatine supplementation on anaerobic working capacity. *J Strength Cond Res* 13 (1999): 135-138.

[63] Stout, JR et al. Effects of 8 weeks of creatine supplementation on exercise performance and fat-free weight in football players during training. *Nutr Res* 19 (1999): 217-225.

[64] Terjung, RL et al. American College of Sports Medicine roundtable. The physiological and health effects of oral creatine supplementation. *Med Sci Sports Exer* 32 (2000): 706-717.

[65] Tipton, KD et al. Post-exercise net protein synthesis in human muscle from orally administered amino acids. *Am J Physiol* 276 (1999): E628.

[66] Tipton, KD and Wolfe, RR. Exercise, protein metabolism, and muscle growth. *Int. J. Sport Nutr Exerc Metab* 11 (2001): 109-32.

[67] Vandenberghe, K et al. Long-term creatine intake is beneficial to muscle performance during resistance training. *J Appl Physiol* 83 (1997): 2055-2063.

[68] Vanderberie, F et al. Effect of creatine on endurance capacity and sprint power in cyclists. *Int J Sports Med* 8 (1998): 2055-2063.

[69] Volek, J et al. Performance and muscle fiber adaptations to creatine supplementation and heavy resistance training. *Med Sci Sports Exerc* 31 (1999): 1147-1156.

[70] Volek, JS and Jackson, C ed. Creatine supplementation and the strength athlete. In *Nutrition and the Strength Athlete* (CRC Press, 2000).

[71] Vukovich, M et al. Body composition in 70-year-old adults responds to dietary beta-hydroxy-beta-methylbutyrate similarly to that of young adults. *J Nutr* 13 (2001): 2049-52.

[72] Vukovich, M et al. The effect of dietary beta-hydroxy-beta-methylbutyrate (HMB) on strength gains and body composition changes in older adults. *Federation of American Societies for Experimental Biology Journal* 11 (1997): A375.

[73] Wallace, M et al. Effects of short-term creatine and sodium phosphate supplementation on body composition, performance and blood chemistry. *Coaching and Sport Science Journal* 2 (1997): 30-34.

[74] Williams, M et al. *Creatine: The power supplement* (Human Kinetics, 1999).

[75] Willoughby, DS et al. Effects of oral creatine and resistance training on myogenic regulatory factor expression. *Med Sci Sports Exerc* 35 (2003): 923-929.

[76] Willoughby, DS et al. Effects of oral creatine and resistance training on myosin heavy chain expression. *Med Sci Sports Exerc* 33 (2001): 1674-1681.

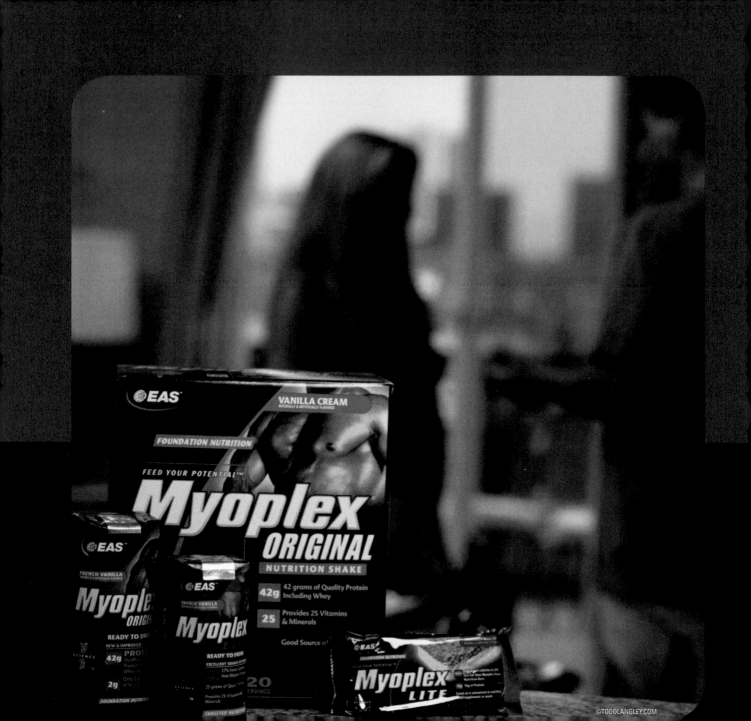

GOAL-SPECIFIC NUTRITION &TRAINING

part four

10 NUTRIENT TIMING

When to Eat and What to Eat for Maximum Performance and Recovery

By Jose Antonio, Ph.D., and Jeff Stout, Ph.D.

If you're training consistently and following a balanced nutrition plan, you're probably ready to take your physique and your performance to the next level. And nutrient timing is probably one of the easiest things you can do to modify your program.

In a nutshell, nutrient timing refers to eating the right nutrients in the right amounts at the right time so as to optimize your performance or physique goals. For you, the goal may be to gain lean body mass, lose body fat or just improve your physique. For an athlete, nutrient timing could make all the difference.

Even if you are not an athlete, and even if you do everything else wrong with your diet, at the very least, do this: Consume a post-workout protein/carb shake right after training.

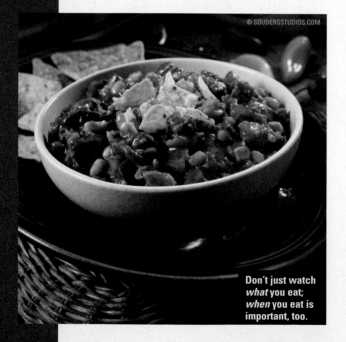

© SOUDERSSTUDIOS.COM

Don't just watch *what* you eat; *when* you eat is important, too.

It's About Recovery

You could summarize the effects of nutrient timing by saying it's really about recovery. Speeding up your recovery could translate into better gains in lean body mass, improved performance and even enhanced weight loss.

According to one study,[1] "an athlete exercising in a carbohydrate-depleted state experiences larger increases in circulating stress hormones and a greater perturbation of several immune function indices. Conversely, consuming carbohydrate during exercise attenuates rises in stress hormones such as cortisol and appears to limit the degree of exercise-induced immunosuppression, at least for non-fatiguing bouts of exercise." This applies to people who engage in prolonged endurance exercise as well as people who are severely restricting carbohydrate intake (i.e., pre-contest dieting).

Nutrient Quality Matters

Before delving into the "when" of nutrient timing, let's discuss the key nutrients and why they work.

Whey and Casein

There are more whey protein-based meal-replacement powders out there than you'd probably care to try. What actually makes whey protein so intriguing are the sub-fractions of various peptides (small proteins) and proteins found within it (e.g., alpha-lactalbumin, beta-lactoglobulin, immunoglobulins and lactoferrin). Each of these sub-fractions may have health benefits.[2] Also, whey is a fast-acting protein that is absorbed quickly and provides the needed amino acids post-exercise; this is critical in expediting the recovery process. For instance, when you eat a large protein meal, you'll get an initial high peak in blood levels of amino acids followed by a rapid decline. On the other hand, if you take the same protein in a slow but continuous fashion (as through a gastric tube), you get a smaller, but more sustained increase in serum amino acids. And even though you may be eating the same quantity of the various amino acids, the time in which they're delivered can have a profound effect on protein synthesis and breakdown. So which is better, a large quick rise followed by a quick drop, or a slow rise that's sustained for a longer period of time? The answer's easy: both.

One study tested the effects of casein or whey protein as a single meal ingested by normal healthy adults.[3] As expected, the whey protein group experienced a quick rise in blood levels of amino acids with a steady decline while the casein group showed a slow increase that was sustained for the seven-hour period. Whole body protein break-down decreased by 34 percent after casein ingestion but not after ingesting whey protein. On the other hand, protein synthesis increased by 68 percent in the whey protein group while the casein group increased by 31 percent. Interestingly, when they examined the amino acid leucine, which is an essential amino acid, they found that leucine balance was better maintained on the casein protein.

What is the reason for the dramatic differences in protein metabolism? Think of cottage cheese, which comes from casein. Whey protein is rapidly emptied from the stomach, whereas casein clots in the stomach and its absorption tends to be much slower. Although casein stimulated protein synthesis less than whey, it had a better effect on inhibiting protein breakdown.

Which is better, casein or whey? It depends on your circumstances. If you are pressed for time and can only get in two or three meals a day, perhaps a combination of whey and casein will work. The whey will produce the quick rise in amino acids while the casein provides the slow sustained increase. If you can eat multiple meals throughout the day (five to six small meals is recommended), it may be best to stick with whey protein. Not only will you get a tremendous rise in protein synthesis, but if you eat whey protein frequently, it could result in sustained high levels of blood amino acids, theoretically leading to an inhibition of protein breakdown. Indeed, even a small amount (2 to 3 grams) of whey repeatedly consumed every 20 minutes over four hours has significant effects on protein gain (measured as leucine deposition).[4] And don't worry about the casein interfering with the whey absorption, or vise versa. Studies have shown the whey and casein fractions are probably absorbed independently without influencing each other's absorption rates.[5] Keep in mind that meal size, calorie level and other non-protein sources in the food may affect your protein's digestion rate.[6]

Leucine

New research has shown that leucine is perhaps the critical amino acid regulating various aspects of intracellular signaling.[7,8] Working synergistically with insulin, leucine is important for enhancing the signal for protein synthesis at the level of "peptide

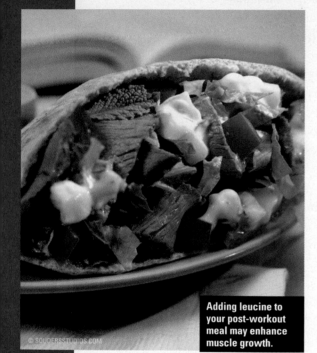

Adding leucine to your post-workout meal may enhance muscle growth.

initiation."[9] Leucine, as well as the other essential amino acids, is important for helping your muscles rebuild and recover after workouts. Leucine by itself, at levels found after eating a meal, plays a critical role in regulating muscle protein synthesis. What's fascinating is that a single leucine-supplemented meal may in fact be sufficient to stimulate muscle protein synthesis for a period of several days; for example, research published in the *Journal of Nutrition* examined whether the acute consumption of leucine feeding persisted over a 10-day period.[10] The results from this investigation showed that a leucine-supplemented meal helped restore postprandial (after eating) muscle protein synthesis in old rats (thus confirming previous studies). Also, in adult rats, chronic daily supplementation with leucine improved the post-absorptive (i.e., no more nutrients are being absorbed from the GI tract) muscle protein synthesis. The researchers speculated that leucine supplementation may be one way to obtain gains in protein without having to necessarily engage in high-protein feeding. Alternatively, it might be worthwhile to add gram levels of leucine to a post-workout meal so as to further enhance the anabolic effect.

Essential Amino Acids

The building blocks of proteins are amino acids. Recent work has shown that essential amino acids plus carbohydrates consumed before exercise resulted in a net phenylalanine uptake that was about 160 percent greater when compared to consuming the same thing post-exercise,[11] translating into a greater potential anabolic effect.

If you're an avid exerciser, it's best that you consume essential amino acids (or the equivalent in mixed protein [about 40 grams of whey protein, for instance] prior to exercise). However, some people prefer not to consume anything prior to training. If that's the case, a post-workout mix of protein (or amino acids), carbohydrates and fat (small amount) will assist you in the recovery process. The consumption of carbohydrates (and protein, for that matter) stimulates insulin secretion from the pancreas. Insulin facilitates the transport of amino acids and glucose into the muscle cell as well as stimulates enzymes responsible for muscle glycogen re-synthesis. In other words, protein—particularly the essential amino acid component—stimulates muscle protein anabolism.

SPORT AND GOAL-SPECIFIC NUTRITION AND TRAINING

Antioxidants—Vitamins E and C

The average athlete consuming a healthy fat diet is more likely to have difficulty consuming enough vitamin E more so than any other vitamin (unless you eat lots of nuts or vegetable oil). Vitamin E supplementation may alleviate some of the free-radical induced muscle damage seen after weight training.[12] Endurance athletes appear to benefit as well. Supplementation of 800 IU vitamin E daily induces a 300 percent elevation (of alpha-tocopherol) in plasma and 53 percent elevation in muscle fibers within about two weeks and appears to be particularly beneficial for Type I (endurance-type) muscle fibers.[13]

Vitamin C supplementation is effective in reducing the incidence of upper respiratory tract infection following prolonged endurance exercise.[14] We know that vitamin C is intimately involved in the repair of connective tissue, and perhaps the repair of damage to the connective tissue component of skeletal muscle can be expedited through extra vitamin C ingestion. Another possible reason involves the antioxidant properties of vitamin C. Vitamin C may act to prevent or alleviate the damage caused by the generation of free radicals subsequent to intense exercise. Thus, vitamin C is a critical micronutrient that athletes should consume, especially after a hard workout.

Do This Before You Work Out!

Though the majority of studies have examined post-workout nutrition, there is intriguing data that suggests a superiority of pre-workout over post-workout supplementation.[15] In this study, scientists compared the anabolic response of consuming an oral essential amino acid plus carbohydrate (EAC) cocktail before versus after heavy resistance exercise. When they measured muscle protein accretion or anabolism over a three-hour period, taking the essential amino acids plus carbohydrates before exercise resulted in about a 160 percent greater uptake compared to consuming it post-exercise. It's possible that the non-essential amino acids are apparently not required to stimulate protein synthesis.

There are more studies on how pre-exercise feedings affect endurance exercise; for instance, the ingestion of one liter of a sports drink one hour prior to a 15-kilometer run followed by a 1.6-kilometer performance run improved performance more so than water alone.[16] Also, ingesting a carbohydrate solution before and during intermittent, high-intensity shuttle running improved performance better than water alone.[17]

You could rightly argue that comparing endurance and strength athletes would be like comparing the white-tailed deer with the mountain lion. Strength athletes do utilize quite a bit of muscle glycogen while they train, although not as much as the endurance athletes. We do know that muscle glycogen is reduced by 30 percent to 40 percent after resistance exercise. So consuming a combination of carbs and protein prior to training is probably a good way to jumpstart the anabolic processes.

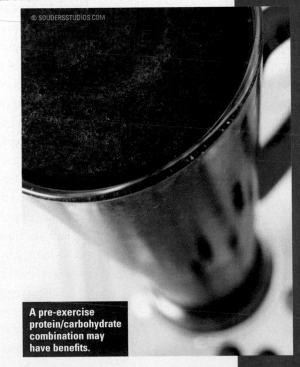

© SOUDERSSTUDIOS.COM

A pre-exercise protein/carbohydrate combination may have benefits.

More studies are needed to verify these findings, but they do raise an important issue. If given a choice, is it better to consume your protein-based shake before or after a workout? First, consuming essential amino acids definitely promotes an anabolic response when taken before or after resistance exercise. The anabolic response just happens to be greater if you consume the essential amino acids prior to exercise. Also, it is apparent that the non-essential amino acids aren't important when it comes to eliciting an anabolic response.

The idea that consuming something prior to exercise has a greater effect is based on the fact that blood flow to working muscles is enhanced while you exercise. It makes sense that if you already have the amino acids and glucose in your system while you're training, then these building blocks can be more easily incorporated into skeletal muscle. Of course, on the practical side, some of us just can't handle having food in our guts before training. Throwing up isn't exactly an anabolic response. For sports such as running or swimming, it's probably not feasible to consume a lot of food or a protein shake before training. Most runners prefer to have a completely empty stomach. On the other hand, if you're a powerlifter, eating a "meal" prior to training may be beneficial. And the prolonged rest periods between sets may keep you from getting sick to your stomach. Basically, if your stomach can handle food or a nutrition shake prior to training, then it's best that you have a pre-workout meal. If you can't handle that, then you must consume a carb-protein shake post-workout. Another idea is to start sipping an amino acid and glucose beverage just before training and continue drinking it throughout the workout. This will ensure that you get the full recovery benefits without having to deal with a bunch of fluid sloshing around in your gut.

During Exercise: Maintaining the Fuel Supply

You also need to give fuel and nutrients to the body while you work out. Carbohydrates and proteins cooperate to boost endurance during exercise and recovery after exercise. It's not that one is good and the other bad; we need both—and we need them together—to optimize performance. Carbohydrates are the primary fuel source for intense exercise, and research shows that consuming a sports drink containing 6 percent to 8 percent carbohydrates plus electrolytes during workouts improves performance and delays fatigue. But newer research has shown that consuming a small amount of protein with carbohydrates during exercise is even better; for instance, a study in the *International Journal of Sport Nutrition and Exercise Metabolism* found that a carbohydrate-protein supplement enhanced endurance performance better than a carbohydrate-containing drink alone.[18] In that study, supplements were consumed immediately before exercise and at 20-minute intervals during exercise. The results were to say the least astounding. The carbohydrate-protein group (CHO-PRO) had a 36 percent and 112 percent greater endurance than the carb-only and placebo groups, respectively.

Although protein is important for the strength athletes, don't think that carbohydrates are just for skinny runners, far from it. Strength athletes need these, too. Studies have found that carbohydrate supplementation can improve exercise performance and decrease the amount of muscle glycogen depletion that normally results from resistance exercises.[19,20]

Jumpstart Post-Workout Anabolic Recovery

According to Tim Ziegenfuss, Ph.D., director of the Exercise Science Laboratory at the Pinnacle Institute of Human Performance in Wadsworth, Ohio, "It is absolutely critical that athletes consume a post-workout protein-carb cocktail right after training; failure to do so will stunt the anabolic process."

Recovery nutrition is an important aspect of performance nutrition. The provision of liquid nutrients after exercise is important for several reasons: First, an anabolic environment is created, as the exercise and insulin signals are both stimulating cellular activity; second, such nutrition can shift the net protein status in a positive direction so that muscle protein is being built in and around the workout; third, muscle recovery is superior due to replenishment of muscle substrates; and fourth, nutrients are rapidly delivered for energy provision when they are most needed.

Timing is everything

There's good timing and there's bad timing. Bad timing? That's when it's Game 6 of the Major League Baseball playoffs, and you interfere with your home team by batting the ball out of the outfielder's glove, preventing a 3rd out. Ouch! That's really bad timing. Good timing? That's when you're speeding down the interstate going 95 miles per hour in your new Benz and you pass a state trooper, who has fallen asleep behind the wheel because of the carbohydrate-induced coma he's suffered after donuts and coffee.

Timing. It applies to exercise as well. After exercise, your body is hungry for nutrients. So what should you feed your muscles? There are three simple rules for optimizing your post-workout recovery:

1 **Drink fluids that contain electrolytes**
Fluid and electrolyte replenishment are perhaps the most important part of recovery. Also, maintaining a well-hydrated state aids your body in burning fat.[21] In other words, drink fluids and burn fat.

CASE STUDY

AN ELITE MIDDLE-DISTANCE RUNNER AND THE ROLE OF POST-WORKOUT NUTRITION

Becki Wells:	29 years old, 5'8"
Weight:	122 pounds to 125 pounds (race weight)
VO$_2$max:	70 ml/kg/min
Body fat:	Between 10 percent and 13 percent (body fat is 8 percent to 10 percent at competitive peak)

Personal best times
800 meters   2:03.7
1,500 meters 4:12.8
Olympic Trials Qualifier at 800 meters and 1,500 meters

As an elite athlete, Becki realizes the importance of training and nutrition. Her body is subjected to workouts that'll make the average bodybuilder curl up in the fetal position.

Weekly workouts
Running: 50 to 60 miles
Weight training: 4 to 5 days per week
Cross-train with swimming and stationary bike 3 to 4 hours per week.

"Instead of focusing on my calorie or fat intake, I am focusing on taking in more protein, I feel that it is helping me recover from workouts more efficiently as well as helping me keep my lean mass; I make it a point to drink a protein shake right after training."

❷ Restore muscle fuel stores by eating carbohydrates and protein

Recent evidence has shown that during the post-exercise period, adding protein to the carbohydrate mix is even better than carbohydrates alone for glycogen repletion, especially during normal training and competition-type exercise.[22,23]

❸ Consume protein/amino acids to repair muscle

Immediately after exercise, a rebuilding process is initiated to repair muscle fibers damaged during your workout. Insulin is a strong stimulus of this muscle-rebuilding process; insulin helps transport glucose and amino acid into the muscle cells or fibers, as well as diminishes the breakdown of muscle protein. This interrelationship between glycogen replenishment, insulin and muscle rebuilding is a cornerstone of muscle recovery. Protein also provides the essential building blocks for muscle repair. The essential amino acid component of protein is critical for muscle repair and recovery.[24]

Proof from the Halls of Science

Five sets of squats, four sets each of leg curls and leg extensions, three sets of walking lunges—not to stop there, you head out to the local track and perform ten 100-meter repeats with a 100-meter rest interval in between. Let's just say your legs are feeling like those on a rubber chicken. If you don't provide your body with the proper nutrition after this painful training session, then you'll be compromising the gains your body can potentially make. Let's look at some recent data on post-workout nutrition.

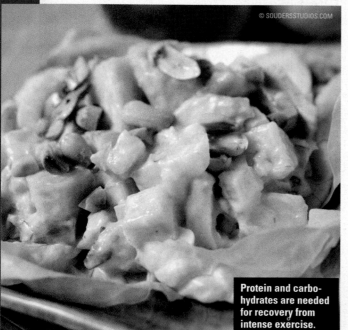

© SOUDERSSTUDIOS.COM

Protein and carbohydrates are needed for recovery from intense exercise.

In a two-part study done at Maastricht University in the Netherlands, scientists examined the effects of a carbohydrate-only drink (1.2 g/kg/hour), and 0, 0.2 or 0.4 g/kg/hour of a protein hydrolysate and amino acid mixture on hormone response.[25] Eight male cyclists were tested under the different dietary conditions in which they consumed these beverages every 30 minutes for five hours after a glycogen-depletion bike ride. They found that the beverages that contained the 0.2 and 0.4 grams of protein produced significant insulin responses compared to the carbohydrate-only trial, suggesting that perhaps the addition of protein to carbohydrates would produce a superior anabolic effect. Additionally, they found that the extra protein was nearly 100 percent more effective at helping muscles refuel or replenish lost glycogen.

Another study had subjects do intense cycling for 2.5 hours, so as to fully deplete their muscle glycogen levels.[26] They supplemented immediately and two hours post-exercise with the following formulas:

- ⌖ **Group 1:** Carb/Protein/Fat (80 grams of carbs, 28 grams of protein, 6 grams of fat)
- ⌖ **Group 2:** Carb/Fat (108 grams of carbs, 6 grams of fat)
- ⌖ **Group 3:** Carb/Fat (80 grams of carbs, 6 grams of fat)

Keep in mind all subjects underwent all three treatments. After four hours of recovery (remember, they consumed this supplement immediately and two hours after exercise), they found that Group 1 had gained the greatest amount of muscle glycogen. The true comparison is really between Groups 1 and 2 since they consumed the same number of calories. If you look at these groups, the only difference is that one group consumed protein instead of carbs—and that group did the best. This study shows that consuming approximately a 500-calorie post-workout meal immediately and two hours after intense exercise is best when it's a mixture of carbs, protein and a touch of fat.

Also, another study compared the consumption of a carb-protein beverage (53 grams of carbs, 14 grams of protein, 1.5 grams of fat, added vitamins, minerals and amino acids) versus the "quintessential sports drink" (21 grams of carbs, zero protein or fat) immediately after exercise and then again at two hours post-exercise.[27] The researchers found that 1) time to exhaustion was 55 percent greater in the carb-protein group, and 2) the amount of muscle glycogen that was stored was 128 percent greater. According to these researchers, "… recovery supplements should be consumed to optimize muscle glycogen synthesis, as well as fluid replacement." Other studies have found similarly good results.[28,29,30,31]

By now it should be crystal clear to you that a combination of protein and carbohydrates is needed for recovery. The hydration beverages on the market are good for just one thing, hydration; they are very poor when it comes to promoting recovery and not quite as good at improving exercise.

Is there an ideal post-workout drink? Interestingly, if you look at the various ratios of carbs to protein, they range as high as 4:1 to as low as 0.7 to 1. Meaning, some studies show you need to consume four times as many carbs as protein, while others show that you need about an equal ratio. According to Sue Kleiner, Ph.D., author of *Power Eating*, you should "… consume roughly 16 to 24 ounces of fluid with about 1.5 grams/kilogram of high-glycemic carbs and 0.5 grams/kilogram of protein." That's about a 3:1 ratio.

Post-Workout Nutrition: Whole Food or Nutritional Supplements?

At a recent sports nutrition conference, a distinguished scientist pointed out (as many scientists have) that there really is no difference between consuming one of these post-workout meal-replacement powders or ready-to-drinks versus eating real food like chicken and potatoes. And you know what, technically, he's probably correct. But that ignores another issue that has nothing to do with science! First, the protein and carbs in a meal-replacement powder (MRP) or ready-to-drink shake (RTD) are real food. Also, there is a convenience factor that makes the RTDs or protein powders a much

tip If you're an endurance athlete, stick to the higher carb-to-protein ratio. If you're a strength athlete, you need a bit more protein. If you're not an athlete, but you're active, a combination of fast-acting protein and high-glycemic index carbohydrates is still your best post-workout bet. Let's face it. There's more to recovery than getting a good night's sleep.

better way of getting nutrients post-exercise. First, let us address the food versus supplements issue. For one thing, there are no direct head-to-head comparisons of meals such as chicken and potatoes versus the equivalent energy and nutrient composition found in a supplement such as a protein-based powder with some carbs. While there are no direct comparisons in the literature, nutritional supplements may be superior for a few reasons:

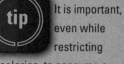

- **They're convenient.** It's a lot easier to consume a ready-to-drink shake or blend protein powder with skim milk and throw in some sliced bananas and strawberries within 15 to 30 minutes post-exercise than to run home and prepare a full-course meal.
- **Essential amino acids** may be the most important single nutrients in kick-starting the anabolic processes. And there are no single foods that are purely essentially amino acids, yet meal-replacement powders and ready-to-drink shakes contain all the essential amino acids that you need.
- **They're easy on the gut.** It would make sense that it's easier to digest a liquid meal that contains high-glycemic sugars and fast-acting protein/essential amino acids than a full meal of chicken and potatoes. "I'm not going to keep a piece of chicken and a potato in my car while I train and then eat this food cold on my way home. It is more convenient to drink a protein shake," says Andy Holmes, former Division II hammer thrower from the University of Nebraska-Kearney.

Nutrient Timing Helps When You Diet

Nutrient timing may help in your quest to improve your physique.[32] In one study, 17 slightly overweight men were put on a 12-week program consisting of mild caloric restriction (17 percent reduction) and a light resistance program utilizing dumbbells. One group ingested a protein supplement (10 grams of protein, 7 grams of carbohydrates, 3.3 grams of fat and one-third the RDA of vitamins and minerals) immediately after exercise. The other group didn't consume a supplement. Protein and calorie intake was the same for both groups; and both groups met their daily RDA for protein. Both groups lost an equal amount of fat. However, the protein-supplemented group maintained muscle while the non-supplemented group lost muscle.

tip Consume a post-workout liquid meal right after training. Make it roughly 250 to 500 calories and be sure it has protein and carbohydrates. The amount of carbohydrates you need with the protein is dependent on your goals. One or two hours later, eat your regular meal, and keep eating well for the rest of the day; 24 hours later ... get back in the gym!

tip It is important, even while restricting calories, to consume a protein-based nutritional supplement after exercise.

Andy Holmes
Former Competitive Hammer Thrower
University of Nebraska-Kearney
Weight: 240 pounds
Body fat: 10 percent

"When trying to gain lean mass and strength there are many factors involved. You can't control genetics, but you can control training, nutrition and recuperation. Keeping this in mind, I try to utilize what advantages I have in these areas and maximize them for the best possible result," says Andy.

Protein is key:

⮞ The idea that one can just eat "normal" and gain weight is absurd. If you want to get big, you have to eat big! This means increasing calories and nutrients to match your goals. When training for lean mass and strength, I find that a diet rich in protein is key. I use about 1.5 to 2.5 grams per pound of body weight. This has shown to be a great standard to go by because it supplies my body with the right amount of protein for my intense training and such extreme stress. I need this protein to not only build, but also repair and renew my body's free amino acid pool.

Pre-workout:

⮞ Protein or amino acids blended with simple carbohydrates 30 minutes before I train has a huge effect on my abilities in the gym. I have a lot more power, endurance, and can put out more effort in the heavier sets and reps. I have made this a way of life with my training, and I would highly recommend it to anyone at any level.

Post-workout:

⮞ About 20 grams of carbs and 40 grams of whey protein. From experience, I know that if I can get these nutrients into my body during that time my body will repair and recuperate adequately. These calories are essential in replacing the ones used during training.

Pre-bed:

⮞ 40 grams of blended protein mixed with extra glutamine 30 minutes prior to sleep.

"I've found the timing of all these nutrients is important. If I am going to the effort to get the most out of my body in the gym, I want to get the most out of the supplements that I take!" adds Andy.

Nighty Night—Fuel While You Sleep

You need to fuel your body while you sleep. This is when your body needs nutrients to facilitate recovery. Let's face it, sleep is the critical window of recovery. If you have a bad night's sleep, you'll pay for it the next day with mediocre workouts and performances. But the drawback is that for eight hours a day, you are literally starving your body, and your body needs a steady stream of nutrients to promote growth and recovery.

Summary and Future Trends

So you want to gain lean body mass, lose fat and improve performance? Then you better pay attention to your watch. If you eat the right nutrients in the right amounts at the right time, you will optimize your performance or physique goals. If you don't utilize nutrient timing, you're ignoring one of the most powerful nutrition tools around.

tips Consume a blended protein (whey, casein, amino acids) to ensure a steady stream of amino acids gets to your growing muscles. In science terms, a combination of the fast (whey and amino acids) and the slow (milk and casein) proteins offer the anabolic and anti-catabolic benefits of both proteins, as well as all those cool bioactive peptides of both.

Key Concepts

1. Nutrient timing can result in a partitioning effect (i.e., gain muscle, lose fat).
2. Recovery is an important aspect of training; nutrient timing expedites recovery.
3. Total energy intake is the most important dietary factor for improving physique and performance.
4. Nutrient quality is as important as timing.
5. High-glycemic carbohydrates are great immediately before, during and immediately after training.
6. Stored carbohydrates are the main fuel source for intense exercise.
7. Whey is a fast-acting protein that is perfect after exercise.
8. Casein is a slow-acting protein that is good prior to sleep.
9. The essential amino acids are perhaps the number one most important macronutrient for expediting recovery and promoting muscle growth.
10. Antioxidants are important for preserving cell membrane integrity.
11. Leucine is a special amino acid that plays an important role in muscle growth.
12. Before you train, consume a mixture of liquid carbs and protein/amino acids: perhaps 10 grams of carbs and 5 grams of protein.
13. During training, consume a sports drink that contains a protein or amino acids.
14. Immediately post-training, consume a combination of carbs and protein.
15. Strength/power athletes should consume relatively more protein than endurance athletes.
16. A nutrition shake or RTD is a better way of getting nutrients post-exercise.
17. Nutrient timing strategies can also help you lose weight.

The Take-Home Message on Nutrient Timing

By now, you are well aware that nutrient timing is as important as fangs to a tiger. No fangs, no food. If there is one thing you need to do above all else, it's that you consume a protein-carb shake right after training. Simple enough? Here's the take-home message on nutrient timing.

1 **Immediately before a workout:** Consume a high-glycemic carbohydrate with just a touch of protein, perhaps something like 10 grams of carbs and 5 grams of whey protein; that way, you won't get an upset stomach but you'll provide fuel for exercise and some amino acids to initiate the recovery process.

2 **During your workout:** Consume a sports drink. In that sports drink, try adding 1 teaspoon of whey protein; the small amount of whey will assist with recovery and the sugar in the sports drink will provide you with extra energy.

3 **Immediately after a workout:** Consume a fast-acting protein, such as whey combined with a high-glycemic carbohydrate; there are various recovery powders that you can buy that do this job well. For some healthy fat, add a teaspoon of flax oil or peanut butter (blend it, of course).

4 **Before going to bed:** Consume cottage cheese or a casein-based protein powder.

The rest of the day is basically a recovery process. Make sure you eat mainly lean protein, unsaturated fats, and high-fiber/low-glycemic index carbs.

Sample Nutrition Plan for a Weight-Training Day

PRE-WORKOUT	DURING	POST-WORKOUT
• **Essential amino acids*** **(EAAs)**–6 grams • **Carbohydrates**–10 grams (mix with water) This can be one scoop of protein powder (EAS® Precision Protein™) blended with water.	• **6-percent carbohydrate-electrolyte drink**. Add 3 to 6 grams of whey protein to mix	• **High-glycemic carbohydrates** (e.g., blend of maltodextrin, sucrose, glucose, fructose)—30 grams • **Whey protein**–30 grams • **Leucine***–3 grams • **EAAs***–3 grams • **Flax seed oil**—1 teaspoon (blend with water or your nutrition shake) • **Creatine**–5 grams (EAS® Phosphagen HP™) This can be in the form of a nutrition shake (EAS Myoplex® Original or Myoplex Lite®).
Consume 30 minutes or less prior to weight training	Drink during training session. Try to consume at least 500 to 1,000 milliliters per hour	Consume immediately post-workout.

DIRECTIONS

*A quality nutrition shake should contain adequate amounts of EAAs and leucine. You can also find supplements at any specialty nutrition store or health food store.

Sample Nutrition Plan for a Cardio Workout Day

PRE-WORKOUT	DURING	POST-WORKOUT
• **6 percent carbohydrate-electrolyte drink** *Add 3 to 6 grams of whey protein to mix	• **6-percent carbohydrate-electrolyte drink.** Add 3 to 6 grams of whey protein to mix	• **High-glycemic carbohydrates**–40 grams • **Whey protein**–20 grams • **EAAs***–3 grams This can be in the form of a nutrition shake (EAS Myoplex® Original or Myoplex Lite®). • **Flax seed oil**—1 teaspoon (blend with water or your nutrition shake)
DIRECTIONS Consume at least 100 calories of the drink **OR** Consume 25 grams of carbohydrate gel 10 to 15 minutes prior to exercise	Consume at least 100 calories of the drink **OR** Consume 25 grams of carbohydrate gel 10 to 15 minutes prior to exercise	Consume immediately post-workout.

*If your stomach can't handle the protein before or during a cardio workout, don't add it.
**A quality nutrition shake should contain adequate amounts of EAAs. You can also find supplements at any specialty nutrition store or health food store.
***If you are following the Body-*for*-LIFE Program, feel free to wait an hour after your cardio exercise before eating.

PRE-BED	RULES FOR THE REST OF THE DAY
• A protein powder that is primarily casein (a "slow" protein) **OR** • Low-fat cottage cheese with a ¼ cup of blueberries	• Don't skip breakfast! Have a lean protein with a low-glycemic carbohydrate (e.g., egg white omelet with oatmeal, skim milk) • Take 1 multivitamin daily • If you're on a low-fat diet, supplement with a teaspoon or two of flax seed oil or all-natural peanut butter • Eat small, frequent meals • Consume at least 1,200 milligrams of calcium
DIRECTIONS Consume one hour prior to bed	

REFERENCES CITED:

[1] Gleeson M et al. Nutritional strategies to minimize exercise-induced immunosuppression in athletes. *Can J Appl Physiol* 26 Suppl:S23-S35, 2001.

[2] Bounous G, Gold P. The biological activity of undenatured dietary whey proteins: role of glutathione. *Clin Invest Med* 14: 296-309, 1991.

[3] Boirie Y et al. Slow and fast dietary proteins differently modulate postprandial protein accretion. *Proc National Acad Sci* 94: 14930-14935, 1997.

[4] Dangin, M., et al. The digestion rate of protein is an independent regulating factor of postprandial protein retention. *Am J Physiol Endocrinol Metab* 280: E340-E348, 2001.

[5] Mahe S et al. Gastrojejunal kinetics and the digestion of 15Nbeta-lactoglobulin and casein in humans:the influence of the nature and quantity of the protein. *Am J Clin Nutr* 63:546-52, 1996.

[6] Dangin, M. et al. Influence of the Protein Digestion Rate on Protein Turnover in Young and Elderly Subjects. *J. Nutr.* 132: 3228S-3233S, 2002.

[7] Anthony JC et al. Signaling pathways involved in translational control of protein synthesis in skeletal muscle by leucine. *J Nutr* 131:856S-860S, 2001.

[8] Anthony JC et al. Orally administered leucine stimulates protein synthesis in skeletal muscle of postabsorptive rats in association with increased eIF4F formation. *J Nutr* 130:139-145, 2000.

[9] Layman DK. Role of leucine in protein metabolism during exercise and recovery. *Can J Appl Physiol* 27:646-63, 2002.

[10] Rieu I et al. Leucine-supplemented meal feeding for ten days beneficially affects postprandial muscle protein synthesis in old rats. *J Nutr* 133:1198-205, 2003.

[11] Tipton KD et al. Timing of amino acid-carbohydrate ingestion alters anabolic response of muscle to resistance exercise. *Am J Physiol* 281:E197-E206, 2001.

[12] Meydani M et al. Protective effect of vitamin E on exercise-induced oxidative damage in young and older adults. *Am J Physiol* 264:R992-8, 1993.

[13] Meydani, M., et al. Muscle uptake of vitamin E and its association with muscle fiber type. *Journal Nutr Biochem* 8(2): 74-78, 1997.

[14] Hemila H. Vitamin C and common cold incidence: a review of studies with subjects under heavy physical stress. *Int J Sports Med* 17:379-83, 1996.

[15] Tipton KD et al. Timing of amino acid-carbohydrate ingestion alters anabolic response of muscle to resistance exercise. *Am J Physiol* 281:E197-E206, 2001.

[16] Millard-Stafford M et al. Pre-exercise carbohydrate-electrolyte ingestion improves one-hour running performance in the heat. *Medicine and Science in Sports and Exercise.* 1994; 26:S196.

[17] Nicholas CW et al. Influence of ingesting a carbohydrate-electrolyte solution on endurance capacity during intermittent, high intensity shuttle running. *Journal of Sports Science.* 13: 283-290, 1996.

[18] Ivy JL et al. Effect of a carbohydrate-protein supplement on endurance performance during exercise of varying intensity. *Int J Sport Nutr Exerc Metab* 13:388-401, 2003.

[19] Haff GG et al. The effects of supplemental carbohydrate ingestion on intermittent isokinetic leg exercise. *J Sports Med Phys Fitness.* 41:216-222, 2001.

[20] Haff GG et al. Carbohydrate supplementation attenuates muscle glycogen loss during acute bouts of resistance exercise. *Int J Sports Nutr Exerc Metab* 10:326-39, 2000.

[21] Bilz S et al. Effects of hypoosmolality on whole body lipolysis in man. *Metabolism* 48:472-6, 1999.

[22] Berardi JM et al. Postexercise muscle glycogen recovery is enhanced with a carbohydrate-protein supplement. Submitted.

[23] Ivy JL et al. Early postexercise muscle glycogen recovery is enhanced with a carbohydrate-protein supplement. *J Appl Physiol* 93:1337-44, 2002.

[24] Rasmussen BB et al. An oral essential amino acid-carbohydrate supplement enhances muscle protein anabolism after resistance exercise. *J Appl Physiol* 88:386-92, 2000.

[25] Van Loon LJ et al. Ingestion of protein hydrolysate and amino acid-carbohydrate mixtures increases postexercise plasma insulin responses in men. *J Nutr* 130:2508-13, 2000.

[26] Ivy JL et al. Early postexercise muscle glycogen recovery is enhanced with a carbohydrate-protein supplement. *J Appl Physiol* 93:1337-44, 2002.

[27] Williams MB et al. Effects of recovery beverages on glycogen restoration and endurance exercise performance. *J Strength Cond Res* 17:12-19, 2003.

11

THE ART OF RECOVERY
Post- and Pre-Workout Strategies and Techniques

By Matt Fitzgerald

Fitness does not increase during workouts. Fitness increases *between* workouts, during periods of relative rest, as the body recovers from and adapts to the stresses of recent exercise. So when it comes to getting the results you seek from exercise, recovery is every bit as important as your workouts themselves.

Many exercisers take the recovery process for granted, assuming that as long as they rest a while between workouts, recovery will take care of itself. While rest is the most important condition of post-workout recovery, *optimal recovery* is not automatic with rest. In order to recover optimally from exercise, you need to fully support the systems that carry out the processes of recovery and adaptation within your body. This support takes many forms, from consuming the right nutrients at the right times, to using light activity to increase circulation, and with it, nutrient delivery and metabolic waste removal. Even the timing and sequencing of your workouts must be done carefully if you wish to truly optimize recovery and thereby maximize the benefits of each workout you perform.[1]

You won't achieve optimal recovery by winging it, as most of us do. You need to have specific knowledge about the various recovery techniques and strategies that can assist you. That's what this chapter is about.

Not Just Compensation: Supercompensation

An individual workout stresses the body by depleting energy supplies, disrupting muscle tissues, changing hormonal patterns and so forth. This type of stress is often referred to as a *training stimulus*. After the workout is completed, the body initiates physiological processes designed to restore homeostasis, or the way the body was before the workout. It replenishes muscle energy stores, builds new muscle proteins, adjusts hormonal patterns and engages in a few other responses. But these recovery mechanisms are so powerful that they have the potential to overshoot the mark of homeostasis; for example, it is common for the body of a strength-trained individual to build more new muscle proteins after a workout is completed than were broken down or damaged during the workout, resulting in net protein accretion in the muscles.

When training stimuli are applied consistently, such "excessive" recovery becomes a regular pattern. Instead of merely recovering from workouts, your body adapts to them.[2] Consequently, your body becomes able to handle greater training stimuli, which, in turn, result in further adaptations. Exercise physiologists use the term "supercompensation" to describe this pattern whereby short-term recovery leads to lasting adaptations.[3]

The goal of recovery is to achieve full compensation, if not supercompensation, with respect to a particular training stimulus before the same stimulus is repeated. If you do not allow yourself sufficient recovery (and here we're talking mainly about rest time) between workouts of a given type, you will not be able to perform the next workout at the same level as the previous one, and instead of building on gains (adaptations), you will only add fatigue to fatigue, breakdown to breakdown. On the other hand, if you allow yourself too much recovery between workouts, your body will pass beyond the supercompensation phase and enter what's called the detraining phase, in which you begin to lose the results you just worked for.[4]

The Rest Question

So you need just the right amount of rest between workouts of the same type—neither too little nor too much. But exactly how much is the right amount? This depends on many factors, including your current conditioning status, the type of training you're doing, your age and the specific nature of the workout you performed most recently. Generally, the younger you are[5], the more experienced you are in exercise[6] and the higher your current level of conditioning, the faster you are able to recover between workouts. Resistance workouts typically require more rest time than aerobic workouts. Also, the higher the intensity level of the workout[7] and the longer it lasts, the more rest time is needed afterward.

If you are just beginning an exercise program, the best way to ensure that you achieve full compensation or supercompensation between workouts is not to work out infrequently but rather to perform easier workouts that do not require as much recovery. Studies show that untrained individuals gain strength fastest when they train each muscle group three times per week.[8] By the same token, advanced bodybuilders might not need to train each muscle group any more often than three times a week, and in certain phases they might train each muscle group only twice a week. Despite their ability to recover more quickly, they will derive greater benefit from performing high-volume, high-intensity workouts that require more recovery time.

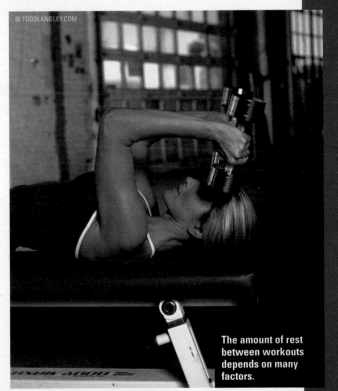

The amount of rest between workouts depends on many factors.

With respect to cardio exercise, beginners should also do manageable workouts rather than infrequent workouts in order to attain complete recovery. An initial weekly schedule of three to five 20-minute walks would be appropriate for a person who has been sedentary but is otherwise in good health. Once a solid foundation has been built, you can take your fitness to the next level either by doing cardio workouts more frequently or by doing more challenging cardio workouts.

However often you choose to work out, and regardless of which types of workouts you do, be sure to arrange your weekly exercise schedule to allow maximum separation between workouts of the same type. Because cardio and resistance workouts stress the body differently, you can still recover from, say, yesterday's cardio workout while doing a resistance workout today. And, obviously, you can continue to recover from Monday's upper-body resistance workout while doing a lower-body resistance workout on Wednesday.

Suppose you choose to perform two moderate-intensity cardio workouts, two high-intensity cardio workouts and three total-body resistance workouts each week. A sensible way to schedule these workouts would be as follows:

MONDAY	TUESDAY	WEDNESDAY	THURSDAY	FRIDAY	SATURDAY	SUNDAY
Resistance Workout	High-Intensity Cardio	Resistance Workout	Low-Intensity Cardio	Resistance Workout	High-Intensity Cardio	Low-Intensity Cardio

In addition to these basic principles, body awareness can guide you very effectively in determining how much rest time to allow yourself between workouts of the same type. Significant levels of fatigue or muscle soreness are good indicators that your body is not yet ready to train again. Both the volume of training your body is able to handle and your ability to judge how much exercise your body can handle will improve over time.

Fueling Recovery

Nutrition is the foundation of post-exercise recovery because it provides the raw materials with which your body can make physical adaptations in response to training. If you take in the right nutrients, in the right amounts, at the right time after workouts, you will recover far more quickly and thoroughly than you will if you don't practice proper nutritional recovery.

Timing is essential with regard to post-exercise nutrition because your body is primed to sponge up needed nutrients at this time; for example, synthesis of muscle glycogen—a form of stored carbohydrate that serves as the body's primary energy source during exercise—proceeds two to three times faster in the two hours immediately following exercise than it does at any other time.

There are three main components of post-exercise muscle recovery; first, it is necessary to restore fluids lost during exercise. When you sweat heavily in a workout, you lose a lot of water as well as vital electrolyte minerals (sodium, chloride, potassium and magnesium). Therefore, it's important to make up the deficit by consuming fluids with electrolytes after exercise. If you do not re-hydrate properly before the next workout, you could experience overheating, muscle cramps and other problems when you do hit the gym again.

The second component of muscle recovery is putting carbohydrate fuel back into the muscles. Again, carbohydrates are the muscles' main fuel source during moderate- to high-intensity exercise. The longer a workout lasts, the lower your muscle fuel supplies become. By using a sports drink containing carbohydrates (and possibly a bit of protein—see Chapter 10 for more on this) during workouts, you can slow down this process. But it's seldom possible to take in carbohydrates during intense exercise as fast as they're burned. So you need to continue taking in carbohydrates after exercise, as well. If you don't get your muscle fuel levels back to normal in time for the next workout, you'll feel weak and fatigued. Studies have demonstrated that individuals who fail to take in adequate carbohydrates during the so-called "muscle recovery window" run a much higher risk of beginning the next day's workout in a glycogen-depleted state.[9]

Finally, the third component of muscle recovery is building new muscle proteins. High-intensity physical activity disrupts and damages some muscle tissues. In addition, some muscle proteins are broken down for energy during hard exercise; therefore, it is essential that you consume protein after workouts to bring your muscles back to full strength. This component of muscle recovery is especially important for those seeking to increase muscle size and strength.

Again, timing is important. During the first hour or two following exercise, the muscles cells are especially insulin receptive. Since insulin is responsible for delivering amino acids (proteins) and glucose (carbohydrates) into the muscle cells, this state of "transient hyperinsulinemia" gives you an opportunity to replenish muscle glycogen stores and build new muscle proteins very rapidly. In one study of this phenomenon performed at Vanderbilt University, 10 healthy adults were subjected to 60 minutes of moderate-intensity exercise. Half the subjects were fed a protein-carbohydrate supplement immediately after completion of the workout. The remaining subjects were fed the same supplement three hours later. Members of the "early" group replenished muscle glycogen three-and-a-half times faster than members of the "late" group. Muscle protein synthesis also proceeded more than three times faster in the early group.[10]

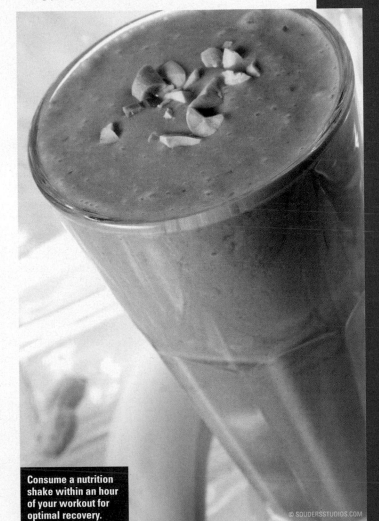

The most convenient way to get all of the nutrition needed for recovery is to drink a nutrition shake containing protein, carbohydrates and electrolytes. These drinks contain exactly what is needed and in the right proportions, without anything extra that might slow down gastric emptying and with it the recovery process. Most people also find them easier to swallow and keep down than solid food immediately after a workout.

If you *are* hungry after your workouts, eating is fine. Just make sure you get all the same nutrients you would get in a quality recovery drink without a lot of extra stuff (fat, excess protein) that might slow down the delivery of nutrients to your muscles. Some nutrition bars are good, convenient recovery foods. In any case, you will need to drink some form of fluid with your meal to meet your body's hydration needs after workouts. For more on post-workout nutrition, turn to Chapter 10.

Consume a nutrition shake within an hour of your workout for optimal recovery.

Preventing and Treating Muscle Soreness

Post-workout muscle soreness, also known as delayed-onset muscle soreness (DOMS), is a normal and unavoidable consequence of strenuous exercise. The only way to completely prevent delayed-onset muscle soreness is to avoid exercise, or do workouts that are too easy to have any beneficial impact on your health and fitness; on the other hand, severe DOMS itself can sabotage your training. Fortunately, there are several legitimate ways of minimizing and treating DOMS and thereby limiting its impact on your training. We'll discuss each of these measures below, but first, a few more words about what DOMS is and what causes it.

FIVE WAYS TO **MINIMIZE** MUSCLE SORENESS

1. Warm up thoroughly at the beginning of every workout. Beginning a workout with light activity warms and lubricates the muscles, making the fibers less prone to tearing during the more intense portion of the session.

2. Know when to say when. Don't push beyond your limits in workouts. Develop a feel for how hard or long your body can go in a workout without being hobbled the next day. Muscle damage and soreness manifest in direct proportion to how much work your muscles do beyond what they are accustomed to.

3. Increase your training workload very gradually. The more slowly you add volume or intensity to your training, the smaller the gap will be between what your muscles are accustomed to and what you require them to do each day and each week.

4. Cool down thoroughly after your high-intensity workouts. Circulation is the primary means by which the muscles repair themselves after intense exercise. Finishing workouts with low-intensity activity keeps circulation levels up without further damaging muscle fibers and thereby kick-starts the recovery process.

5. Paradoxically, one of the most effective ways to minimize DOMS is actually to cause it, in small amounts, with a controlled application of eccentric training. Also known as "doing negatives," eccentric training is a type of weight lifting that focuses on the lowering portion of the movement, rather than the actual lifting portion, usually with a very heavy weight. Research has shown that doing a small amount of eccentric training provides a protective effect against future muscle damage and soreness from strength training.[11] The only downside to eccentric training is that you need a partner's help to do it safely.

What Causes Delayed-Onset Muscle Soreness?

In 1902, the first doctor to study DOMS hypothesized that it was associated with the microscopic tearing of muscle fibers during unaccustomed physical activity (that is, activity that is either more intense or more prolonged than one normally does). Subsequent study has confirmed that such "mechanical stress" is indeed the primary cause of muscle soreness after exercise. The mechanisms are complicated, however, and although a great deal of light has been shed on them in recent years, there remains more to be learned. Here's what we do know.

It seems that eccentric muscle contractions cause the most muscle fiber damage. In an eccentric contraction, the muscle lengthens as it contracts (for example, during the lowering phase of a biceps curl) instead of shortening as in a concentric contraction or staying the same length as in an isometric contraction. The muscle is really being pulled in two directions at once during an eccentric contraction, like a tug of war, so it's easy to see the potential for tearing. Also, it appears that during eccentric contractions, fewer muscle fibers are recruited than when the same muscle produces the same amount of force concentrically, so there is greater strain on individual muscle fibers in an eccentric contraction.

When a muscle fiber is strained too far, the surface membrane breaks open and some of its chemical contents spill out, damaging other muscle tissue, activating nerve fibers and initiating an inflammation response. The soreness itself is probably associated with inflammation more than it is with the actual damage, resulting in soreness that takes many hours to develop and often does not peak until two to three days after the workout. In addition to pain, other symptoms are loss of strength, stiffness and decreased range of motion. While DOMS does not constitute a serious injury in itself,

FIVE WAYS TO **TREAT** MUSCLE SORENESS

1. Get a sports massage. While massage is not quite the magic medicine that many mind-body types claim it is, some research shows that it does increase circulation and is helpful in breaking up muscular adhesions.[12,13]

2. Ice your sore areas, or take an ice bath if you can stand it. Cold treatments are among the best ways of reducing inflammation without inhibiting tissue repair. Combining a cold treatment with compression of the sore muscle, for example with a neoprene sleeve, is even more effective.[14]

3. Get in some light activity between hard workouts. Studies show that performing low-intensity exercise such as walking and stretching on the day after a hard workout can accelerate recovery from DOMS.[15] Such light activity, known as active recovery, increases circulation, upon which muscle tissue repair depends, without causing new tissue damage.

4. Maintain a diet high in antioxidants. There is some evidence that oxygen radicals play a role in the cellular damage that follows the rupture of muscle fibers during exercise. Antioxidant vitamins and enzymes are needed to limit this damage. Vitamins C and E are especially effective in defending against oxidative damage to muscle tissues.[16] Good dietary sources of vitamin C are citrus fruits, melon and berries. Vegetable oils, nuts, dark green vegetables and whole grains are rich in vitamin E.

5. Use an anti-inflammatory medication such as Ibuprofen only occasionally, in cases of extreme discomfort. Long-term chronic dependence on such medications may result in damage to the liver and kidneys and reduce your body's ability to handle inflammation on its own. When soreness borders on the intolerable, try using one of the newer sports creams that have anti-inflammatory properties. But always bear in mind that no medication accelerates muscle tissue healing, and that training hard with lingering muscle damage—even if the pain is covered up—will only cause further damage.

overtaxing a damaged muscle by returning to intense training too quickly can lead to permanent damage.

Note that there seems to be little connection between the acute muscle soreness you're feeling during and immediately after workouts and the soreness you wake up with the next morning. Acute soreness is associated with the buildup of metabolic wastes in fatigued muscles and dissipates within hours as these wastes are flushed away. Typically, acute soreness affects different muscles than DOMS, which is concentrated in those muscles that have done the most eccentric work.

Too Much of a Good Thing: Avoiding Overtraining

Most exercisers have heard of overtraining, also known as overreaching, but few have an accurate understanding of what it is. Often, overreaching is confused with *overtraining syndrome*, which is a phenomenon unto itself. Overtraining syndrome is a fairly serious condition characterized by a decrease in performance capacity and other symptoms resulting from chronic failure to achieve adequate post-exercise re-

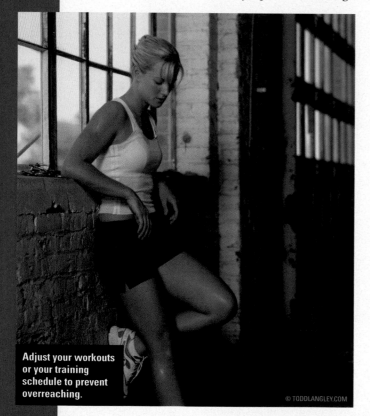

Adjust your workouts or your training schedule to prevent overreaching.

© TODDLANGLEY.COM

covery or from maintaining a training workload that is beyond the athlete's absorption capacity for a long period of time.[17] Often a loss of enthusiasm for training is seen, as well.

The first observed symptom of overtraining is usually an unexpected leveling off and subsequent diminishment of performance. One or more of a long list of additional symptoms may also appear. These include insomnia, irritability, chronic fatigue, loss of appetite, headaches, weight loss and nausea. In most cases, the athlete must drastically reduce training for a prolonged period of time in order to return to normal functioning.

Overtraining syndrome is rare except among athletes of a very high level of conditioning, because only such athletes can work too much and/or rest too little long enough for overtraining syndrome to develop.[18] Average exercisers tend to break down (i.e., get sick or injured) quickly when they do more exercise than their body is able to absorb, and therefore they do not enter the kind of irreversible tailspin that is associated with overtraining syndrome.

However, the first sign of overreaching is the same as that of overtraining syndrome: diminishing performance. If you experience an unexpected setback in your workout performances that cannot be explained by a factor such as *undertraining*, there's a good chance you're overreaching. Don't panic. You'll bounce back in no time if you adjust your training schedule, and perhaps also your workouts themselves, to give your body greater opportunity to absorb training stimuli, and if you get serious about practicing the various supplemental recovery techniques discussed in this chapter.

Supplements for Recovery

There are four key nutritional supplements that can greatly enhance your body's recovery from exercise by boosting the various systems involved in recovery processes. Here they are.

CREATINE

Creatine phosphate is an indirect source of energy present in muscle cells and used to fuel maximum- and near-maximum-intensity efforts. It can be manufactured from its constituent amino acids in the liver and obtained through dietary consumption of creatine, which is found in animal foods such as beef. But creatine supplementation can significantly increase the amount of creatine phosphate that is stored in the muscles. And when the muscles store greater amounts of creatine phosphate, they can work at higher intensities for longer periods of time, thus increasing the training effect of strength workouts. Literally dozens of studies have demonstrated the effectiveness of creatine supplementation.[19]

Recommended Dosage:
The preferred form of creatine supplementation is creatine monohydrate, because it is the best delivery system for the nutrient. Start out by taking 5 grams four times a day, for five days. Then stick to a maintenance dose of 5 grams, one time a day, preferably after your workout.

GLUTAMINE

Individuals who participate in strenuous exercise have an elevated risk of contracting viral infections. There is evidence that cells of the immune system are less able to mount a defense against infections after hard workouts. Although there are many nutrients that have a beneficial effect on the immune system, one of the most important appears to be glutamine. Glutamine is the most abundant amino acid in muscle cells and has been shown to be an important fuel for certain types of immune cells. Glutamine levels have been shown to decrease in relation to extreme exercise and overtraining,[20] so supplementation is often recommended to those who regularly participate in strenuous exercise.

In one study to determine whether glutamine supplementation could help provide immune system support, 200 runners and rowers consumed either a glutamine-containing drink or placebo drink. The percentage of athletes who reported no infections was 81 percent in the glutamine group and 49 percent in the placebo drink. The author suggested that providing glutamine increases the availability of glutamine for key cells of the immune system.[21]

Recommended Dosage:
The recommended dosage for glutamine supplementation is between 10 and 15 grams daily.

HMB

Beta-hydroxy beta-methylbutyrate, or HMB, is a compound that is consumed in the diet and produced in the body from proteins containing the amino acid leucine. There is some evidence that HMB reduces proteolysis, or muscle breakdown, following strenuous exercise. Many strength and speed athletes use the HMB supplement because they find that it reduces recovery time and allows them to exercise more intensely and thus gain muscle size and strength more quickly. Clinical studies of the effects of HMB have produced mixed results, but a recent meta-analysis of these studies suggested that HMB does have a positive effect on strength and lean muscle mass.[22]

Recommended Dosage:
The recommended dosage for HMB supplementation is 3 grams per day. Take 1 gram before three of your daily meals.

L-CARNITINE

A natural compound with both vitamin-like and amino acid-like properties, L-carnitine is supplied in the diet by meats and is also manufactured in the liver and kidneys. Its primary function in the body is to transport fatty acids across cell membranes so they can be metabolized in the mitochondria. A growing number of athletes and exercisers take L-carnitine supplements to enhance post-workout recovery because there is mounting evidence that it reduces exercise-induced muscle tissue damage.[23] In a recent study, L-carnitine supplementation not only significantly reduced exercise-induced muscle damage but also greatly increased blood concentrations of one of the primary hormones involved in muscle building (IGHFB-3).[24]

Recommended Dosage:
The recommended dosage for L-carnitine supplementation is 2 grams per day.

Sleep and Recovery

Any influence that compromises health also compromises exercise performance, and sleep deprivation is no exception. Sleep provides essential support for a variety of post-exercise recovery processes. Lack of sufficient sleep reduces the body's ability to process glucose and therefore to produce energy. It also heightens levels of cortisol, which attacks muscle tissue and must be suppressed in order for proper post-workout tissue repair to occur; in addition, human growth hormone, the anabolic (i.e., muscle-building) hormone that plays the biggest role in rebuilding tissue after exercise, requires sleep for full activation. So the less sleep you get, the less usable muscle you wake up with.[25] Sleep loss also weakens the immune system by reducing the activity of interleukins, a group of molecules involved in signaling between cells of the immune system.

Sleep experts believe that perhaps a majority of adults in our society are chronically sleep deprived.[26] While individual sleep needs can vary widely, the well-known eight-hour standard seems to be about right for most adults. Those who regularly engage in strenuous exercise often need slightly more sleep than others. According to the latest surveys, the average American adult now sleeps less than seven hours a night during the workweek. Among fitness enthusiasts, such night-in, night-out deprivation will take the edge off your performance at the very least and could lead to greater health issues over time.

REFERENCES CITED:

[1] Fleck, S and Kraemer, W. *Designing Strength Training Programs* (Third Edition). (Human Kinetics, 2004).

[2] Ahtiainen, JP, Pakarinen, A, Alen, M, Kraemer, WJ and Hakkinen, K. Muscle hypertrophy, hormonal adaptations and strength development during strength training in strength-trained and untrained men. *Europ J of Appl Phys* May 7 (2003).

[3] Bompa, TO. *Periodization: Theory and Methodology of Training* (Human Kinetics, 1999).

[4] Gibala, MJ, MacDougall, JD and Sale, DG. The effects of tapering on strength performance in trained athletes. *Int J of Sports Med* 15.8 (1994): 492-497.

[5] Rowland, T. Developmental aspects of physiological function relating to aerobic exercise in children. *Sports Med* 10.4 (1990): 253-266.

[6] Noakes, T. *Lore of Running* (Human Kinetics, 2004).

[7] Zatsiorsky, V. *Sci and Pract of Strength Train* (Human Kinetics, 1995).

[8] Rhea, MR, Alvar, BA, Burkett, LN and Ball, SD. A meta-analysis to determine the dose response for strength development. *Med and Sci in Sports and Ex* 35 (2003): 456-464.

[9] Roy, BD, Luttmer, K, Bosman, MJ and Tarnopolsky, MS. The influence of post-exercise macronutrient intake on energy balance and protein metabolism in active females participating in endurance training. *Int J of Sport Nutr and Ex Metab* 12 (2002): 172-188.

[10] Levenhagen, DL et al. Post-exercise nutrient intake timing in humans is critical to recovery of leg glucose and protein homeostasis. *Am J of Physi, Endoc and Metab* 280 (2001): E982-E993.

[11] Hyatt, JPK and Clarkson, PM. Creatine kinase release and clearance using mm variants following repeated bouts of eccentric exercise. *Med and Sci in Sports and Ex* 30: 1059-1065.

[12] Tiidus, PM. Manual massage and recovery of muscle function following exercise: a literature review. *J of Ortho Sports Phys Therapy* 25.2 (1997): 107-112.

[13] Tiidus, PM and Shoemaker, JK. Effleurage massage, muscle blood flow and long-term post-exercise strength recovery. *Int J of Sports Med* 16.7 (1995): 478-483.

[14] Eston, R and Peters, D. Effects of cold water immersion on the symptoms of exercise-induced muscle damage. *J of Sports Sci* (1999): 231-8.

[15] Sayers, SP, Clarkson, PM and Lee, J. Activity and immobilization after eccentric exercise: I. Recovery of muscle function. *Med and Sci in Sports and Ex* (2000): 1587-1592.

[16] Meydanit, M et al. Protective effect of vitamin E on exercise-induced oxidative damage in young and older adults. *Am J of Phys* 264 (1993): R992-R998.

[17] Fleck, J and Kraemer, W. The overtraining syndrome. *National Strength and Conditioning Assoc Journ*. August/September (1982): 50-51.

[18] Fry, RW, Morton, AR, and Keast, D. Overtraining in athletes. An update. *Sports Med* 12 (1991): 32-65.

[19] Nissen, SL and Sharp, RL. Effects of dietary supplements on lean mass and strength gains with resistance exercise. *Scandinavian J of Med and Sci in Sports* 13.4 (2003): 272.

[20] Smith, DJ and Norris, SR. Changes in glutamine and glutamate concentrations for tracking training tolerance. *Med and Sci in Sports and Ex* 32.3 (2000): 684-9.

[21] Castell, LM and Newsholme, EA. The effects of oral glutamine supplementation on athletes after prolonged, exhaustive exercise. *Nutr* 13.7-8 (1997): 738-42.

[22] Panton, LB et al. Nutritional supplementation of the leucine metabolite beta-hydroxy-beta-methylbutyrate (HMB) during resistance training. *Nutr* 16.9 (2000): 734-9.

[23] Maggini, S et al. L-carnitine supplementation results in improved recovery after strenuous exercise. *Annals of Nutr and Metab* 44.2 (2002): 86.

[24] Kraemer, WJ et al. The effects of L-carnitine L-tartrate supplementation on hormonal responses to resistance exercise and recovery. *Jl of Strength and Conditioning Res* 17.3 (2003): 455-62.

[25] Godfrey, RJ, Madgwick, Z and Whyte, GP. The exercise-induced growth hormone response in athletes. *Sports Med* 33.8 (2003): 599-613.

[26] Bonnet, MH and Arand, DL. We are chronically sleep deprived. *Sleep* 18.10 (1995): 908-11.

12 THE WINNING GAME
Change Your Mind and You *Can* Change Your Body

By Victoria L. Freeman, Ph.D.

What happens in your mind is inextricably linked to what happens in your body. We know, for example, that meditation can change brain activity and improve immune response.[1] Even the often-skeptical medical community is embracing the power of the mind-body connection. Consider that in 2003, the National Center for Complementary and Alternative Medicine joined with 15 other National Institutes of Health entities to launch a multimillion dollar mind-body research initiative.[2] Clearly this is not a fly-by-night concept.

"The idea of your body following your mind is really the foundation of health," says Juli Compton, M.S., a licensed counselor and wellness coach. People usually want to jump into behavior changes too fast, like going from doing no exercise to jogging several days a week or from eating fast food every day to never eating it, but Compton says if you do that, your chances of long-term success are pretty slim. "Even though it takes a little longer on the front end, you've got to figure out what health and fitness mean to you on a personal level and get educated about your choices," she says.

There is no silver bullet, no bottle of magic. Yes, there are plenty of fitness quick fixes out there, but they won't last. "Do your mental homework and make the changes in your mind first, then you'll see lasting changes in your body," says Compton.

And remember, you don't just wake up one day with a body that stops traffic. It takes time to undo the damage you've done and rebuild. Just as your body transforms gradually, so does your mind. James Prochaska, Ph.D., psychology professor and co-author of *Changing for Good: A Revolutionary Six-Stage Program for Overcoming Bad Habits and Moving Your Life Positively Forward* (Quill, 2002), has identified mental stages that people naturally go through as they leave unhealthy

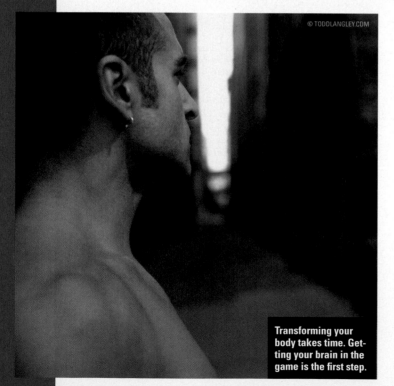

© TODDLANGLEY.COM

Transforming your body takes time. Getting your brain in the game is the first step.

SPORT AND GOAL-SPECIFIC NUTRITION AND TRAINING

habits behind and adopt healthier ones. Below is the technical name of each stage followed by a more friendly description that captures the essence of each point in the journey. The stages we will discuss go like this:

1) Pre-contemplation or "I won't" or "I can't"
2) Contemplation or "I may"
3) Preparation or "I will"
4) Action or "I am"
5) Maintenance or "I still am"

We'll use the friendly names from here on out, and we'll talk a lot more about these stages in an upcoming section.

One of the most exciting discoveries Prochaska and his colleagues made as they studied people struggling with challenges like smoking, alcoholism, weight control and exercise is that different strategies and types of goals are more effective at some stages than others; for example, if you're still in the "I won't" or "I can't" stage, it means you're not convinced that fitness is all it's cracked up to be or that it's worth the effort. At that

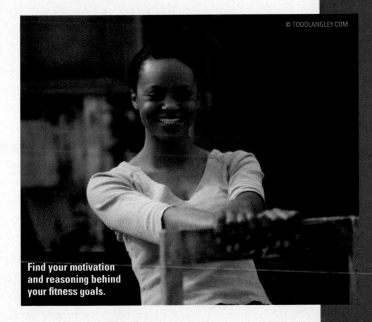

© TODDLANGLEY.COM

Find your motivation and reasoning behind your fitness goals.

point, it's a bit premature to set a goal of jogging three days a week. You'd be much more successful in the long run if you first look at the pros and cons of beginning an exercise program, figure out what you would enjoy doing and take an honest look at what will motivate you to stay with it. In order to move from "I won't" to "I am," there's a lot that has to happen in your head. In other words, we're back to that idea of mental homework.

On the flipside, if you're already at "I am," meaning you've already been exercising or eating well for a while but you just want to try something new or fine tune, going all the way back to those early decisions is unnecessary and will slow your progress. The further along in the change process you get, the more effective are exercise goals like jogging three days a week or nutrition goals like limiting your fast food consumption to one day a week.

"Is all this stage stuff really necessary? Can't I just start trying some things?" you may be asking yourself. Sure you can. Most people do. And most people fail. Action-oriented change programs (or those in which people begin immediately to change a behavior like overeating or smoking without paying attention to where their heads are in the process) typically have 1 percent to 5 percent long-term participation rates. In contrast, those programs in which people determine which stage of change they're in, match their beginning strategies to their stage, and modify goals and strategies as they go result in 50 percent to 85 percent participation.[5]

The stages of change combined with goal-setting strategies are even cornerstones for successful health and fitness coaching programs like Wellcoaches (www.wellcoaches.com). Founder and CEO of Wellcoaches Corporation, Margaret Moore says, "We've found that helping people understand where they are in the change process and develop appropriate goals makes a big difference in their success. Coaches can speed up the process for many people, but readiness to take action is not about the coach, it's about the client."

What does this mean to you? It means if you're serious about getting healthy and fit and staying that way, there are a couple of things to hang your hat on. The first is that to insure your new healthy habits last, you've got to do the mental work before the physical work. The second is that if you want to get to the finish line faster, match your beginning goals directly to the stage of change you're in and modify them as you "graduate" from one stage to the next. On paper it's really not that complicated. It's *doing* it that's tough.

At the end of the day, winning the mind game boils down to three steps: First, decide where you want to go and why; second, figure out where you are now (your stage of change); and third, chart your course (or set your goals) and get moving!

Where Do You Want To Go and Why?

Do you know where you're headed with your fitness plan? If you don't, how will you know when you get there? And how will you know what road to take?

Before a marathoner takes his or her first step in a race, you can bet they know where they're headed. The finish line is the vision or the ultimate goal. And while things may happen to change the outcome, they probably also have a time to finish the race in mind.

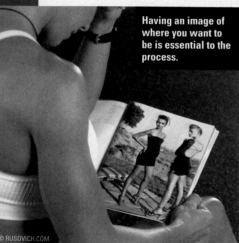
Having an image of where you want to be is essential to the process.

A fitness vision is like that. It's your destination point. It's what you ultimately want your health and fitness to look like. When you get *there*, you know you've arrived. "Most people have created visions for their life in some area, like their careers. They can picture themselves in the job of their dreams and that picture is a powerful force for moving forward," says Compton. "But for some reason, many of us are less likely to be as disciplined about our health."

The same envisioning process that propels you toward professional nirvana can be the wind beneath your fitness wings, too. What does a fitness vision look like? They're as varied as the number of people trying to get fit. Some want to lose weight, some want to tone up, some want to improve sport performance and others just want to feel better. Only you know what you want to achieve and what will make the most positive impact in your life. Let's take a look at a few examples of fitness visions with different destinations and timeframes.

> - In the next six months, I want to lose 3 inches off my waist.
> - By the end of 12 weeks, I want to lose 10 pounds and firm up my thighs and butt.
> - By next summer, I want to be able to jog 3 miles nonstop.

What's your vision? If you aren't sure, answering this question will help: From a fitness perspective, what do you want to achieve or how do you want to change in the next three months, six months or year?

Then once you've answered the "what" and "when," you need to answer the "why." Knowing why you want to do something tells you the motivation behind your action. And that motivation is what will keep you going when challenges come up (and they always do, for all of us). "If I had to pick one thing that will make or break a fitness transformation, it's your motivation or the reason you're doing this in the first place," says Gabrielle Highstein, Ph.D., R.N., instructor at the Division of Health Behavior Research at Washington University School of Medicine and faculty member of Well-coaches, Inc. "You've got to dig deeply enough to find that personal, passionate reason for making this commitment, or you won't weather the storm."

So go back to your first vision statement now and add the word "because" at the end, then complete the sentence. Here's what our first examples look like with motivation added.

> ⬈ In the next six months, I want to lose 3 inches off my waist because I want to see my abs and be able to wear my favorite trousers again.
> ⬈ By the end of 12 weeks, I want to lose 10 pounds and firm up my thighs and butt because I want to look good in a two-piece bathing suit for our vacation.
> ⬈ By next summer, I want to be able to jog 3 miles nonstop because I want to run a 5K.

As you can see, adding motivation to your vision makes it much more personal and relevant to your life. Your motivation is your ace in the hole—it's what gives you a reason to stay on track when life throws you a curve ball.

Where Are You Now?

When you're plotting the fastest and most efficient way to reach a road trip destination, what do you do? Most likely you work on connecting two reference points, right? One is where you're going and the other is where you're starting from. We've talked about where you want to go. It's time to figure out where you are now.

Remember the stages of change we discussed earlier? Here's where we start putting those to good use. "Once you understand the stages and the overall process of changing a behavior, you can apply it to any area of your life—career, personal relationships and definitely fitness," says Highstein.

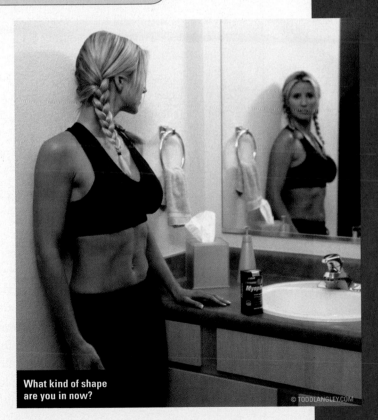

What kind of shape are you in now?

People are a lot more likely to give themselves a break and be willing to hang in there when they fully understand the road they're traveling, Highstein says. It's like knowing all the twists and turns and bumps in the road ahead of time. Getting prepared is a whole lot easier that way.

So let's take a look at each stage and how one leads to the next. As you read through them ask yourself, "Does this sound like me?"

1. I won't or I can't

People in this stage not only can't see the solution, they can't even see the problem. They have no intention of making health or fitness changes due to one of two reasons. Either they don't think they need to (I won't) or they don't think they're capable of it (I can't).

People in the "I won't" stage have not accepted why they need to change and will generally fight to maintain their ignorance, says Prochaska; for example, think of all the readily available information on the negative health effects of smoking and obesity. Yet there are 10 million smokers who refuse to stop,[4] and a startling 64 percent of the American population remains overweight.[5] Here's a group deeply entrenched in denial.

If life seems too out of control and you simply can't see a way to add anything else to your weekly agenda, you're probably at the "I can't" stage. For these folks, the number one excuse for not taking care of themselves is lack of time. And there's another group of "I can't" people—those who have tried repeatedly and failed to get in shape may feel so depressed and dejected that they truly believe they aren't capable of succeeding. While they may have accepted the importance of fitness and health, they feel paralyzed by their current circumstances.

Stages of Change Self-Evaluation

Answer yes or no to the following statements. If you answer yes, your stage follows in parentheses.

1. I achieved my original vision more than six months ago. **(I still am)**
2. I've taken action toward my vision within the past six months, but I'm still not there yet. **(I am)**
3. I'm intending to take action soon, like in the next month. **(I will)**
4. I'm intending to take action sometime, but it may be as much as six months away. **(I may)**
5. I'm not intending to take action any time in the foreseeable future either because I'm not interested or because I'm too overwhelmed. **(I won't or I can't)**

Source: Adapted from the Transtheoretical Model developed by Dr. James Prochaska and presented in *Changing for Good: A Revolutionary Six-Stage Program for Overcoming Bad Habits and Moving Your Life Positively Forward* (Quill Publishers, 2002, page 68). Printed with permission of author.

---

2. I may

When you know there's a problem you want to change and you've begun considering how to go about it, you're at the "I may" stage. "I may" people want to understand why and how they got to this point, but they're usually still several months away from taking a serious action step.

The hallmark characteristic of this stage is when you know what changes you want to make and even have some thoughts on how to get there, but you aren't quite ready to go yet. People can spend a long time talking about and thinking about making a change like exercise or healthy eating, but when push comes to shove, they don't have a good enough reason to get out of their old routines and the bottom line commitment just isn't there. What's missing is the driving force to propel them out of their rut and down the healthy road.

3. I will

Tension starts to build in the "I will" stage and when you get this far, you're planning to make the commitment and take action within a short time, maybe as soon as a few days. A big step for this stage is to declare your commitment out loud. Tell someone who can support you, "I'm starting my exercise program this coming Monday."

But before you take your first action step, make sure you have a plan in place. Figure out what time of day, which days of the week, and what exercise activity will best fit your needs. Or what healthier foods you'll substitute for those fast food pit stops.

It's not uncommon at this point to feel a little ambivalent or torn about your decision. That's OK. Just use your time to develop a solid plan of action that includes back-up options when things go awry. More on back-up plans later.

4. I am

This is it, the moment of truth. When you can say "I am," it means you've made the commitment and taken action. You're actually working out or you've cleaned all the junk food out of your house and eaten healthy meals instead.

This stage is the busiest time. People at this point often say it's the stage that requires the most time and energy because they're making real alterations in their lifestyle.

The danger here, though, is that many people equate taking action with successful behavior change. But those of us who have started and stopped an exercise program or eaten healthy for a couple of weeks—only to blow it in one weekend—get discouraged and give up. Just remember that there's a big difference between having a few good days and actually achieving a long-term fitness vision.

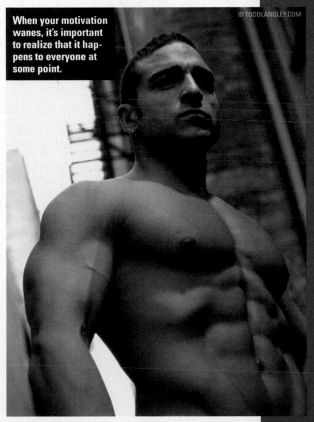

When your motivation wanes, it's important to realize that it happens to everyone at some point.

© TODDLANGLEY.COM

5. I still am

Those proud warriors who stick it out this long see real rewards for their efforts. Fat melts away, toned muscle takes its place and performance skills improve. But even though on some level you can declare victory, this stage is not without challenges.

How many people do you know who have lost the same 20 pounds or the same 5 inches time after time? They start out all gung ho and may even reach their goals, but then something happens. Motivation wanes, they get a new job, have a baby or get injured, and suddenly all the gains they worked so hard to achieve are gone and they're back to the drawing board, or back at "I won't," "I can't" or "I may." Psychologists call this problem a behavior relapse, and it's so common that we're going to spend some more time talking about how to prevent or successfully recover from it in the next section when we discuss goal setting.

So which stage are you in now? If you still aren't sure, spend a few minutes completing the self-evaluation exercise, then come back and join us.

It's Time To Chart Your Course

At this point, you know where you are and you know where you're headed. What's left is to chart your course between here and there, and goal setting is the best way to do that. "Too often people want to arrive without making the journey," says Gary Ryan Blair, founder of The GoalsGuy Learning Systems, Inc. (www.goalsguy.com) and author of numerous books on goal setting. "But that's not how it works."

There is no such thing as fitness magic and none of us has a guarantee that we'll be successful, but goal setting greatly increases your probability for success. "In Vegas," Blair says, "the odds are always with the house and there's not much you can do about that, but thankfully life is different from Vegas. In life, there are many things you can do to stack the deck in your favor, and goal setting is one of the best."

Goals are what bridge the gap between where you are now and your ultimate vision for the future. They're like mile markers that you check off to make sure you're headed in the right direction. You've probably heard about short-term and long-term goals, but chances are you haven't set goals specifically designed to move you from one level of fitness commitment to the next. That's what we'll do here.

If you recall at the beginning of this chapter, we talked about how at different points in your fitness journey, different goals are more effective than others. Even though lasting fitness combines mental and physical work throughout the process, experience and research both tell us that in the early stages mental goals are especially important, whereas down the road more action-oriented goals are often your best bet.

In just a minute we'll take a closer look at different kinds of goals for each stage of change. But first, let's spend a little bit of time talking about goal setting in general. What distinguishes a good goal from a bad goal?

Goal Setting—What Works, What Doesn't

The great thing about sports, says Blair, is that you always know the score and how much time is left. As a result, there's always a sense of urgency to get things done. A good goal is a lot like that—it lights a fire in you to get moving.

Blair says the most important characteristics of a good goal are that it is specific, measurable and time bound. Saying you want to get in shape is not specific or measurable or time bound. What does "in shape" mean? How do you know when you're there? How do you measure being "in shape"? And when do you plan to do this? It's much more motivating to say, "I will lose two inches off my waist in the next three months." That you can measure. That creates a sense of urgency.

Here are more examples of bad goals made good:

- **Instead of:** I'm going to start eating healthier.
- **Try this:** By the end of this month I will be eating fast food only one day a week.

Or

- **Instead of:** I'm going to start working out.
- **Say this:** I'm going to walk for 30 minutes on Monday, Wednesday and Friday of next week.

Or

- **Instead of:** I want to get stronger.
- **Say this:** I will increase my bench press max from 175 pounds to 200 pounds in the next three months.

Big difference, huh? A good goal tells you exactly where you're headed and when, so it's easy to gauge your progress and make adjustments if necessary.

One more point about goals: Your vision is your long-term goal, and it's probably at least six months to a year away. That's too far off to instill that critical sense of urgency, and besides, you'll need some check points along the way to gauge your progress and keep you on track.

Blair recommends creating an additional mid-term goal and several weekly or bi-weekly goals leading up to it. Once you've successfully reached your mid-point (which will probably mean you're at "I am"), start again with weekly or bi-weekly goals until you achieve your vision. Break the time up in whatever chunks work best for you, but the whole idea is to look at the process in specific, manageable steps and celebrate your achievements along the way.

Key Concepts to Remember

1. If you want to make lasting changes in your body, you've got to spend the time and effort to get your mind committed to the idea first.

2. Remember that neither mental nor physical change will happen overnight. They both occur in stages.

3. The stages-of-change concept illustrates the process we naturally go through as we exchange unhealthy habits for healthy ones.

4. Developing a fitness vision defines your endpoint or your ultimate goal and gives you something to work toward. It should include your motivating reason(s) for making this commitment.

5. Knowing which stage of change you're in now enables you to create effective mid-term and short-term goals that will bridge the gap between where you are and where you want to go.

6. Once you know your destination and your starting point, and you've charted your path, it's time to get going.

7. Challenges and setbacks are a normal part of the process. Prepare yourself ahead of time and develop back-up plans to keep yourself on track.

Here's an example of a vision, a mid-term and a short-term goal.

- ◆ **Vision:** Within the next six months, I will lose 20 pounds and 3 inches off my waist.
- ◆ **Mid-term Goal:** At the end of 12 weeks, I will have lost 10 pounds and 1 ½ inches off my waist.
- ◆ **Short-term Goal:** I will lose at least 1 pound this week by walking three days for a minimum of 30 minutes each and limiting my fast food intake to two days.

As you can see from the above example, your short-term goals are the ones that contain the actual behaviors you'll change or the steps you'll take to get where you want to go.

Match Your Goals To Your Stage of Change

Prochaska says that efficient change depends on doing the right things at the right time. So what is the right thing for where you are now, and how do you apply goal-setting techniques to your stage of change? Let's take each stage in turn and look at goals appropriate for each.

I won't or I can't

Very definitely in the "I won't" category, David, age 42, has high blood pressure and is 30 pounds overweight, but he doesn't think exercise is important in his life. He's busy climbing the corporate ladder and can't be bothered with that fitness nonsense.

At age 33, Beverly has tried every fad diet known to man (and woman) and failed at every one of them. A classic example of "I can't," she's convinced she's destined to carry around the extra 20 pounds she's lost and gained back numerous times. So she's decided the extra weight isn't really that bad and she might as well eat whatever she wants. At least food makes her happy, for a while.

If you recall, folks at this stage haven't yet accepted there's a problem that needs fixing. At this point, goals should be focused on mental homework that defines the problem and makes the impossible seem possible. You've most likely heard that knowledge is power, and it's never more true than it is here.

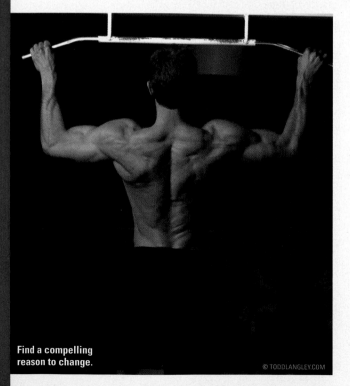

Find a compelling reason to change.

© TODDLANGLEY.COM

GOAL TIPS:

If you can relate to David, forcing yourself into exercising three days a week is destined to fail. Instead, how about reading a magazine article showing the health consequences of high blood pressure and talking to your doctor about the link between exercise, weight loss and blood pressure?

If you see yourself in Beverly, deciding to eat nothing but fruit starting tomorrow will not get you very far. A much more effective goal for this stage would be to read a credible review of fad diets so you'll understand why no one can succeed with them.

The bottom line is to set a goal of gathering the information necessary to convince your head you truly need to make a change, *and* that it's possible to succeed. Read, talk to doctors, friends, spouses—whatever it takes to raise your awareness of the changes you need to make and why.

SAMPLE GOALS:

➤ This week, I will read the article on exercise, weight loss and blood pressure that my doctor gave me during my last physical, and I'll talk to Brent about the weight he lost during his heart attack recovery.

➤ I'll start reading *Body-for-LIFE* by Bill Phillips to learn about people who have successfully lost weight.

➤ Before this weekend, I'll read that review on fad diets that Stephanie told me about.

I may

Janine is 38 years old and works about 60 hours a week as a CEO of a medium-sized corporation. When the subject is work, she's about as disciplined and accomplished as they come. But she's forgotten about her body and its needs, and now it's 40 pounds later and with high cholesterol to boot. Janine knows she needs to do something about her weight and health, and she's told herself several times she will … someday when things slow down at work.

There's still a considerable amount of mental work required at the "I may" stage. While you may have identified the problem and even kicked around some possible solutions, the thing that's missing is the deeply powerful and personal reason to get going.

What Is Your Fitness Personality?

Knowing your responses to the following five questions will help you select exercise activities that fit your personality style, and that, in turn, will increase your enjoyment. If you find that some types of exercise come up repeatedly in your answers, consider trying those first.

1 Do you tend to be more introverted or extroverted?
Introverted = Solo walking, jogging, weight training, yoga, pilates
Extroverted = Golf, group exercise classes, team sports

2 Do you like to be spontaneous or prefer a high degree of control over your environment?
Spontaneous = Racquet sports, team sports, surfing
Controlled = Weight training, cardio machines, yoga, pilates, golf, swimming

3 Are you more internally motivated (do things for self-satisfaction) or externally motivated (for the benefits rather than the experience)?
Internal – Walk or jog on a treadmill, cycle for fun, swim for fun, yoga or pilates for the experience itself
External = Exercise to lose weight, participate in group exercise classes for social interaction, compete in fitness contests, lift weights for body results

4 Do you enjoy more aggressive, forceful activities or less aggressive ones?
Aggressive = Kick-boxing, racquet sports, martial arts
Nonaggressive = Yoga, walking, dance

5 Do you tend to be an adventurous thrill-seeker or do you avoid risk?
Adventurous = Rock climbing, hang gliding, alpine skiing, mountain biking, martial arts
Risk-avoiding = Walking, jogging, stairstepper, weight training, yoga, swimming

Source: Adapted from the sport-personality congruence model developed by James Gavin, Ph.D. and presented in *The Exercise Habit* (Leisure Press, 1992). Printed with permission of author.

Without the internal "aha" experience to shift their motivation into high gear, people in this stage can go on forever. Sometimes it takes a heart attack, stroke or some other major health event to light a fire under these folks, but wouldn't it be better if you simply spend some time honestly examining your body and life and identifying your super-charged reason for change?

GOAL TIPS:

Decide what it will take to get you headed in the fitness direction. Maybe it's an upcoming high school reunion, maybe you or one of your kids is getting married soon and you're thinking about how you'll look in all those pictures. Whatever it is, the reason has to be deeply personal and relevant to your life. Until you have that internal driving force on your side, any physical action goals are destined to fail.

SAMPLE GOALS:

By next Monday, I'll create a pros and cons list related to making a fitness commitment, including all the reasons to get in shape that I'm really passionate about and all the reasons to put it off. If the pros for making a change are greater, I'll be ready to move on. (If they aren't greater, you either aren't being honest with yourself or you need more information.)

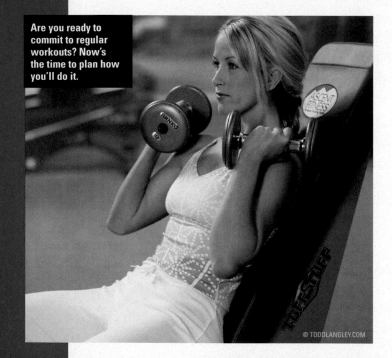

Are you ready to commit to regular workouts? Now's the time to plan how you'll do it.

© TODDLANGLEY.COM

I will

After toying with the idea of getting in shape, Richard decides at age 48 the time has come. The moment of truth came when he took his kids on a camping and hiking trip for the weekend. By the middle of the first day he was too tired to move, so he decided to start working out the very next week. He even joined a gym and bought some exercise clothes.

On his first day over his lunch hour, Richard arrives at the gym and stares at all the equipment. He realizes he has no idea what he should do, or wants to do, and all the trainers are busy helping other people. He's running out of time, so he fiddles around on a few pieces of equipment, gets frustrated and leaves.

At this stage, you're ready to make the commitment and you need to say it out loud to someone who can support your effort; however, it's not uncommon to continue feeling a bit of nagging uncertainty about your decision because you still aren't completely past the mental homework. Now's the time for planning exactly what you'll do and when you'll do it. Remember the old adage—if you fail to plan, you plan to fail.

GOAL TIPS:

Plan, plan, plan. If your mission includes exercise, decide what activities you'll do and learn anything you need to about them before getting started. Did you know research has shown that people who do activities that match their personality tend to enjoy exercise more and stay with it longer?[3] If you aren't sure what kind of exercise will fan your flame, see "What is Your Fitness Personality?" previously in this chapter. Then pick your workout days and plan whatever adjustments necessary in your schedule to insure success.

If you intend to tackle nutrition, what specific changes are you going to make? And for what meals on which days? If you're eliminating some unhealthy foods from your diet, what healthy alternatives will you replace them with and why? Do you even have those good foods in the house? Better go shopping!

SAMPLE GOALS:

- Within the next week, I'll create an exercise plan I can live with, adjust my schedule to accommodate it and make an appointment with a trainer at the gym to learn the equipment for my first workout.
- Within the next week, I'll make a list of all the foods I need to take healthy sack lunches to work and go buy them.

I am

At 30, Samantha finds herself at the end of her first month of regular exercise. After years of starting and stopping, she finally gave the mental homework a try, and it worked! Thinking back on the last month, she realizes there were two things that really helped her stay on track. One was getting her workout clothes ready the night before and setting her gym bag by the door to the garage—couldn't miss it that way! And another was giving herself little weekly rewards for a job well done. One week her reward was a new pair of exercise shoes, another week she took off from work early on Friday and went to a movie with a friend.

It Can Be Done—Here's Proof!

At age 50, Gary, an accounting software salesman, is witnessing first-hand the power of working through stages of change to adopt a healthy lifestyle. A year ago Gary was having a triple cheeseburger and biggie fries for lunch, M&Ms in the afternoon and whatever struck his fancy for dinner. "I always made New Year's resolutions to get in shape," says Gary, "but I never did my homework to set specific goals and gather the information I needed for a real commitment." Then a combination of events converged to thrust him from his longstanding "I may" position to "I am."

His wife made the fitness commitment, started working with a wellness coach and saw great results. Then some close friends were diagnosed with diabetes and heart disease, and Gary realized that unless he changed his ways in a hurry he was headed down the same road, especially given the history of diabetes and heart disease in his family.

He says, "Even though I knew I needed to do something about my weight and physical condition years ago, I just couldn't get going. But when all these things happened so close together, I finally decided it was time." Gary started working with the same coach who had helped his wife.

He says doing a lot of reading and planning in the beginning, as well as learning how to set very specific goals, has greatly contributed to his success. "My goals have definitely changed over time as I've learned more and made more progress," he says. "You can't just say, 'I want to lose weight.' Your goals have to be very detailed and you have to continually monitor your progress," Gary says.

"I've lost 28 pounds so far by walking for 30 minutes three times a week and cutting out sugary snacks, and while I still have a few pounds to go I know I'll get there. I understand what I have to do now, and I'm testing out new changes in my diet and exercise strategies to see how my body reacts," says Gary. "The biggest thing with all of this is that you have to decide to do it for yourself, not for someone else."

This is the first stage that's more physical than mental work (although your head isn't totally out of the game here either). Now is when you actually do those workouts instead of camping out on the couch and substitute whole-grain toast and low-fat yogurt for your old ritual of morning donuts. Just remember you aren't out of the woods yet because your changes are still too new to be habit-forming.

GOAL TIPS:

This is the action stage, so completing your scheduled workouts or sticking with your nutrition plan are obvious goals. But along with those, set a goal of developing some cues to support your efforts, like Samantha did with her gym bag. Another example of a cue: If you know that you can't resist the double caramel sundae at a certain ice cream shop, don't go! And we all need a reward for our efforts now and then. Set another goal to create an incentive (other than food) that you can plan to celebrate your accomplishments.

SAMPLE GOALS:

- I'll lift weights for 30 minutes on Tuesday, Thursday and Saturday of this week, and when I succeed I'll take Sunday to do that fishing trip I've been dying to go on.
- I know Thursdays are crazy at work, so I'll set my Palm Pilot to remind me of my workout at 4:30 p.m.

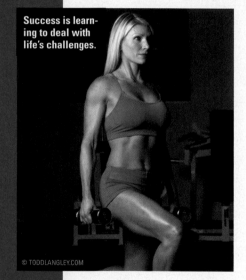

Success is learning to deal with life's challenges.

© TODDLANGLEY.COM

I still am

Just in time for her 28th birthday, Rachel finally arrived at her goal weight of 125 pounds, down from 165 pounds only a year ago. By reviving her high school love of swimming, adding in some weight training and limiting her desserts to one day a week, she was finally there.

All of Rachel's newfound energy and confidence paid off at work, too. When her boss transferred to another department, he recommended Rachel as his replacement. The bad news is that management was more demanding than Rachel bargained for, and now, six months later at 155 pounds she's trying to figure out what went wrong.

Even after several months of success or even if you're already an accomplished athlete, there will still be challenges like work responsibilities or injury that rear their ugly heads and threaten your commitment. The best way to prevent relapse, or falling off the wagon, is to plan ahead for setbacks and challenges. No one is immune, so always have a workout and nutrition plan B. And hey, if you don't succeed with plan B, just pick yourself up, dust yourself off, figure out how the train wreck happened and move on.

GOAL TIPS:

Make a list of all the challenges that can come up to derail your fitness plan on a weekly basis, then create plan B for each challenge. Consider things like last minute meetings, injuries or days when your motivation takes a plunge.

SAMPLE GOALS:

- By the end of this week, I'll have a back-up exercise plan for nights when I have to work late. (Some examples are switching your workout to morning or walking the stairs at work.)

- I'm going to take some healthy snacks like whole-grain crackers, dried fruit and nutrition bars to work next Monday, so the next time I have to stay late I won't binge on vending machine garbage.
- I'll read up on typical injuries and rehab for my sport this weekend so I'll be ready to switch gears just in case.
- By this coming Friday, I'll have a "break the mold" workout planned for days when I really don't feel like exercising. (Some ideas are following a new exercise video or going on a bike ride with the kids.)

Wrap Up

In case you haven't noticed yet, the fitness battle is won in your head first. And while it isn't rocket science on paper, the daily doing is hard work. If it were easy, everyone would be a perfect 10, and we all know that isn't the case.

Be prepared to take one step forward and two steps back. If you get off track, forgive yourself and keep going. No one is perfect. We all make mistakes. The key is to figure out what went wrong and prevent it from happening again. If you really get stuck and can't see your way out, consider hiring a fitness or wellness coach from a reputable organization like Wellcoaches, Inc. (www.wellcoaches.com). They're specialists in goal setting and guiding people through the stages of change. They might give you the extra push you need to get over the hump.

One last thing: You may want to redefine success. Most of us say things to ourselves like, "Yeah, I've lost 5 pounds, but I still have another 20 to go. I'm not even close yet." Or "After a whole month, I've only lost 1 inch off my waist. I've still got three more to go. Am I ever going to get there?"

You may not get there with that kind of negative self-talk. Five pounds is a lot of fat. Have you ever seen what 5 pounds of pure fat looks like? And 1 inch off your waist is a big difference—that's a whole size. Rather than beating yourself up for not doing it faster, why not try patting yourself on the back for every step forward you take. The road to success is paved with 1,000 steps. I can't remember who said that, but it's surely appropriate here.

And speaking of steps, are you ready to take a big one? We've created a tear-out worksheet that will walk you through the whole process … you guessed it, step by step. Just turn to the Appendix and fill in the blanks.

So what happens next when you achieve your vision (and you will if you follow this program)? That's easy. You create a new vision and do it all again. Eleanor Roosevelt once said that when you cease to grow, you begin to die. Did she mean physically, mentally or spiritually? Perhaps she was referring to all three.

> **tip**
> The best way to prevent relapse, or falling off the wagon, is to plan ahead for setbacks and challenges. No one is immune, so always have a workout and nutrition plan B.

REFERENCES CITED:

[1] *Complementary and Alternative Medicine at the NIH (newsletter)* 10.3 (Summer 2003) p. 2.

[2] Davidson, RJ et al. Alterations in brain and immune function produced by mindfulness meditation. *Psychosomatic Medicine* 65.4 (2003): 564-570.

[3] Gavin, J. *The Exercise Habit* (Leisure Press, 1992).

[4] *National Health and Nutrition Examination Survey.* Centers for Disease Control and Prevention National Center for Health Statistics, 2000.

[5] Prochaska, J et al. *Changing for Good: A Revolutionary Six-Stage Program for Overcoming Bad Habits and Moving Your Life Positively Forward* (Quill, 2002).

13 THE IRON GAME
The Basic Fundamentals of Weight Training

By Charles Staley, B.Sc., M.S.S.

When properly performed, resistance training (otherwise known as weight training or weight lifting) has a proven track record of providing fast, safe results as compared to other forms of exercise. Depending on the type of resistance training you use, these results can mean everything from muscle gain or fat loss; increased strength and power; enhanced sports performance; and injury prevention and rehabilitation. In fact, it's hard to find any other single activity that can provide so many benefits with such a minimum investment of time, effort, energy and equipment.

Despite these benefits, many exercisers (both novice and experienced alike) often find themselves confused and frustrated as they encounter apparently conflicting advice from books, magazines, TV shows and personal trainers. Some of the more common questions include the following:

> "How many times a week should I train?"
>
> "Should I use machines or free weights?"
>
> "Should I do one set, three sets or 10 sets?"
>
> "Should I lift slowly or explosively?"
>
> "How can I tighten up my lower abs?"
>
> "I can't get sore—what do I do?"

The list goes on, but chances are you've asked some of these questions yourself. This chapter will greatly speed up your learning curve and put you on the path to greater understanding and better results. So with that, here's an overview of what this chapter will cover:

- The primary principles of successful resistance training and why you need to understand them.
- Successful lifting and loading strategies, such as pyramids, EDT, ladders, compensatory acceleration training (CAT) and others.
- Practical program-design concepts (e.g., setting up the "weekly split"; determining

the ideal number of sets and reps; determining the proper number of exercises per session; and so forth.)
- A sample resistance training program that employs the above-mentioned principles, concepts and strategies.
- Finally, this chapter will provide some invaluable books, videos, Web sites and other resources that will enable you to continue your education.

TRAINING PRINCIPLES

Principles are the foundation of knowledge and practice. Whenever you find yourself confused or have a question about resistance training, these principles will provide the answer. Principles do not lack practicality as many people wrongly assume. Think you already know this stuff? This chapter has some unique insights that even advanced lifters can benefit from!

The Principle Of Progressive Overload

The principle of progressive overload is the "Mother" principle, the bedrock upon which all other principles depend. If your resistance training program doesn't abide by this principle, it isn't really resistance training.

The Story Of Milo

Some of you may have heard of the story of the Greek athlete Milo of Crotona, famous for his feats of strength. The entire field of resistance training is founded on and explained by this simple story. Basically, Milo was a young man who dedicated his life to becoming stronger. Milo took a very young calf and lifted it up onto his shoulders once a day, every day. As the calf grew, Milo found himself lifting a gradually heavier load every day, until eventually, he could lift a full-grown steer.

Milo's little experiment demonstrated the fact that the human body, like any living system, is *adaptable*. This means that the body can change itself in order to cope with new stresses that it might encounter. If you lie out in the sun, you'll get a tan (or a sunburn if you lie out too long). If you use a wrench every day, you'll get calluses (or blisters if you do too much too soon). Similarly, if you contract your muscles against a greater resistance than they are used to, they'll grow bigger and/or stronger. (Later in the chapter you'll see how you can tweak your resistance training program so your gains involve mostly increased muscle mass, or strength, speed or power without much extra muscle mass.)

That's the principle of progressive overload in a nutshell: Simply expose your body to progressively greater and greater challenges, and it will adapt accordingly. In resistance training, there are a number of ways you can employ the overload principle, and all of them can and will work. They include lifting a heavier weight, lifting the same weight for more reps or for more sets, lifting a weight over a greater range of motion, lifting the weight slower or faster or lifting a weight in an unaccustomed manner (for example, performing ab crunches on a Swiss ball instead of on the floor).

tip

How To Apply the Principle of Progressive Overload

- Lift heavier weights
- Lift the same weight for more reps
- Lift a weight over a greater range of motion
- Lift a weight slower or faster

SPORT AND GOAL-SPECIFIC NUTRITION AND TRAINING

Understanding the Intensity-Volume Relationship

Generally, there are two aspects of what's called "the training load" that you can manipulate over the course of a training cycle: intensity and volume.

❶ INTENSITY:

Intensity simply means the absolute difficulty of the resistance you're using. You can also think of it as the "quality" of the load. In resistance training, intensity is usually expressed as a percentage of "1RM" (or "one rep max"). Your 1RM is defined as the most weight you can lift for one rep (but not two). So for example, if you can squat 200 pounds for one rep, and today you've decided to lift 160 pounds for 5 sets of 5 reps, you'd be using 80 percent of your current 1RM for that exercise. If next week you decide you're going to attempt to use 170 pounds for the same sets and reps, you'd be using 85 percent of 1RM.

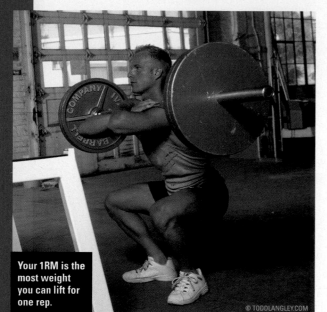

Your 1RM is the most weight you can lift for one rep.

© TODDLANGLEY.COM

Basing your weights on 1RMs has benefits as well as drawbacks: It's seemingly precise and methodical; however, there is a problem—your 1RMs are likely to vary quite a bit over the course of a day, week or month. Another problem is that 1RM testing is potentially dangerous, especially for beginners who may lack the technical precision and experience to handle maximum weights.

Fortunately, there is an easier way for most lifters to respect the overload principle in their training: simply lift the heaviest weight possible in correct form for the set/rep format you're using. Going back to the earlier example, if you squat 160 pounds for 5 sets of 5, and the last set was very difficult to complete, then in all probability you created a good training stimulus for your body, regardless of what the actual percentage of 1RM you were using. When you repeat that workout, you should try to use slightly more weight for the same sets and reps, or you can attempt slightly more total work with the same weight—perhaps 6 sets of 5 reps. In either case, you've created a slightly greater challenge for your body. There are many ways to apply this principle (and we'll cover them in more detail later on).

Whichever method you choose to use in your own training, there are some fairly established relationships between load intensity and the primary result you'll experience from your training. Table 1 explains these relationships.

❷ VOLUME:

Training volume simply refers to the *amount* of work that you perform in a given time period. You could track your volume for a single workout, or for one week or for a month's worth of training. While intensity is the *quality* of your training, volume is the *quantity*. Successful resistance training requires progressive increases in both intensity and volume at one point or another, but rarely at the same time. If your training is high quality, it won't be high quantity, and vice versa. Think of it this way: You can't run a marathon at 100-meter sprint speed, nor can you perform 8 reps with your 1RM. So, as a general rule, the heavier the load, the less total work you'll perform with it.

As you might expect, there are a few additional factors to consider:

 New challenges to your body must be *gradually* progressive. If you can currently curl 95 pounds for three sets of 12 repetitions, and you perform this workout once every five days, you shouldn't try to increase the load or the reps per set by more than maybe 5 percent per workout—doing so is unnecessary and invites the possibility of injury.

 Your progress (which could mean lean muscle gains and/or strength increases) won't continue at the same rate throughout your lifting career. Progress will be fast at the beginning and will gradually slow down as you become more experienced. It's not unusual for a beginner to double his or her strength in a handful of months, but once you've been in the game for several years, you'll be lucky to experience even a tenth of that progress in the same time frame. That's great news for beginners, and for you advanced lifters, it just means you'll need to get a bit sneakier to coax a bit more from your body.

 As you might expect, if you reduce your training intensity and/or volume, or if you remove them altogether, your body's adaptations will eventually disappear. This is sometimes called "The Principle Of Reversibility." Put another way: "Use it or lose it." In essence, if you want to be stronger and/or more muscular, you've got to train hard and adopt smart nutritional practices.

The Principle of Specificity

The principle of specificity simply means that a specific type of training will yield a specific result. There are a lot of applications of this principle—some are obvious, some are not. Here are a few obvious examples of the specificity principle in action:

 If you want to get stronger without getting bigger, you need to emphasize low reps and heavy weights.

 If you want bigger arms, you need to emphasize arm exercises in your training.

 If you want better muscular endurance, you need to use high-repetition protocols in your workouts.

 If you want a bigger bench press, you need to concentrate on that specific exercise.

Now, a less obvious example of the specificity principle: Some muscles, such as the hamstrings, are composed of primarily fast twitch muscle fibers; therefore, the principle of specificity would suggest that you train these muscles using heavy weight and/or maximum speed, since fast twitch fibers are more responsive to high-tension stresses.

SPORT AND GOAL-SPECIFIC NUTRITION AND TRAINING

Table 1: The Relationship Between Training Load and Primary Training Effect

REPETITION BRACKET	APPROXIMATE PERCENT OF 1RM	PRIMARY ADAPTATION
1 - 5 reps	85 - 100	strength
6 - 8 reps	77.5 - 85	strength/mass gains
9 - 12 reps	70 - 77.5	mass gains
13 - 20 reps	60 - 70	strength endurance

The relationships in this table assume that the reps performed are done with the largest possible weight; for example, 1 to 5 reps equates to 85 to 100 percent of 1RM only if maximum weights are used. If you did 5 reps but 10 were possible, you'd use about 75 percent of 1RM.

These numbers are only approximations, but they serve as a good starting point; for example, even low repetitions can lead to significant muscle size gains if enough sets are performed.

"Strength" in this case refers to an increase in "1RM" strength without a significant increase in size. "Mass gains" refers to increases in muscle size without a significant increase in strength. "Strength endurance" refers to the ability to lift moderate weights for many repetitions despite fatigue.

Beginners tend to adapt more generally, whereas advanced lifters tend to adapt more specifically. This means that for beginners, almost any repetition bracket will tend to lead to increases in all of these attributes, whereas advanced exercisers will tend to experience only the adaptations noted above.

The Principle of Variation

The principle of variation means that you must periodically change your workout or your body will reduce its adaptive response. Bottom line: Your progress stagnates. There are many ways to change your training choices, including using different exercises, split construction, training techniques, training frequency and loading parameters.

The Principle of Individuality

Despite the reliability of the previously discussed principles, the principle of individuality must be considered when putting your training program together.

Everyone who performs the sample program provided later in the chapter will experience a slightly different result. And to complicate things a bit more, if those same people again perform that same program five years from now, they'll get a whole new batch of slightly different results because *people's bodies change over time.*

Think about it. If you perform a particular program for the next 12 weeks, you become fitter (this might mean stronger, or it could also mean leaner, more flexible, etc.). So if you then use exactly the same program again, your body is better prepared to deal with that challenge; therefore, it won't react as strongly the second time around. This fact has lead to the popular saying "all programs become less and less effective every time you use them."

Time-Tested Training Principles

The Principle Of Primary Constraints: This principle simply refers to the fact that continuous progress depends upon identifying and then eliminating your weakest correctable link, or the "bottleneck" in your overall training. You can apply this principle across many levels; for example, one often hears the question, "What's more important, training or diet?" If your training is well thought out and you're disciplined in the gym, but you're eating Cap'n Crunch® for breakfast, then for you, diet is the most important element to focus on, since it has more room for improvement. Hopefully the point is made that a strength overused becomes a weakness, so spend your time on muscle groups, athletic qualities, habit patterns and so on that are weak in relation to everything else.

The Principle Of Fatigue Management: Many of us mistakenly judge the value of a workout by how much it hurts or by how sore it leaves us, but in order to create a training effect, you have to perform a certain amount of work (hence the term "workout"). "X" amount of work leads to "x" amount of training effect; for example, if you ride your bike for a mile at a certain speed, you burn a certain amount of calories, creating an impact on the endocrine and metabolic processes and so forth. On a muscular level, if you expose a muscle to a certain amount of work, it will lead to a loss of intra-muscular cellular proteins, which are subsequently not only replaced, but in fact, replaced in spades. So just in case you decide to do it again, you'll have just a bit more muscle to make things easier for your body.

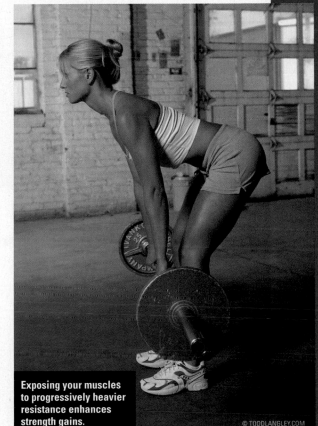

Exposing your muscles to progressively heavier resistance enhances strength gains.

© TODDLANGLEY.COM

Here are three strategies for inreasing your ability to perform as much work as possible over the course of a training session:

❶ Fatigue Management Strategy #1: Increased rest intervals: Since fatigue accumulates over the course of a workout, it makes little sense to use the same rest interval between every set. A better approach is to take shorter rests between early sets and longer rests between later sets.

2 Fatigue Management Strategy #2: Use antagonistic pairings: Muscles work in pairs. As one muscle contracts to flex a joint (such as the biceps of the upper arm), then its antagonistic partner (the triceps in this example) must elongate and relax to permit the contraction. If both muscles contract simultaneously, no movement can take place, meaning when one muscle contracts, its antagonistic partner is recovering. You can take advantage of this phenomenon by performing your exercises in antagonistic pairs—biceps with triceps, quads with hamstrings, pecs with lats and so forth. This technique allows you to perform more work in the same period of time and also ensures balanced muscle development around your joints.

3 Fatigue Management Strategy #3: Minimize redundancy: Once you've worked a muscle group or a motor quality sufficiently, move on to the next task, or get out of the gym. It's common to see people working the same muscle with five to six different exercises in the same workout. What purpose does it serve to do barbell bench presses followed by dumbbell bench presses followed by Smith bench presses? If you feel a pressing need to do so many exercises, increase the number of workouts instead.

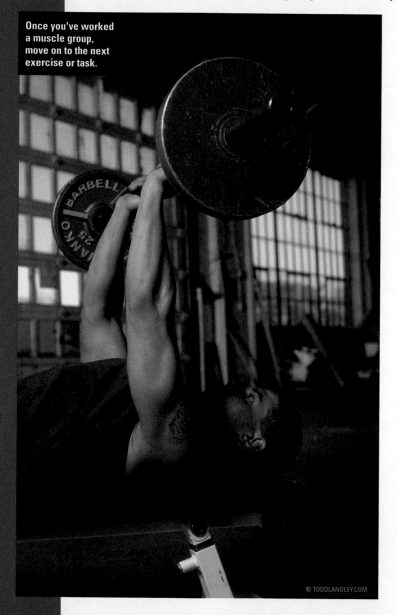

Once you've worked a muscle group, move on to the next exercise or task.

© TODDLANGLEY.COM

CHARLES STALEY'S FIVE STEP METHOD FOR CREATING YOUR OWN RESISTANCE TRAINING PROGRAMS

It's time to create an effective weekly training "split," including determining exercise selection, selection of loading strategies and optional set/rep protocols. This is where we get into questions like:

"What exercises should I use?"

"How many sets should I use for each exercise?"

"How many reps per set should I perform?"

"How much rest should I take between sets?"

"How often should I train?"

Step One: List the Muscles You Plan To Train on a Weekly Basis

Most people will train all muscle groups, but some people, due to injuries, equipment restrictions or other factors, may omit one or more major muscle group. For the purposes of this discussion, let's assume you'll be training your whole body. Your list will look like this:

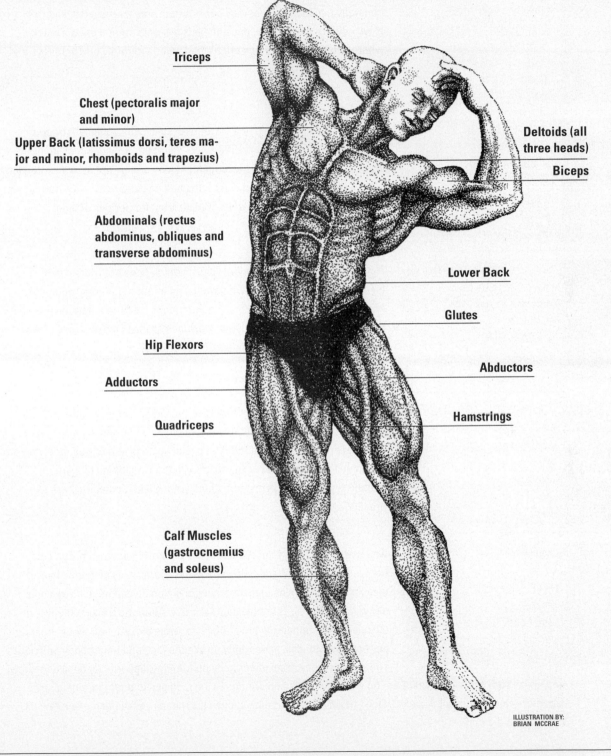

Triceps

Chest (pectoralis major and minor)

Upper Back (latissimus dorsi, teres major and minor, rhomboids and trapezius)

Abdominals (rectus abdominus, obliques and transverse abdominus)

Hip Flexors

Adductors

Quadriceps

Calf Muscles (gastrocnemius and soleus)

Deltoids (all three heads)

Biceps

Lower Back

Glutes

Abductors

Hamstrings

ILLUSTRATION BY:
BRIAN MCCRAE

Step Two: Assign Each Muscle Group to a Day of the Week

There are many possible ways to do this—here are a few examples to get you started:

Monday:	pecs, lats, shoulders
Tuesday:	quads and hamstrings
Wednesday:	off
Thursday:	biceps and triceps
Friday:	off
Saturday:	calves and abs
Sunday:	off

Notes: In this split, you're lifting four days a week. Larger muscle groups generally need longer recovery periods than smaller muscles, and this is why quads, hamstrings, pecs and lats are only trained once a week, whereas biceps and triceps are trained twice—directly on Thursdays and indirectly on Mondays.

Monday:	quads and hamstrings
Tuesday:	off
Wednesday:	biceps and triceps
Thursday:	off
Friday:	pecs, lats, shoulders
Saturday:	off
Sunday:	off

Notes: This is an example of a "three-day split" with a similar structure to the first split. The primary difference is that this split contains no direct work for abs or calves. This arrangement may or may not be warranted for your particular situation, but if your abs and calves are already strong and well developed it may work quite well, at least for periods of time.

Monday:	quads, hamstrings and abs
Tuesday:	off
Wednesday:	pecs and biceps
Thursday:	off
Friday:	lats and triceps
Saturday:	shoulders
Sunday:	off

Notes: Here we have a four-day split, in which pecs are trained with biceps on one day, and lats with triceps on another day. The rationale? Most pec exercises heavily involve the triceps, and the antagonists of the triceps are your biceps. Similarly, most lat exercises make strong use of the biceps, which are antagonistic to the triceps.

Monday:	whole body
Tuesday:	off
Wednesday:	whole body
Thursday:	off
Friday:	whole body
Saturday:	off
Sunday:	off

Notes: "Whole body training" refers to the use of large, "multi-joint" exercises such as squats, bench presses, deadlifts, chin-ups, dips and so on. These exercises challenge large muscular regions and for the most part eliminate the need for direct exercises for the smaller muscle groups. This method is ideal for athletes and others whose time and energy are at a premium.

Monday:	upper body
Tuesday:	cardio
Wednesday:	lower body
Thursday:	cardio
Friday:	upper body
Saturday:	cardio
Sunday:	off

Notes: Weight train intensely, for no more than 46 minutes, three times per week: Monday, Wednesday and Friday. Perform 20 minutes of aerobic exercise, first thing in the morning on an empty stomach three times per week: Tuesday, Thursday and Saturday. Alternate training the major muscles of the upper and lower body; for example, the first week, train upper body on Monday, lower body on Wednesday and upper body on Friday. The second week, train lower body on Monday, upper body on Wednesday and lower body on Friday. There are no absolute rights and wrongs when it comes to putting training splits together—many possibilities exist. Don't be afraid to be creative, even if it means you might make a few mistakes along the way.

Step Three: Assign Exercises For Each Muscle Group

Once you've constructed a split, designate exercises for each muscle group. Using one of the splits we looked at earlier, here is an example:

Notes about the exercises selected for this example:

1 A common question at this point might be "How do I know how many exercises I should do for a muscle group in one workout?" As you might expect, the answer will vary, but in general, larger, more complex muscles (such as pecs, lats and the leg muscles) benefit from as many as two (and less commonly, three) exercises during each session. Smaller, less-complex muscles (such as biceps, triceps and calves) profit from one to two exercises per session. Notice the two pec exercises on the Wednesday workout—the bench presses utilize a barbell and the arms extend perpendicular to the torso, whereas the incline presses use dumbbells and a different arm-extension angle. That's an example of "minimizing redundancy" in program design. Look at the other days in this cycle and you'll notice the same principle in use.

2 Notice the alternation between lower body days and upper body days in the above split. This is an effective and commonly used pattern.

3 You'll notice that abs are trained only once a week here, and you may be wondering why. Although there could be a good rationale for doing this in certain situations, it's also important to realize that there is no single, ideal training split—all splits have positive and negative aspects. It's recommended that you create a new training split every four to eight weeks (or after 12 weeks if you're doing the Body-*for*-LIFE Program) as a way to increase the benefits and minimize the drawbacks of whatever split you're using.

4 You may also notice that there is minimal use of machines in the above example. In general (although there are exceptions) free weights provide a more complete, more intense and arguably healthier training effect as opposed to machines.

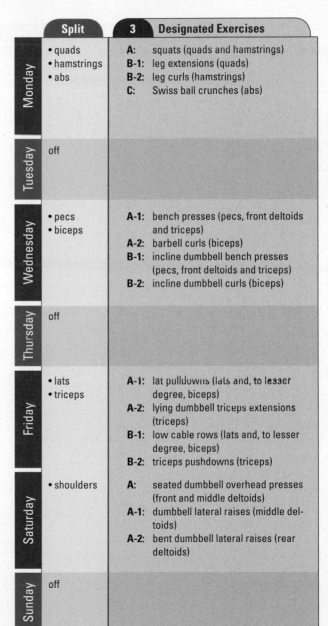

Split	3	Designated Exercises
Monday	• quads • hamstrings • abs	**A:** squats (quads and hamstrings) **B-1:** leg extensions (quads) **B-2:** leg curls (hamstrings) **C:** Swiss ball crunches (abs)
Tuesday	off	
Wednesday	• pecs • biceps	**A-1:** bench presses (pecs, front deltoids and triceps) **A-2:** barbell curls (biceps) **B-1:** incline dumbbell bench presses (pecs, front deltoids and triceps) **B-2:** incline dumbbell curls (biceps)
Thursday	off	
Friday	• lats • triceps	**A-1:** lat pulldowns (lats and, to lesser degree, biceps) **A-2:** lying dumbbell triceps extensions (triceps) **B-1:** low cable rows (lats and, to lesser degree, biceps) **B-2:** triceps pushdowns (triceps)
Saturday	• shoulders	**A:** seated dumbbell overhead presses (front and middle deltoids) **A-1:** dumbbell lateral raises (middle deltoids) **A-2:** bent dumbbell lateral raises (rear deltoids)
Sunday	off	

Step Four: Determine Loading Parameters for the Selected Exercises

Now that we've assigned exercises for the muscle groups we're training, it's time to assign "loading parameters," which simply mean the selection of sets, reps, rest intervals and intensity ranges for the exercises you're performing.

Using the same split we've been working with, here are two examples of loading parameters: one for strength development as the primary desired outcome and the other for muscle mass gain as the expected outcome.

A Hypothetical Example of Loading Parameters for Strength Development

	Split	3 Designated Exercises	4 Loading for Strength Development
Monday	• quads • hamstrings • abs	**A:** squats (quads and hamstrings) **B-1:** leg extensions (quads) **B-2:** leg curls (hamstrings) **C:** Swiss ball crunches (abs)	6 sets of 2 reps with 3-minute rests between sets 3 sets of 5 reps with 2.5-minute rests between sets 3 sets of 5 reps with 2.5-minute rests between sets 2 sets of 12 reps with 2.5-minute rests between sets
Tuesday	off		
Wednesday	• pecs • biceps	**A-1:** bench presses (pecs, front deltoids and triceps) **A-2:** barbell curls (biceps) **B-1:** incline dumbbell bench presses (pecs, front deltoids and triceps) **B-2:** incline dumbbell curls (biceps)	6 sets of 2 reps with 3-minute rests between sets 3 sets of 5 reps with 2.5-minute rests between sets 3 sets of 5 reps with 2.5-minute rests between sets 3 sets of 8 reps with 2.5-minute rests between sets
Thursday	off		
Friday	• lats • triceps	**A-1:** lat pulldowns (lats and, to lesser degree, biceps) **A-2:** lying dumbbell triceps extensions (triceps) **B-1:** low cable rows (lats and, to lesser degree, biceps) **B-2:** triceps pushdowns (triceps)	6 sets of 2 reps with 3-minute rests between sets 3 sets of 5 reps with 2.5-minute rests between sets 3 sets of 5 reps with 2.5-minute rests between sets 3 sets of 8 reps with 2.5-minute rests between sets
Saturday	• shoulders	**A:** seated dumbbell overhead presses (front and middle deltoids) **A-1:** dumbbell lateral raises (middle deltoids) **A-2:** bent dumbbell lateral raises (rear deltoids)	6 sets of 2 reps with 3-minute rests between sets 2 sets of 10 reps with 2.5-minute rests between sets 2 sets of 10 reps with 2.5-minute rests between sets
Sunday	off		

A Hypothetical Example of Loading Parameters for Muscle Mass Development

	Split	3 Designated Exercises	4 Loading for Muscle Mass Development
Monday	• quads • hamstrings • abs	**A:** squats (quads and hamstrings) **B-1:** leg extensions (quads) **B-2:** leg curls (hamstrings) **C:** Swiss ball crunches (abs)	4 sets of 8-10 reps with 2.5-minute rests between sets 4 sets of 8-10 reps with 2.5-minute rests between sets 4 sets of 8-10 reps with 2.5-minute rests between sets 4 sets of 8-10 reps with 2.5-minute rests between sets
Tuesday	off		
Wednesday	• pecs • biceps	**A-1:** bench presses (pecs, front deltoids, and triceps) **A-2:** barbell curls (biceps) **B-1:** incline dumbbell bench presses (pecs, front deltoids and triceps) **B-2:** incline dumbbell curls (biceps)	4 sets of 8-10 reps with 2.5-minute rests between sets 4 sets of 8-10 reps with 2.5-minute rests between sets 2 sets of 10-12 reps with 2.5-minute rests between sets 2 sets of 10-12 reps with 2.5-minute rests between sets
Thursday	off		
Friday	• lats • triceps	**A-1:** lat pulldowns (lats and, to lesser degree, biceps) **A-2:** lying dumbbell triceps extensions (triceps) **B-1:** low cable rows (lats and, to lesser degree, biceps) **B-2:** triceps pushdowns (triceps)	4 sets of 8-10 reps with 2.5-minute rests between sets 4 sets of 10-12 reps with 2.5-minute rests between sets 2 sets of 10-12 reps with 2.5-minute rests between sets 2 sets of 10-12 reps with 2.5-minute rests between sets
Saturday	• shoulders	**A:** seated dumbbell overhead presses (front and middle deltoids) **A-1:** dumbbell lateral raises (middle deltoids) **A-2:** bent dumbbell lateral raises (rear deltoids)	4 sets of 8-10 reps with 2.5-minute rests between sets 2 sets of 10-12 reps with 2.5-minute rests between sets 2 sets of 10-12 reps with 2.5-minute rests between sets
Sunday	off		

Notes on the Loading Parameters Selected for Both Examples:

❶ The alphanumeric designation used in these examples shows which exercises are performed alone, and which ones are supersetted. When, for example, you see "A-1" and "A-2" it means that these exercises are performed together (one set of A-1, followed by one set of A-2, etc., until all sets are completed).

❷ The primary thing to notice here is that, in general, the cycle designed for strength development relies more on heavier weight and lower repetition sets with longer rests between sets as compared to the muscle mass cycle.

SPORT AND GOAL-SPECIFIC NUTRITION AND TRAINING

3 Don't become too focused on the exact numbers here. Four sets of 8 will lead to a very similar result as 4 sets of 7 or 4 sets of 9.

4 You may also notice that on the strength cycle above, not all of the exercises use low reps and heavy weights. Some muscle groups and exercises cannot be safely trained using these loading parameters. Lateral raises are an example of this.

5 Despite the examples, muscle mass can indeed be achieved through heavier weight protocols, if enough total work is performed.

6 Since strength is largely foundational to muscle size, and since you would eventually lose strength if you always trained for muscle mass, it's a smart idea to alternate between three- to six-week cycles devoted to strength development and four- to six-week cycles dedicated to lean mass development.

7 There are "fixed" rest intervals in the examples so you'll have a general sense of how much rest you should expect to need between sets, but as mentioned earlier, it makes a lot more sense to rest a bit less between early sets and a bit longer between later sets.

Step Five: Develop a Progression Strategy

The fifth and final step in creating successful resistance training programs is to find a way to increase the training stress from workout to workout. Do you simply use more weight each time? And if so, how much? Or do you add more reps? Or both?

In reality, any or all of these methods are perfectly valid, depending on the goal at hand. What follows are the most commonly used methods with my commentary on each:

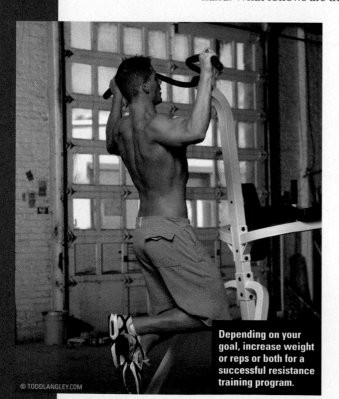

Depending on your goal, increase weight or reps or both for a successful resistance training program.

© TODDLANGLEY.COM

Gradually increase weight, keeping sets, reps and rest periods constant: This is a very common and effective strategy. It's a simple, clean way to keep track of your progress.

Gradually increase the number of reps per set while keeping the weigh constant: This method is another sound approach—perhaps more applicable to muscle training than it is for strength development.

Keep weight, sets and reps constant while gradually reducing rests between sets: This method works by increasing the density (or work/rest ratio) of your workouts. It's particularly effective for body composition objectives.

One last suggestion regarding progression: whichever method(s) you use, don't go all out on the first week of a new training cycle. Chances are you'll be using new and/or unfamiliar exercises, meaning you'll derive a training effect from the novelty of the change in your exercise menu. It's not necessary to push on the first week—you'll probably be sore even from a moderate effort on week one. You can try using four-week cycles, each with a new exercise menu, while remembering to really exert yourself at the maximum *only* on the last week of each cycle.

A TOOLBOX OF LIFTING SYSTEMS AND TECHNIQUES

Sets and Reps Method: This is the "bread and butter" and perhaps oldest of all methods. In essence, the goal is to perform a predetermined number of sets and reps with the same weight for every set. A common example of the sets and reps method is three sets of 10 reps, also known as the Delorme method. Any set/rep format may be used, however, from 3x3 to 1x100. The advantages of this method are simplicity and ease of documenting the workout.

Escalating Density Training (EDT): EDT is my own proprietary training system, based on the principles of fatigue management. EDT training involves discrete periods of time (called "PR Zones"), in which all sets and reps are to be completed. Typically, two antagonistic exercises (such as a quadriceps exercise and a hamstring exercise) are performed together, back to back, within a single PR Zone. Once you've identified your antagonistic exercises, the following instructions should be followed:

- After warming up for each exercise, select a load that approximates your 10RM ability (meaning, a weight you can lift 10, but not 11 times) for each exercise. Ideally, the weight used for each exercise should be equally difficult.

- Sets, reps and rest intervals: EDT training (the format employed in this program) does not use "fixed" set/rep patterns or rest intervals. Here's how it works: Begin each PR Zone by performing sets of 5 with very short (10- to 15-second) rests. As you begin to fatigue, you'll increase your rest intervals as you drop down to sets of four, then three, then two, and as the time limit approaches, you might crank out a few singles in an effort to accomplish as many repetitions as possible in the time allotted.

- Forget about training to failure. Try to do half of what is possible (e.g., 5 reps with a 10RM weight) at the beginning of the time frame. As the end of the PR Zone approaches, however, you'll find yourself working at or near failure as you attempt to break your rep record, but don't "try" to go to failure.

- Progression: Unless otherwise noted, each time you repeat the same workout, your objective is to simply perform more total repetitions in the same time frame. As soon as you can increase the total number of reps by 20 percent or more, start the next workout with 5 percent more weight and start over. Similarly, if you manage to improve upon your last performance for the same workout by 40 percent, then you'll increase your weights by 10 percent on the next workout.

- Biomechanics: The cornerstone of EDT is based on the concept of doing gradually more and more work in the same unit of time from workout to workout; therefore, it's critical that your exercise biomechanics (i.e., technique) are consistent on every workout. If you perform strict curls on one workout and loose form the next, you aren't really doing more work (for the arms at least!).

⊘ Crowd control: If you're performing EDT workouts during "rush hour" in a crowded commercial gym, you may occasionally have problems with other gym members interrupting the pace of your workout by using one of your exercise stations while you're performing another exercise. If someone asks to use your station, one effective strategy is to just look at your watch and say "I'll be done in 4 (or whatever) minutes, if that's OK." More often than not, they'll walk away thinking, "Wow, that guy has a plan!" Now, despite these measures, you may still occasionally run into problems. If this happens, simply extend the PR Zone as long as it takes to get your reps in. Part of the beauty of EDT is its precision, but on the other hand, don't get unnecessarily freaked out if you occasionally need to extend a PR Zone by a few minutes to get your reps in. The point is, you did the work; you'll get the results.

Ladder Method: The ladder method is a highly effective training method popularized by Pavel Tsatsouline: Choose a load that can be lifted for six to seven reps. Start with one rep, then two reps for the second set, three reps for the next set, and so on, until you're one to two reps away from failure. Then start a new ladder, starting again with one rep, then two reps, etc. It should look something like the example on the left:

Rest periods are completely intuitive; just rack up as many total reps as possible in the allotted time period. One big advantage of this method is that your warm-up sets are integrated into the workout itself. You just walk into the gym and get right into your first ladder.

Pyramids: Pyramids have been around forever, but many people were first exposed to this method through Bill Phillips' best-selling book, *Body-for-LIFE*. Pyramids involve performing several sets, with each successive set involving more weight and correspondingly fewer reps. A typical example for a trainee capable of a 315-pound 1RM might look like the Pyramid Method example on the left:

Often, pyramids also involve a "descending" component, in which one or more "back-off" sets are performed after the heaviest weight has been reached. See the example on the next page.

The rationale behind these sets is that your nervous system will be "primed" from the heavy weights lifted in the fourth and fifth sets, allowing even more reps than normal on the back-off sets. The advantage of the pyramid system is that the earlier sets serve as a warm-up for the later sets; however, one potential problem is that you may run the risk of creating too much fatigue on the way up the pyramid, hampering your performance on the heaviest sets.

To adapt Phillips' pyramid to your own workouts, use this set/rep scheme. Keep in mind that Phillips recommends increasing the weight of your lifts based on an effort scale of one (lowest) to 10 (highest). Start your first set with an effort level of five and work your way up with every set. With your sixth and final set, choose an exercise that

Ladder Method	
Set One:	one rep
Set Two:	two reps
Set Three:	three reps
Set Four:	four reps
Set Five:	five reps
Set Six:	one rep
Set Seven:	two reps
Set Eight:	three reps
Set Nine:	four reps
Set Ten:	one rep

Pyramid Method (example for a trainee capable of a 315-pound 1RM)	
Set One:	205x12
Set Two:	225x10
Set Three:	245x8
Set Four:	265x6
Set Five:	285x4
Set Six:	245x10
Set Seven:	205x15

SPORT AND GOAL-SPECIFIC NUTRITION AND TRAINING

Example Pyramid Workout: Dumbbell Bench Presses						
Set	40x12	50x10	60x8	70x6	60x12	40x12
Minutes between sets	1	1	1	1	1	0
Intensity level	5	6	7	8	9	10

Wait two minutes before moving to another body part/muscle group.

corresponds to the current body part. For our purposes, we'll look at dumbbell bench presses for five sets, concluding with dumbbell flyes for the final set.

Drop Sets: Drop setting involves lifting a given weight for as many reps as possible, and then quickly reducing the weight (which is often done by a training partner) and then completing as many additional reps as possible with the newly reduced weight. Sometimes lifters will use as many as three or four "drops" when utilizing this method. For example:

245x8 (quickly reduce weight to 205)
205x6 (quickly reduce weight to 175)
175x4

Drop sets are very popular among bodybuilders because of the marked pain and soreness they create and is exactly why they are not advised for athletes—the post-exercise muscle soreness tends to greatly impair fine-motor skills in many sport events. One variation of the drop-set method, popularized by strength coach Charles Poliquin, is called the "1-6 method." This method involves lifting a very heavy (but not necessarily maximum) weight for one rep, and then reducing the weight enough to permit a second set of six reps with almost no rest between the two sets. This method is superior to strength development and results in less soreness, making it a better choice for most athletes.

Forced Reps: Forced reps is a very similar concept to drop sets. The main difference is that when using forced reps, the lifter completes as many reps as possible with a given weight, and then continues with the help of a partner who manually assists the lifter as she/he continues the set; for example, you might perform eight reps with 205 pounds (which for this example would be your "8RM weight"), at which point you complete perhaps another four reps with the help of a partner.

Supersets: Supersets involve the use of two or more exercises, performed back to back in a circuit. In some cases, the exercises involve different muscle groups, while in other cases, several exercises for the same muscle group are performed.

Negatives: Negative-only training involves performing your reps so the negative (or lowering) portion of each rep is emphasized. This is usually accomplished with the help of a partner, who provides strong manual assistance to lighten the concentric (or lifting) portion of the rep. Muscles are stronger eccentrically than they are concentrically, so this technique allows for heavier weight than what could otherwise be lifted. A common use for this method is the performance of negative-only pull-ups, which are often used in cases in which the exerciser cannot complete any repetitions concentrically. One caution, however: Eccentric exercise creates considerably more soreness than mixed (concentric-eccentric) work.

Static Training: Static training (more commonly known as isometrics) was very popular in the 1960s but has fallen out of favor over the past several decades. It involves contracting a muscle against an immovable object. Like all training methods and techniques, static training has both pros and cons. In the pro category, static training allows for larger than usual contractions and requires less time and equipment than other methods. In the con category, however, when you use static training, it's impossible to quantify how hard you're contracting or how much work you're actually doing. Also, strength increases are only at and around the exact joint angles used during the static exercise used, and muscle mass generally does not increase when static methods are used exclusively.

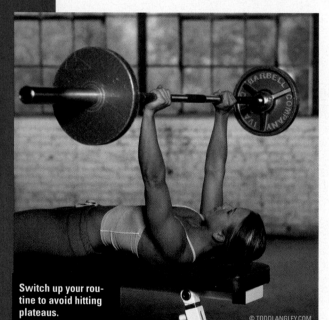

Switch up your routine to avoid hitting plateaus.

© TODDLANGLEY.COM

Mixed-Regimen Method: The mixed-regimen method is a mix of both dynamic and static methods. A common application would be performing a squat in the following way: Take your stance and lower to the bottom position. Then hold for 5 seconds. Next, ascend halfway up, hold for another five seconds, and then return to the starting position.

Partial Range of Motion: A popular method of strength development, especially among strength athletes, is to perform various exercises only through a partial range of motion; for example, one might perform bench presses through only the top half of the full range of motion (the strongest part of the full range). One could also use the weakest range—moving the bar from the chest to halfway to full lockout. These manipulations, when applied sparingly and intelligently, can jolt the body out of a performance plateau.

Compensatory Acceleration Training (CAT): CAT training is a distinct form of accelerative lifting coined by Fred Hatfield. It refers to speeding up movement in such a way so that improved leverages are created; for example, when ascending out of a deep squat position, mechanical leverage begins to improve once past the "sticking point." This improving leverage reduces the tension on the working muscles, and in turn, the training stimulus is compromised. Deliberately accelerating through these movement paths increases muscular tensions. CAT technique takes time to master, because the acceleration must continue past the sticking point, yet end before the antagonist muscles are triggered into decelerating the movement in an effort to prevent joint hyperextension or loss of control. This "braking" action would be antagonistic to normal coordination patterns involved with common athletic skills such as hitting, throwing, jumping and kicking.

Ballistic Training: William Kraemer, perhaps America's most respected and prolific strength researcher, uses the term "ballistic training" to describe movements that are "accelerative, of high velocity, and with projection into free space." Ballistic training involves plyometrics, modified Olympic lifting, jumping, throwing and striking movements (such as punching or kicking a heavy bag). Kraemer argues that in traditional barbell training, a significant portion of the movement path (specifically, the end of the concentric phase) is spent decelerating the bar, a protective response assumed by the antagonists to maintain joint integrity (in upper body movements such as bench pressing) or to prevent the athlete from leaving the ground in exercises such as the squat. If Kraemer's contention is correct, one would choose to gradually reduce the volume of traditional barbell drills as the training cycle progresses, in favor of ballistic exercises that lack this deceleration phase, making them easier to learn and more coordination specific for most athletes.

Plyometric Training: Although plyometrics are overused and misused by many people in their quest for the "magic pill" solution to their training problems, plyometric drills can be a valuable component of a speed-strength development program, as well as for general fitness enhancement. Plyometric workouts must be designed with sufficient recovery periods to ensure that fatigue does not take the elasticity out of the athlete's movements, since it is this repeated "elastic" neuromuscular control of impact that provides the training effect.

CONCLUDING COMMENTS

Think of your resistance training experience as a journey rather than a destination. Your participation should not depend entirely on the secondary rewards. You may find that the weight room is a laboratory of the mind, and many people find that some of their most creative and uplifting moments occur during lifting sessions. Resistance training is a process of self-discovery and personal excellence.

Helpful Resources

Bill Pearl's *Key's To The Inner Universe*: the largest single collection of resistance training exercises (and how to perform them correctly) you'll ever find. Available from www.billpearl.com.

Dragon Door Discussion Forum: Intelligent discussion on all forms of training and physical conditioning by Pavel Tsatsouline and colleagues. Visit: www.DragonDoor.com

Integrated Sport Solutions: Coach Staley's home base for his unique products and services. Visit: www.IntegratedSportSolutions.com

The Ultimate Guide To Massive Arms: Charles Staley's best-selling treatise on escalating Density Training. This book details arm training but the principles and techniques are easy to apply to any body part. Available in paper bound or e-book version. Available through www.EDTScrets.com.

Charles Staley's Private Coaching Group: Join my inner circle and enjoy our weekly calling hours, conference calls, high-profile guest interviews, online forum, free seats to Boot Camps and much more. Please visit www.StaleyTrainingSystems.com

Testosterone.Net: "Muscle With Attitude." Entertaining, cutting-edge articles on training and nutrition. Visit: www.Testosterone.Net.

14 GOING THE EXTRA MILE

Guidelines for Cardio Exercise and Sample Workouts

By Matt Fitzgerald

Cardio exercise can be loosely defined as any sustained activity of sufficient intensity to strengthen the cardiorespiratory system when repeated consistently. One of the virtues of cardio exercise is that a wide range of activities meet these criteria, from walking to chopping wood; consequently, just about anyone can find at least one form of cardio exercise he or she enjoys. You can also make cardio training fun by purposely taking advantage of the variety of options through cross-training—that is, by routinely practicing two or more cardio activities.

The benefits of cardio exercise are wide-ranging. Perhaps its most important benefit is that, in burning large amounts of calories, cardio exercise causes the body to shed excess fat and to keep it off; in fact, according to a study conducted by the National Weight Control Registry, cardio exercise is the strongest predictor of success in maintaining large weight losses—stronger than any single dietary factor.[1] So cardio exercise not only makes us look better and feel better about ourselves, but it also greatly reduces our risk for various health problems that are related to being overweight, such as diabetes[2], high blood pressure[3], certain cancers[4,5] and stroke.[6]

Regular cardio exercise has also been proven to reduce stress[7], increase performance in everyday activities[8], improve sleep[9] and even improve memory and cognitive functioning.[10] In short, if you're not getting cardio exercise, you're not really living!

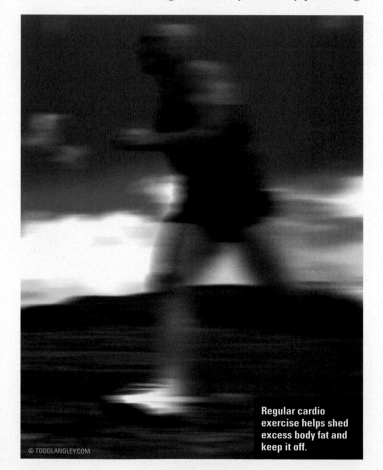

Regular cardio exercise helps shed excess body fat and keep it off.

© TODDLANGLEY.COM

Options Aplenty

As we've suggested already, the first step is to find one or more forms of cardio exercise that you enjoy. The following information will help to guide you in selecting activities that are right for you.

Indoor Activities

Five types of cardio exercise machines are now standard equipment in most fitness facilities: elliptical trainers, rowing machines, stair climbers, stationary bikes and treadmills. Here's how they compare:

⊘ ELLIPTICAL TRAINER

Benefits: The elliptical trainer was designed to emulate the running motion and the fitness benefits of running without impact. Using the elliptical trainer is therefore an excellent cross-training activity for those who like to run but want to protect their lower extremities from the overuse injuries that are common among runners.

Quick Tip: Using a higher resistance or incline level increases the muscle-toning effect of using an elliptical trainer, while increasing your tempo increases the calorie-burning effect.

⊘ ROWING MACHINE

Benefits: The rowing machine provides the best total-body workout of any cardio machine, combining a decent calorie burn with a high level of resistance for muscle toning. It is also the only cardio machine that develops the muscles of the upper body to any significant degree.

Quick Tip: In your first rowing workouts, focus entirely on learning proper technique, advises U.S. Olympic Rowing Coach Mike Teti. "The most common mistake is doing all the work with your upper body," he says. Concentrate instead on transferring the force from your thighs to your core musculature to your upper body with each stroke.

⊘ STAIR CLIMBER

Benefits: The stair climber is an excellent overall lower-body muscle toner. If your butt cheeks are now a pair of marshmallows, and you'd like to turn them into a couple of firm loaves of rye bread, use a stair climber!

Quick Tip: Avoid leaning on the stair climber's handrails, as many people do. You burn fewer calories this way and it puts too much strain on your lower back. Always stand upright and use the handrails only for balance. Another common form flaw is taking giant steps, which can strain the knees. Regardless of the resistance level you're using, take normal steps.

> **tip**
>
> **Cardio Exercise Will Help You:**
> - Lose fat
> - Reduce stress
> - Increase performance
> - Improve sleep
> - Improve memory
> - Improve cognitive functioning

STATIONARY BIKE

Benefits: The stationary bike offers an excellent combination of rapid calorie burning and lower-body muscular development.

Quick Tip: It's very important to adjust the seat height correctly when using the stationary bike. Incorrect setup can lead to knee and lower back pain. Set the seat so there is a very slight bend in your knee when the pedal is at the bottom of its rotation. In addition, always use the toe straps, as these allow you to generate force more evenly throughout the pedal stroke for a more comprehensive muscle-toning effect.

TREADMILL

Benefits: The good old treadmill is unsurpassed as a means of frying the lard off your middle.

Quick Tip: Because treadmill running is a high-impact activity, if you're just beginning a treadmill running program, start off by mainly walking. Gradually increase the portion of the workout you spend running from one session to the next until you're running straight through.

Outdoor Activities

Going nowhere on a machine in a crowded, stuffy gym can become rather dull. Actually moving forward while exercising in the freedom of the outdoors (when weather permits) is usually more fun. Five great outdoor cardio options are walking and hiking, running, inline skating, bicycling and swimming (which can also be done in an indoor facility).

WALKING AND HIKING

Benefits: Walking and hiking are the most accessible forms of exercise in the dual sense that nearly all of us know how to perform these activities, and they can be done almost anywhere and at any time. There is minimal technique to learn, the risk of injury is low, and it is possible to start very slowly with walking and hiking. For these reasons, they are popular choices among beginning exercisers of all ages.

But don't be fooled: walking and hiking can provide as intense a workout as you want. By maintaining good form and a brisk pace, you can very easily achieve the heart rate level (60 percent to 80 percent of maximum) that is ideal for fat burning. Add in some hills and walking and hiking become even more effective.

Getting Started: If you've been doing most or all of your cardio training indoors, be cautious when making the transition to outdoor walking and hiking. Even though they are fairly low-impact activities, walking and hiking do carry some risk of overuse injuries for beginners. To avoid these problems, work out on soft surfaces as much as possible, ease your way into longer walks or hikes and wear properly fitting shoes. Stretching and strengthening the calves and ankles with resistance exercises also help.

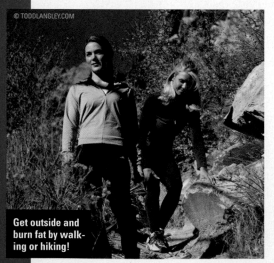

© TODDLANGLEY.COM

Get outside and burn fat by walking or hiking!

As for technique, "Entire books have been written about walking technique, but the best advice can be summed up in two words: walk naturally," says Dave McGovern, author of *Marathon Walking*. "Stand up straight, don't swing your arms wildly or take very long strides, and you'll do just fine." When climbing hills, maintain your rhythm and shorten your stride. Going downhill, lengthen your stride and maintain your rhythm.

Be sure to wear clothing that is designed for outdoor exercise (such as tights, jogging tops, etc.). Many walkers and hikers dress for the mall and are either uncomfortable or wind up lollygagging.

Staying Healthy

Overuse injuries such as runner's knee and lower back pain are all too common among regular cardio exercisers. There are four main causes of these injuries, according to John Connors, M.D., a podiatrist who treats many of the world's top distance runners. By being aware of these factors and taking steps to avoid them, you can greatly reduce your chances of getting hurt.

1 Too much too soon

At any given time, your body can safely handle only slightly more exertion than it is accustomed to, and it always needs recovery time in order to grow accustomed to increasing levels of exertion. This is true whether you're a former couch potato who's just beginning to exercise or an Ironman triathlete. So be patient, take it one step at a time and listen to your body.

2 Improper technique

Improper technique in any cardio activity can put undue stress on joints, bones and soft tissues and lead to injury. Swimmer's shoulder is a classic example of an overuse injury that can be avoided by learning proper technique. Whichever cardio activities you participate in, take the time to learn good form from an authoritative source such as a coach or book.

3 Muscle imbalances

Muscular imbalances contribute to many overuse injuries. Most individuals have tendencies toward certain imbalances due to their individual build, past injuries and lifestyle. Repetitive movements such as running also tend to create and exacerbate imbalances. The best way to bring your muscles into balance is through stretching and functional strength training. In particular, you want to focus on stretching muscles that have become shortened and tightened and strengthening important stabilizing muscles that are underdeveloped. A good personal trainer or physical therapist can help you diagnose your particular imbalances and suggest corrective stretches and strengthening exercises.

4 Improper selection and use of equipment

In order to avoid injuries it is also necessary that you use the right gear as it is meant to be used; for example, if your feet overpronate when you run, it is essential that you wear a stability or motion control running shoe to prevent the many injuries that can result from excessive foot roll. Again, rely on experts to guide you in the selection and proper use of equipment.

RUNNING

Benefits: "Running is the simplest sport," says Deena Kastor, American record holder for the marathon. "You don't need fancy equipment or facilities to do it. All you need is a pair of shoes and your own two legs, and you can do it anywhere in the world. And it's also one of the healthiest sports to do for weight loss, cardiovascular fitness and overall health."

Staying Motivated

Let's face it: cardio exercise can get to be a little monotonous. But if you practice a few proven motivational techniques, you can keep your enthusiasm level high at most times, and you'll certainly avoid the all-too-common pitfall of quitting your program outright due to boredom. Try these five motivational tricks:

1 Set goals

Goal setting is one of the most powerful motivational tools. Goals fuel your training with a sense of purpose and even urgency and also give you opportunities to experience the "intrinsic motivator" that is the joy of achieving goals. Set both long-term goals (e.g., "lose 10 pounds by my birthday") and short-term goals (e.g., "burn 2,000 calories through cardio exercise this week). The best goals are SMART—that is, Specific, Measurable, Achievable, Relevant and Time-bound.

2 Train seasonally

Variety is inherently more enjoyable and motivating than monotony; for this reason, you might want to train differently at different times of year. "For instance, you could establish four phases of the year that would include base building, strength/speed, peaking/competing, and rest/recovery," suggests JoAnn Dahlkoetter, Ph.D., a sports psychologist and author of *Your Performing Edge*. "Each stage can bring you up to a higher level of fitness, or you can divide the year into different types of training or participating in different activities."

3 Schedule breaks

Sometimes the best way to get motivated for exercise is to *not* exercise. "Short, medium and long breaks are all necessary to maintain your motivation levels," says Dahlkoetter. "Try taking a one-day break from training each week and take three days once a month. Then allow a week's rest after each major phase of your training (every three months). Take two to four weeks off once per year." Taking scheduled breaks from training will help you avoid taking those disastrous *unscheduled* breaks that result from burnout.

4 Train with others

We humans are social animals. Why not take advantage of your social nature by exercising as often as possible in the company of others? Working out with a partner or in a group is almost always more fun than doing it alone, and it also tends to increase one's commitment to scheduled workouts.

5 Reward yourself

You can enhance the motivational power of goals by attaching little rewards to them; for example, don't let yourself buy that new pair of shoes you've been coveting until you've achieved your target of 20 workouts this month.

Getting Started: Overuse injuries are extremely common in running, due in large part to the high-impact nature of the activity. To avoid them, build your running volume very gradually so your bones, muscles and joints have the opportunity to adapt to the stress. Also, choose your shoes carefully. Kastor recommends having a knowledgeable running shoe expert analyze your stride in order to match you with the right shoe. Also, use your running shoes for running only and replace them every 300 miles to 400 miles. Varying the types of surfaces you run on can prevent injuries, too.

🡒 INLINE SKATING

Benefits: One of the newer forms of cardio exercise, inline skating is also one of the most enjoyable, especially for women. "It's a lot like dancing," says Eddy Matzger, a world-class inline speed skater who leads inline workshops around the world (www.skatecentral.com). "It teaches body awareness better than any other form of exercise I've tried, and I've tried them all."

It's also a great workout. Inline skating falls right between running and bicycling in terms of energy expenditure, and it provides excellent conditioning for the muscles of the butt and thighs.

Getting Started: Wearing the wrong skates can spoil your inline experience as soon as it begins. Avoid this disappointment by purchasing high-quality skates designed for fitness skating. When you try them on, they should be snug but not constricting and should provide some ankle mobility. To avoid blisters, wear running socks with moisture-wicking properties and break in your new skates gradually.

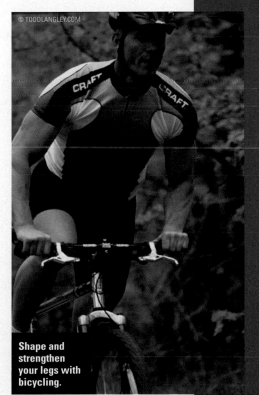

© TODDLANGLEY.COM

Shape and strengthen your legs with bicycling.

Technique is everything in inline skating. "It's all about learning balance and using gravity instead of fighting it," says Matzger. One great way to learn balance is to practice gliding on one skate at a time, perhaps while pushing a shopping cart around a parking lot. Matzger also recommends the interesting practice of wearing your skates for everyday activities like working and doing laundry. "It sounds funny but it's actually a very effective way to get comfortable on skates," he says.

The other important thing to learn is how to stop. "There are at least five ways to slow down or stop on inline skates," says Matzger. Have an experienced skater teach them to you one at a time, beginning with whichever one comes most naturally. Most metropolitan areas have inline clubs that offer the perfect environment in which to learn stopping and other techniques.

Once you're confident that you can slow down and stop when you need to, you can begin to cover some real ground on skates and get a serious workout on them; however, it is best to avoid rough surfaces, steeper hills, and high-traffic areas until—and unless—you become a true expert.

🡒 BICYCLING

Benefits: "The big advantage of outdoor cycling over indoor cardio machines is the balance factor," says Gale Bernhardt, an endurance coach and author of *The Female Cyclist.* "When you're forced to balance in addition to moving forward, your body uses more muscle fibers and burns more calories." In addition to stripping away fat and developing a strong heart and lungs, bicycling also shapes and tones the legs better than any other form of cardio exercise. Additionally, because there is no impact, the risk of injury is low.

Getting Started: You can't bicycle without a bike. There are a few basic varieties to choose from; which bike is best for you depends on the kind of riding you plan to do. Mountain bikes have sturdy frames, thick, knobby tires and a front shock absorber on many models. If you plan to do any amount of off-road riding, choose one of these (they work just fine on pavement, as well). If you plan to ride on the road and want a bike you can really move on, get a traditional road bike. These are light and aerodynamic; hence they are well suited to going far and fast. If you're interested in a more casual, comfortable ride, consider a cruiser, with its upright riding position and cushy seat.

Beyond type, the most important factor in bike selection is fit. Have a knowledgeable professional match you with the right size and make any necessary adjustments. Also essential are a good helmet and cycling shorts. While cycling shorts make a big difference, do expect some minor crotch discomfort as your body adjusts to bearing weight in this area when riding.

Make sure to ride your bike in safe areas. The best way to choose your routes is to go where the cyclists in your area like to go—be it a park, a road with a good bike lane, or a quiet neighborhood. When mountain biking, always investigate the trails you choose before riding them.

To get the best workout, learn how to shift gears so you always maintain a cadence of 80 to 90 pedal strokes per minute, except on hills. Also, always carry water (or a sports drink) and a spare tire, and know how to change it. (It's easy.)

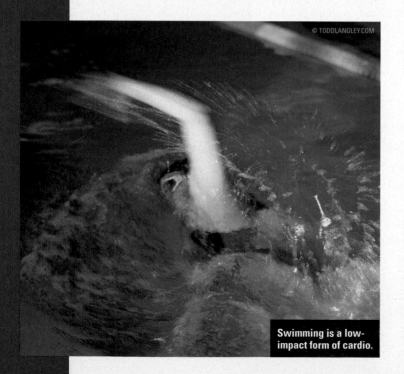

© TODDLANGLEY.COM

Swimming is a low-impact form of cardio.

🧭 SWIMMING

Benefits: Swimming is one of the few forms of cardio exercise that works primarily the muscles of the upper body. It is also the only non-weight-bearing form of cardio exercise (besides other water-based activities like pool running), so it's a great training option for those with injuries to the lower extremities or for times when your legs are sore.

Getting Started: Learning proper freestyle swimming technique is often quite challenging for beginners. The most effective way to learn is to join a local masters swim group. "It's motivating to be around other people (especially if they are faster), and you will have a coach there to tell you what to do, both for a workout, as well as to improve your technique," says Alex Kostich, a champion open-water swimmer.

SPORT AND GOAL-SPECIFIC NUTRITION AND TRAINING

To find a masters swimming group in your area, log onto www.usms.org and click on "Places to Swim," or call United States Masters Swimming at 800-550-SWIM.

Guidelines for Cardio Exercise

Before beginning any kind of cardio exercise regimen, you should consult with your physician and have a physical. The three fundamental variables of cardio exercise are frequency, duration and intensity. Together, the frequency and duration of workouts determine your time commitment to cardio exercise. For the average person, the goal is to achieve optimal body composition and basic cardiorespiratory fitness with the minimum amount of cardio exercise. In order to minimize your time commitment, you need to manipulate the intensity of your cardio workouts in the most effective way possible.

It's About Energy

In exercise, intensity refers to the rate at which your body is *currently* producing energy in relation to the *maximum* rate your body is able to produce energy for a specific activity. There are almost infinite degrees of intensity; for example, suppose you are running five miles an hour. If you increase your pace just slightly, to 5.1 miles an hour, your body is producing a little more energy and is therefore working at a higher intensity.

Intensity is important because it is the primary determinant of how your body adapts to exercise. By training at a certain intensity level, your body responds over time in such a way as to become better able to train at that same intensity level. The more time you spend at that level, the more pronounced these adaptations become, up to a limit.

So it's important to know which training intensities are connected to which results. Once you have this knowledge, you can emphasize the training intensities that lead to the results you seek.

How Hard Is Hard?

There is no absolute measure of intensity in cardio exercise. You can measure intensity by VO_2 max (your maximum rate of oxygen consumption), maximum speed, maximum heart rate or other variables, and you will get different answers from each.

What is the most practical way to measure and control intensity during cardio workouts? The answer is body awareness. There are specific sensory cues, or body signals, associated with each level of exercise intensity. You can use these to perform each type of cardio workout at the appropriate intensity and get the best results from it. Use the following table for guidance:

Intensity Level	Body Signal
Aerobic Intensity	Your breathing is elevated but controlled. You could speak one full sentence without gasping.
Threshold Intensity	The effort feels comfortably hard. If you picked up the pace even a little bit, you would start to suffer!
Sprint Intensity	You feel you are moving at the fastest pace you can maintain for the designated interval (10 - 60 seconds).

THREE RANGES

Although there are innumerable degrees of intensity, there are just three general intensity ranges that you'll want to target in workouts. In the aerobic intensity range, the aerobic energy system primarily is trained. At "threshold" intensity, the first anaerobic system primarily (called anaerobic glycolysis) is trained. And at "sprint" intensity, the second anaerobic system (the creatine phosphate system) is trained. Each leads to its own set of beneficial adaptations, so your program should include all of them. Let's look at them one by one.

Aerobic Intensity

In aerobic metabolism, oxygen is used to break down primarily fatty acids and carbohydrates (in the form of muscle glycogen and blood glucose) to release energy. The aerobic system produces harmless byproducts (carbon dioxide, water and heat). For this reason, and because the supply of its energy substrates is great, aerobic-intensity exercise can continue for relatively long periods of time, especially in well-conditioned individuals. But because aerobic metabolism is relatively slow, this energy system is inadequate to support extremely high-intensity efforts.

Exercising at aerobic intensity results in many positive adaptations. It strengthens the heart and the entire cardiorespiratory system, not only benefiting your overall health but also enhancing performance in all sports, every form of exercise and any life activity you can name. Aerobic conditioning is truly the foundation of fitness.

Aerobic intensity exercise also increases your endurance, so you can sustain activity for longer periods of time. It does this by increasing your body's fat-burning efficiency and glucose storage capacity. Aerobic intensity exercise is also an excellent means of improving body composition because the rate of fat-burning peaks in the middle of this intensity range.

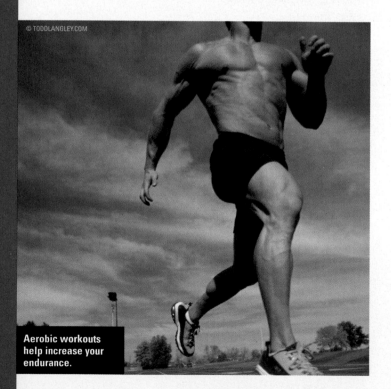

© TODDLANGLEY.COM

Aerobic workouts help increase your endurance.

Also, because aerobic intensity exercise can be maintained much longer than exercise at higher intensities, its overall calorie-burning potential is greater.

Threshold Intensity

In anaerobic glycolysis, glucose is broken down for energy without the use of oxygen. This process is faster than aerobic metabolism, so it can support higher intensity efforts; however, anaerobic glycolysis produces metabolic waste products that inhibit muscle contractions, resulting in exhaustion. The aerobic system can use these waste products as fuels, but when exercise intensity crosses a certain threshold, wastes are produced faster than they can be used. They then accumulate in the muscles, which begin to "burn" and feel weak, and pretty soon you're pooped.

Working out at or near this threshold also carries significant benefits. To begin with, it simply enhances the cardiovascular benefits that come from aerobic training. It also enhances positive changes in body composition, but in this regard it's even more efficient than aerobic training because calories are burned faster at threshold intensity than at aerobic intensity.

For more serious exercisers and athletes, threshold intensity training greatly enhances the body's ability to recover between hard efforts in a workout or competition. This allows you to do more advanced workouts and get a more pronounced effect from them.

Sprint Intensity

The second anaerobic energy system, the creatine phosphate system, fuels maximum and near-maximum efforts such as sprints and heavy weight lifting. Only tiny amounts of creatine phosphate are stored in the muscles, so this energy system cannot support efforts lasting longer than 15 seconds.

Sprint-intensity workouts burn more calories per minute than all workouts of lesser intensity. They are also an excellent supplement to strength training because they condition the same energy system and develop the same muscle fibers.

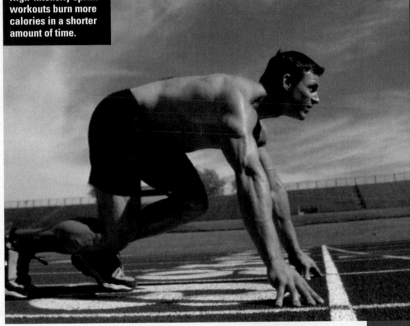

© TODDLANGLEY.COM

High-intensity sprint workouts burn more calories in a shorter amount of time.

The Workouts

One of the most common mistakes made in cardio exercise is that of doing the same workout every time. In order to improve your results, you should cycle through workouts that emphasize different intensity levels. Here are five workouts you should incorporate into your cardio training program.

AEROBIC WORKOUT:

In your modality of choice (jogging, elliptical trainer, etc.), maintain a steady pace for 20 to 40 minutes. The first and last few minutes should be very easy. The middle portion of the workout should be performed at an effort level of roughly seven on a 1 to 10 scale.

ENDURANCE WORKOUT:

The endurance workout is simply an extended aerobic workout. As such, it strengthens the aerobic energy system and enhances your body's fat-burning efficiency. As with the aerobic workout, warm up and then maintain a steady, moderate intensity, but continue for at least 40 and up to 60 minutes.

Why would you want to do longer aerobic workouts if your goal is to minimize your time commitment to cardio training? By doing a longer aerobic workout once a week, you can do shorter cardio workouts the rest of the week without sacrificing fitness. This is a useful strategy for those who are very busy during the week and have more time for exercise on the weekends.

⊙ THRESHOLD WORKOUT

The threshold workout trains your body to work comfortably and efficiently at higher levels of intensity. Warm up for five minutes and then perform two to three intervals of eight to 12 minutes at a comfortably hard intensity. Return to warm-up intensity for a few minutes between intervals. Cool down for five minutes.

● SPEED WORKOUT

The speed workout enhances your body's ability to buffer and transport the metabolic waste products of high-intensity exercise. Warm up for five minutes and then perform six to 10 intervals lasting 90 seconds each at a hard intensity. Return to warm-up intensity for two to three minutes between intervals. Cool down for five minutes.

● 20-MINUTE AEROBIC SOLUTION

Designed by Bill Phillips, this is a super-efficient workout format based on constantly varying intensity. Divide the 20-minute total workout duration into 20 separate 1-minute blocks. Using a 1-10 intensity scale, progress through the workout as follows:

Minute	1	2	3	4	5	6	7	8	9	10	11	12	13	14	15	16	17	18	19	20
Intensity	5	5	6	7	8	9	6	7	8	9	6	7	8	9	6	7	8	9	10	5

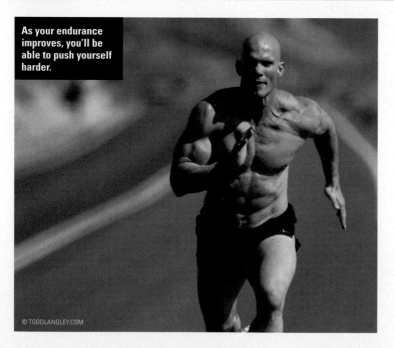

As your endurance improves, you'll be able to push yourself harder.

© TODDLANGLEY.COM

Your Cardio Program

If your primary goal for cardio exercise is to optimize your body composition with the minimum time investment, you should do three to four cardio workouts per week. If you're just starting out, do only short aerobic intensity workouts for a few weeks.

Once you've established a solid foundation of aerobic fitness, begin cycling through all five of the above-described cardio workout types repeatedly. Continual variation is the key to continual improvement.

Start off with manageable workouts of each type and make them gradually more challenging until you're carrying the overall training load that's needed to yield the results you seek. Stick with it and you *will* get the results you seek!

REFERENCES CITED:

[1] Klem, ML, Wing, RR, McGuire, MT, Seagle, HM and Hill, JO. A descriptive study of individuals successful at long-term maintenance of substantial weight loss. *American Journal of Clinical Nutrition* 66 (1997): 239-246.

[2] Helmrich, SP, Ragland, DR, Leung, RW and Paffenbarger, RS. Physical activity and reduced occurrence of non-insulin-dependent diabetes mellitus: a population-based cohort study. *American Journal of Epidemiology* 145 (1991): 301-308.

[3] Blair, SN et al. Influences of cardiorespiratory fitness and other precursors on cardiovascular disease and all-cause mortality in men and women. *Journal of the American Medical Association* 276 (1996): 205-210.

[4] Oliviera, SA, Kohl, HW, Trichopoulos, D and Blair, SN. The association between cardiorespiratory fitness and prostate cancer. *Medicine and Science in Sports and Exercise* 28 (1996): 97-104.

[5] Thune, I, Brenn, T, Lund, E and Gaard, M. Physical activity and the risk of breast cancer. *New England Journal of Medicine* 336 (1997): 1269-1275.

[6] Abbott, RD, Rodriguez, BL, Burchfiel, CM, and Curb, JD. Physical activity in older middle-aged men and reduced risk of stroke: The Honolulu Heart Program. *American Journal of Epidemiology* 139 (1994): 881-893.

[7] Cramer, SR, Nieman, DC and Lee, JW. The effects of moderate exercise training on psychological well-being and mood state in women. *Journal of Psychosomatic Research* 35 (1991): 437-449.

[8] Ourania, M, Yvoni, H, Christos, K and Ionannis, T. Effects of a physical activity program: The study of selected physical abilities among elderly women. *Journal of Gerontology and Nursing* 29.7 (2003): 50-5.

[9] Kubitz, KA, Landers, DM, Petruzzello, SJ and Han, M. The effects of acute and chronic exercise on sleep: A meta-analytic review. *Sports Medicine* 21 (1996): 277-291.

[10] Pierce, TW, Madden, DJ, Siegel, WC and Blumenthal, JA. Effects of aerobic exercise on cognitive and psychosocial functioning in patients with mild hypertension. *Health Psychology* 12.4 (1993): 286-91.

GLOSSARY OF TERMS

ADP (Adenosine Diphosphate): This is an important chemical involved in the energy production of a cell. ADP is formed when ATP is broken down within the mitochondria (the cells' "furnaces") to provide energy for muscular contraction. In order to recreate ATP and replenish cellular energy stores, ADP must combine with creatine phosphate.

Aerobic: This means "requiring oxygen." Aerobic metabolism occurs during low-intensity, long-duration exercises, like jogging.

Aerobic Metabolism: Oxygen is used to break down primarily fatty acids and carbohydrates to release energy.

Alanine: A non-essential amino acid. It is an important source of energy for the muscles, the brain and the central nervous system. It helps in the metabolism of sugars and organic acids. It also strengthens the immune system by producing antibodies. Found in meat, poultry, fish, eggs and dairy products.

Alkaloid: Any of various organic compounds normally with basic chemical properties and usually containing at least one nitrogen atom in a heterocyclic ring, occurring chiefly in many vascular plants and some fungi. Many alkaloids, such as nicotine, quinine, cocaine and morphine, are known for their poisonous or medicinal attributes.

Amino Acids: A group of nitrogen-containing, carbon-based organic compounds that serve as the building blocks from which protein (and muscle) is made.

Anabolic: This term refers to promoting anabolism which is the actual building process of tissues, mainly muscle, in the body. This might occur through the body's own natural reactions to muscular work and proper nutrition or through the introduction of drugs. Anabolism occurs by taking substances from the blood that are essential for growth and repair and using them to stimulate reactions that produce tissue synthesis.

Anabolism: The building up of tissue mass.

Anaerobic: This word means "without oxygen." Anaerobic metabolism in muscle tissue occurs during explosive activities like weight lifting or sprinting.

Anaerobic Glycolysis: Glucose is broken down for energy without the use of oxygen. This process is faster than aerobic metabolism, so it can support higher intensity efforts.

Anti-Catabolism: The halting of cellular breakdown in the body. A number of effective nutritional supplements such as glutamine, AKG and HMB may help promote anti-catabolism. Slowing down the breakdown of protein tips the scales of protein metabolism in favor of new muscle growth.

Antioxidants: These minimize tissue oxidation and help control free radicals and their nasty effects.

Anti-Proteolysis: A specific type of anti-catabolism: namely, the slowing or halting of protein (muscle) breakdown in the body.

Arginine: A non-essential amino acid. It holds a reputation for keeping the heart in good shape. It also performs numerous vital functions like facilitating the healing of wounds and promoting the secretion of key hormones such as insulin, glucagons and growth hormone. Found in meats, poultry, fish, dairy products, chocolate and nuts.

Asparagine: A non-essential amino acid. It is required by the nervous system to maintain equilibrium and is also required for amino acid transformation from one form to the other and is achieved in the liver. Found in dairy, beef, poultry and eggs.

Aspartic Acid: A non-essential amino acid. Recent studies have shown that aspartic acid may increase resistance to fatigue and increase endurance.

Assimilation: This is the process by which foods are absorbed and utilized by the body.

ATP (Adenosine Triphosphate): This is a high-energy molecule stored in muscle and other cells in the body. When a muscle cell needs energy to contract, ATP is broken down in to ADP to provide this energy. ATP can be thought of as the actual fuel that makes muscles move. Oxygen and glucose contribute to the formation of ATP. Many distributors of the supplements alleged to be performance-enhancing or ergogenic aids claim the supplements increase oxygen or glucose delivery to the cells. This would, in turn, increase the usable fuel in the form of ATP, increasing the duration of muscular endurance.

Ballistic Training: Involves plyometrics, modified Olympic lifting, jumping, throwing and striking movements (such as punching or kicking a heavy bag).

Banaba Leaf: Is a native plant of the Phillipines. It is used as a folk medicine there among diabetics to help them control their blood sugar levels.

Beta-alanine: An amino acid produced naturally in the body and found in foods such as chicken.

Beta-hydroxy beta-methylbutyrate (HMB): A compound that is consumed in the diet and produced in the body from proteins containing the amino acid leucine. HMB reduces muscle breakdown following strenuous exercise.

Bioenergetic: The replenishment of your metabolic fuel, stored glycogen as well as adenosine triphosphate (ATP) and phosphocreatine (PCr)—two main fuels for anaerobic exercise.

Biological Value (BV): A measure of protein quality, assessed by how well a given food or food mixture supports nitrogen retention in humans.

Body Composition: The percentage of your body composed of fat versus lean mass. Very sensitive methods of body composition measurements, including DEXA, can actually subdivide body composition into more specific categories, such as percentage of bone mineral, body water, hair, etc.

Branched-Chain Amino Acids (BCAAs): These are leucine, isoleucine and valine. BCAAs are considered essential amino acids because human beings cannot survive unless these amino acids are present in the diet. BCAAs are needed for the maintenance of muscle tissue and appear to preserve muscle stores of glycogen (a storage form of carbohydrate that can be converted into energy). BCAAs also help prevent muscle protein breakdown during exercise.

Buffer: A substance that minimizes changes in hydrogen-ion concentration (pH). Buffers such as sodium phosphate are used by athletes to help reduce lactic-acid buildup during strenuous exercise.

Caffeine: A bitter alkaloid found in coffee and tea that is responsible for their stimulating effects. May help promote fat loss.

Calcium: An element taken in through the diet that is essential for a variety of bodily functions, such as neurotransmission, muscle contraction and proper heart function. Imbalances of calcium can lead to many health problems. Found in dairy products. May help promote fat loss.

Calories: An energy-producing unit that is contained in food and released upon oxidation by the body.

Capsaicin: The ingredient in chili peppers that causes heat. Found primarily in the seeds and membranes.

Carbohydrates: These are organic compounds containing carbon, hydrogen and oxygen. They're a very effective fuel source for the body. The different types of carbohydrates include starches, sugars and fibers and are classified into three groups—monosaccharides, disaccharides and polysaccharides. Carbohydrates contain four calories per gram. Glucose—blood sugar—is a carbohydrate used by every cell in the body as fuel.

Carnosine: Neutralizes acid buildup in your muscles, and it accounts for up to 60 percent of your body's natural lactic acid buffering action. The more carnosine your muscles hold, the longer you'll be able to delay the accumulation of lactic acid in your muscles during intense exercise and the longer you'll be able to exercise at peak levels.

Casein: The main protein in milk. Found in meal-replacement powders, protein powders, cottage cheese and ready-to-drinks. It's a slow-acting protein because it "clots" in your stomach, making absorption slower.

Catabolic: This is the opposite of anabolic. It means the breakdown of tissue. Catabolic states occur with disease, infection, injury, intense training, strict dieting and immobilization. Catabolic conditions are not conducive to lean muscle mass gains; in fact, they typically cause a loss of lean muscle mass.

Catabolism: This refers to the breakdown or loss of muscle and other bodily tissues.

Catecholamines: Any of a group of amines derived from catechol that have important physiological effects as neurotransmitters and hormones and include epinephrine, norepinephrine and dopamine.

Cellulose: A type of fiber that cannot be digested.

Chitosan: Made up of the ground-up, powdered shells of marine crustaceans. It is supposed to bind to dietary fat, preventing digestion, absorption and storage, but it is unlikely it has any significant effect on fat loss.

Cholesterol: This is a type of lipid that, although most widely known as a "bad fat" implicated in promoting heart disease and stroke, is a vital component in the production of many steroid hormones in the body. It also plays a vital role in proper cell-membrane structure and functioning. It's a substrate for bile-acid synthesis, as well as sex hormone and vitamin D synthesis. There are different types of cholesterol: namely, HDL and LDL (HDL being the "good" form and LDL being the "bad" form).

Chromium: An essential trace element required for normal carbohydrate and fat metabolism and is required for optimal insulin activity and maintenance of normal blood glucose levels.

Colostrum: A component of breast milk that is found at its highest concentration two to three days after giving birth. It's a rich source of protein, antibodies and growth factors.

Conjugated Linoleic Acid (CLA): Helps in the reduction of body fat storage, increases lean body mass and protects against cardiovascular disease and certain cancers. It reduces the body's fat storage abilities by regulating several enzymes involved in fat metabolism.

Compensatory Acceleration Training (CAT): Speeding up movement in such a way so improved leverages are created.

Complete Proteins: These are proteins that contain all the essential amino acids in the right balance.

Cortisol: This is one of the primary catabolic hormones in the body needed to survive. However, catabolism, or the breakdown of body tissue, is not the only function of cortisol. It is typically secreted in response to physical trauma or prolonged stress. Its functions include controlling inflammation, increasing muscular catabolism and glycolysis (the energy-yielding conversion of glucose to lactic acid), suppressing immune response and maintaining normal vascular circulation and renal function, among other functions. Suppressing cortisol production at key times during the day may help bodybuilders avoid excess muscle breakdown.

Creatine Phosphate (CP): This is an inorganic phosphate molecule that binds with ADP to form ATP. Supplementing with creatine monohydrate helps increase CP reserves in muscles, which is good.

Cystine: A non-essential amino acid. Cystine is also critical to the metabolism of a number of essential biochemicals including coenzyme A, heparin, biotin, lipoic acid and glutathione. It is an important precursor to glutathione, one of the body's most effective antioxidants. Found in most high-protein foods such as wheat germ, oat flakes, cottage cheese, yogurt, pork, sausage meat, chicken, turkey and duck.

Daily Value (DV): A blanket value that encompasses the average nutritional needs of most healthy individuals within all of the various RDAs. Daily value is also a suggested daily intake levels for nutrients.

Deficiency: A sub-optimal level of one or more nutrients that are essential for good health, most often seen with vitamins. Many natural supplements that are marketed to athletes as ergogenic aids are effective at enhancing performance if an individual is efficient in that nutrient. A deficiency can be caused by poor nutrition, increased bodily demands (especially from intense training) or both.

Degradation: The breaking down of tissue mass.

Delayed-Onset Muscle Soreness (DOMS): The microscopic tearing of muscle fibers during activity that is either more intense or more prolonged than one normally does.

Dietary Induced Thermogenesis (DIT): Every time a meal is eaten, the body burns energy in order to process the food eaten; this increase in energy is called DIT.

Disaccharide: A carbohydrate compound made up of two sugars. Examples are sucrose (table sugar), lactose (milk sugar) and maltose.

Docosahexaenoic Acid (DHA): A healthy fat. DHA has been shown to reduce levels of blood triglycerides. DHA alone appears to be just as effective as fish oils, which contain both DHA and eicosapentaenoic acid (EPA), in beneficially lowering triglyceride levels in people at risk for heart disease.

Drop Sets: Lifting a given weight for as many reps as possible and then quickly reducing the weight (done with a partner) and completing as many additional reps as possible with the newly reduced weight.

DSHEA: A term which stands for the "Dietary Supplement Health and Education Act of 1994." This law was established by Congress and states that "dietary supplements" are defined as: vitamins, minerals, herbs or other botanicals (except tobacco), amino acids, any "dietary substance for use by man to supplement the diet by increasing the total dietary intake," and "a concentration, metabolite, constituent, extract or combination of any of the above-listed ingredients."

Eicosapentaenoic Acid (EPA): It's an excellent and healthy fat. It's also one of several omega-3 fatty acids used by the body. Our main dietary sources of EPA are cold water fish such as wild salmon. Increased intake of EPA has been shown to be beneficial in coronary heart disease, high blood pressure and inflammatory disorders such as rheumatoid arthritis.

Electrolytes: Substances that, in a solution, are capable of conducting electricity. These charged particles are present throughout the body and are involved in many activities such as regulating the distribution of water inside and outside cells in the body. Examples include the bulk minerals, potassium, sodium and chloride.

Energy: The capacity to do work. The energy in food is chemical energy: It can be converted to mechanical, electrical or heat energy. Energy is sometimes measured in "calories."

Enzyme: A protein molecule that acts as a "helper" in thousands of chemical reactions in the body, including: digestion of food, hormone production, muscle-cell repair.

Epigalloctechin Gallate (EGCG): EGCG has the ability to enhance thermogenesis (the burning of calories in the body) by inhibiting the enzyme that breaks down catecholamines.

Essential Amino Acids (EAAs): Amino acids not made by the body that must be obtained through the diet. Can be found in animal-based protein such as beef, pork, chicken and milk proteins such as whey, casein and eggs.

Essential Fatty Acids (EFAs): Fats that our bodies can't make that we must obtain through our diets. These fats (which include linoleic and linolenic acid) are very important to hormone production, as well as cellular synthesis and integrity. Good sources of these fats are flax seed oil and safflower oil.

Fat: One of the macronutrients. Fat contains nine calories per gram; it has the most calories of all the macronutrients. Dietary fats may also be referred to as lipids or triglycerides. Fats serve a variety of functions in the body; they act as structural components for all cell membranes, as well as supply necessary chemical substrates for hormone production. There are two types of fat—saturated "bad " fat and unsaturated "good" fat.

Fat-Free Mass (FFM): This refers to all portions of body tissues not containing fat. These tissues include all skeletal bones and muscles, skin, organs and body water, as well as hair, blood and lymph. Fat-free mass is a term used frequently in the texts of clinical studies. Often, an increase in fat-free mass equals an increase in skeletal muscle.

FDA (Food and Drug Administration): A government organization that ensures that the food we eat is safe and wholesome, that the cosmetics we use won't harm us and that medicines, medical devices and radiation-emitting consumer products such as microwave ovens are safe and effective.

Food Guide Pyramid (FGP): Illustrates the research-based food guidance system developed by the USDA. The Pyramid is based on USDA's research on what foods Americans eat, what nutrients are in these foods and how to make the best food choices for you. The Pyramid is an outline of what to eat each day. It's a general guide that allows you to choose a healthful diet that's right for you.

Forced Reps: When using forced reps, the lifter completes as many reps as possible with a given weight and continues with the help of a partner who manually assists the lifter as he/she continues the set.

Free Radicals: Highly reactive molecules possessing unpaired electrons that are produced during metabolism of food and energy production and are believed to contribute to the molecular damage and death of vital body cells. Free radicals may be a factor in aging or disease and may ultimately contribute to death. Antioxidants help neutralize free radicals.

Fructose: The main type of sugar found in fruit. It's sweeter than sucrose (table sugar) and has a low glycemic index (GI). In other words, eating fructose won't cause nearly as dramatic a release of insulin as glucose (dextrose). Eating a high-fructose diet may increase blood fats. Because of its low glycemic index and because it's metabolized mostly in the liver, fructose is often used as a sugar substitute for diabetics.

Glucagon: A hormone that is responsible for helping maintain proper blood sugar levels. When blood sugar levels go too low, glucagon activates glucose production in the liver, as well as regulates the release of glycogen from muscle cells. Eventually it may cause the catabolism of muscle cell proteins for glucose. This is considered a catabolic hormone.

Glucose: The simplest sugar molecule. It's also the main sugar found in blood and is used as a basic fuel for the body. When you eat complex carbs, they're broken down by the body into glucose. Glucose is also found in various fruits but not in as high concentrations as sucrose and fructose, two other sugars. However, when too much glucose is eaten, it's converted to fatty acids and triglycerides by the liver and adipose (fatty) tissue. Due to its quick absorption by the body, it's often used as an invigorating and strengthening agent in many medicinal formulations. It will cause the body to release a rapid and large amount of insulin to counteract the large influx of sugar.

Glutamic Acid: A non-essential amino acid that the body uses to build proteins. This amino acid is important in the metabolism of sugars and fats and aids in transportation of potassium across the blood-brain barrier. Found in meat, poultry, fish, eggs and dairy products.

Glutamine: The most abundant amino acid in muscle cells and has been show to be an important fuel for certain types of immune cells. Glutamine levels have been shown to decrease in relation to extreme exercise and overtraining; supplementation is often recommended to those who regularly participate in strenuous exercise. Found in beans, meats, fish, poultry and dairy products.

Glycemic Index (GI): This is a measure of the extent to which a food raises the blood sugar (glucose) level as compared with white bread, which has a GI of 100. Glucose (dextrose) scores a 138, brown rice an 81, and fructose (fruit sugar) is all the way down at 31.

Glycine: A non-essential amino acid. Glycine helps trigger the release of oxygen to the cell-making process and is important in the body's manufacture of hormones responsible for a strong immune system. It also helps build up glycogen levels. Found in many foods high in protein, such as fish, meat, beans and dairy.

Glycogen: This is the principal storage form of carbohydrate energy (glucose), which is reserved in muscles and in the liver. When muscles are full of glycogen, they look and feel full/pumped.

Glycolysis: The process of breaking carbohydrates or glucose down to make energy.

Growth Hormone (GH): A hormone that is naturally released by the pituitary gland; it is an anabolic hormone. GH promotes muscle growth and the breakdown of body fat for energy. GH levels are high in children and in teens but diminish greatly after age 20. Some sports supplements are supposed to increase the amount of GH that is naturally released in the body, and therefore create an anabolic state and increase fat burning in the athlete. Unfortunately, most have little effect.

HDL: This stands for "high-density lipoprotein." It's one of the subcategories of cholesterol—typically thought of as the "good" cholesterol. HDL cholesterol is the form that is typically used to clear fats from the system, therefore not lending itself to the formation of plaque in the arteries that can cause heart attacks. It may be possible to raise HDL cholesterol levels by ingesting quality unsaturated fats like flax seed oil. Exercise has also been shown to increase HDL levels.

Histidine: An essential amino acid. Histidine has been used in treatment of rheumatoid arthritis, allergic diseases, ulcers and anemia. Found in dairy products, meat, poultry and fish.

HMB (beta-hydroxy beta-methylbutyrate): A compound that is consumed in the diet and produced in the body from proteins containing the amino acid leucine. HMB reduces muscle breakdown following strenuous exercise.

Hormones: Substances in the body that are very important to bodybuilders. Two important hormone-producing organs are the pituitary gland and the testes. Hormones regulate various biological processes through their ability to activate or deactivate enzymes. Examples of this regulation are the effect of the testosterone hormone on the enzymatic activity relating to protein production of muscle cells. Other hormones, such as insulin and glucagon, control blood sugar levels and energy storage in the body. Hormones can be made of proteins.

Hydroxycitric Acid (HCA): Is a compound extracted from the skin of a native Indian fruit called Garcinia cambogia. HCA may decrease the production and storage of new fat cells, even if blood sugar levels get too high.

Hyponutremia: When the body's sodium levels are decreased to the point of illness.

Incomplete Proteins: Proteins that lack or are low in one or more of the essential amino acids.

Insulin: An anabolic hormone secreted by the pancreas that aids the body in maintaining proper blood sugar levels and promoting glycogen storage. Insulin secretion speeds the movement of nutrients through the blood stream and into muscle for growth. When chronically elevated, as with a high-carbohydrate diet, insulin can cause fat gain. However, short bursts of insulin, caused by consuming high-glycemic carbs, may help enhance the uptake of nutrients like creatine and glutamine by muscle cells.

Intensity: The absolute difficulty of the amount of resistance. The "quality" of the load.

Interleukins: A group of molecules involved in signaling between cells of the immune system.

Isoleucine: An essential amino acid. Isoleucine promotes muscle recovery after physical exercise. It's needed for the formation of hemoglobin, as well as assisting with regulation of blood sugar levels and energy levels. Found in almonds, chicken, eggs, fish, lentils, meat, etc.

Ketones: Organic chemical compounds resulting from the breakdown of triglycerides. They are used as an energy source in the body during very low-carbohydrate diets.

Ketosis: An increase in the production of ketones.

Lactic Acid: This is a molecule produced from glucose during anaerobic metabolism. When oxygen becomes available, lactic acid can be completely broken down to carbon dioxide and water. Lactic-acid buildup is a primary cause of muscle fatigue. Supplements that limit lactic-acid buildup may enhance athletic performance.

L-Carnitine: Supplied in the diet by meats and manufactured in the liver and kidneys. It transports fatty acids across cell membranes so they can be metabolized in the mitochondria. Athletes take this to enhance post-workout recovery because evidence shows it reduces exercise-induced muscle tissue damage.

LDL: This stands for "low-density lipoprotein" and is a subcategory of cholesterol, typically thought of as the "bad" cholesterol. LDL is the type of cholesterol that circulates throughout the blood stream and may cause heart disease. Levels of LDL cholesterol can be elevated by ingestion of saturated fats and a lack of exercise.

Lean Body Mass (LBM): Another term that describes fat-free mass (see fat-free mass).

Leptin: A protein-based hormone secreted primarily from fat cells and it holds the key to lasting fat loss. It's a master control hormone—it has the ability to control a wide variety of other hormones below it.

Leucine: An essential amino acid. Leucine is an essential building block of protein in all tissues that is found in all dietary protein. It regulates protein synthesis and protein breakdown. Leucine is also important for post-exercise. Taking supplemental leucine before and after intense training and between meals can help normalize glutimine levels in both the blood serum and muscle, thereby promoting anti-catabolic muscle metabolism, as well as supporting immune function.

Linoleic Acid: An essential fatty acid and, more specifically, an omega-6 polyunsaturated fatty acid. Good sources of this fatty acid are safflower oil and soybean oil.

Linolenic Acid: An essential fatty acid and, more precisely, an omega-3 polyunsaturated fatty acid. It is found in high concentrations in flax seed oil.

Lipid: This is simply another name for dietary fats or triglycerides.

Lipolysis: The breakdown of fat.

Loading Parameters: The selection of sets, reps, rest intervals and intensity ranges for the exercises you're performing.

Lysine: An essential amino acid. Supplementation of lysine is one of the best options available for the treatment of herpes simplex virus infections, especially in oral forms. Found in cheese, eggs, soy products, fish, lima beans, milk and potatoes.

Macronutrients: The nutrients that we ingest in large (macro means "big") quantities on a regular basis. These include proteins, carbohydrates, fats and water. All of these macronutrients are necessary to sustain life.

Meal-Replacement Powders (MRPs): A category of supplements that contain protein, carbohydrates, vitamins, minerals and other key nutrients that are used to replace a regular-food meal for purposes of weight loss, weight gain or increasing dietary nutrient intake.

Medium Chain Triglycerides (MCTs): A shortened version of a long chain triglyceride (LCT) that may help burn fat.

Metabolic Rate: This refers to the rate the body converts energy stores into working energy. In other words, it's how fast the "whole system" runs. The metabolic rate is controlled by a number of factors, including muscle mass (the greater your muscle mass, the greater your metabolic rate), caloric intake, exercise and use of stimulant or depressant chemicals.

Metabolism: A frequently used term that refers to the utilization of nutrients by the body for both anabolic and catabolic processes. It's the process by which substances come into the body and the rate at which they are utilized.

Methionine: An essential amino acid. Methionine assists in the breakdown of fats, thus helping to prevent a buildup of fat in the liver and arteries that might obstruct blood flow to the brain, heart and kidneys. It's a good source of sulfur, which inactivates free radicals. Found in beans, eggs, fish, garlic, lentils and meat.

Micronutrients: Dietary nutrients that we ingest in

relatively small (micro means "small") amounts compared to macronutrients. Examples of micronutrients include vitamins and minerals. Many micronutrients are essential dietary nutrients that perform vital functions in the body. Micronutrients are typically ingested in gram quantities or less.

Minerals: Naturally occurring, inorganic substances that are essential for human life and play a role in many vital metabolic processes.

Mixed-Regimen Method: The mixed-regimen method is a mix of both dynamic and static methods. An example would be performing a squat in the following way: Take a stance and lower to the bottom position. Then hold for five seconds. Next, ascend halfway up, hold for another five seconds, and then return to the starting position.

Monosaccharide: A simple carbohydrate made up of one sugar molecule. Examples are glucose and fructose.

Monounsaturated fats (MUFAs): Healthy fats found in nuts, avocados and oils.

Muscle Fatigue: The failure of a muscle to continue to perform work, caused by muscle ATP depletion. Lactic-acid buildup also plays a role in muscle fatigue. Some natural supplements marketed to athletes have the ability to postpone muscle fatigue, thus increasing the work potential of the muscle—one of the most potent is creatine, which increases the availability of ATP, which is used for energy.

Myocyte: This means "muscle cell."

Negatives: Negative-only training involves performing reps so the negative (or lowering) portion of each rep is emphasized.

Nutrients: These are components of food that help nourish the body: that is, they provide energy or serve as "building materials." These nutrients include carbohydrates, fats, proteins, vitamins, minerals, water, etc.

Omega-3: A name for a certain fatty acid. The "3" designates where the first double-bond is located in the fatty acid carbon chain. Linolenic acid is an example of an omega-3 fatty acid.

Omega-6: Another name for a fatty acid. Omega-6 refers to the first double-bond on a fatty acid chain that is located at the sixth carbon acid. Linoleic acid is an example of an omega-6 fatty acid.

Optimal Nutrition: The best possible nutrition, distinct from merely adequate nutrition that is characterized by no overt deficiency. This term describes people free from marginal deficiencies, imbalances and toxicities and who are not at risk for such. All athletes making an effort to increase muscle growth naturally must try to achieve optimal nutrition. In many cases, this requires supplementation of protein, vitamins and minerals and possibly other conditionally essential nutrients such as glutamine and creatine.

Overtraining Syndrome: A decrease in performance capacity and other symptoms resulting from chronic failure to achieve adequate post-exercise recovery or from maintaining a training workload that is beyond the athlete's absorption capacity for a long period of time.

Partial Range of Motion: A popular method of strength development to perform various exercises only through a partial range of motion; for example, one might perform bench presses through only the top half of the full range of motion (the strongest part of the full range).

Performance Nutrition Pyramid (PNP): This nutrition pyramid takes all of the latest research into account, including the Glycemic Index of carbs, proper nutrient timing and combining and the value of essential fatty acids. In order to support both optimal body composition and muscular growth and function, a macronutrient ratio of 40 percent protein, 40 percent carbs and 20 percent fat is recommended with the PNP.

PCr (phosphocreatine): Increasing levels of PCr in muscles cells is important for maintaining energy and strength during heavy bouts of repeated lifting.

Phaseolamin: An extract from white kidney beans. Phaseolamin inhibits alpha-amylase (the enzyme that breaks down starches in the stomach) for some time, but until recently commercial products containing phaseolamin were too weak to work in the body.

Phenylalanine: An essential amino acid. Phenylalanine helps to alleviate the symptoms of premenstrual syndrome (PMS) and various types of chronic pain. It also prevents weight gain by suppressing appetite. Found in meat and cheese.

Phosphates: May help exercise performance through their ability to buffer lactic acid, improve the body's ability to deliver oxygen to contracting muscles and enhance the cardiovascular system's ability to deliver more nutrients to the muscle, which is important for muscle growth.

Phosphorus: A highly concentrated mineral in bone matter. It's used to create strong bones and teeth.

Phytochemical: This term means "plant chemical." It's used to refer to a broad spectrum of bioactive plant compounds that are typically used in herbal preparations and a variety of other nutrition supplements.

Plyometric Training: Plyometric drills can be a valuable component of a speed-strength development program, as well as for general fitness enhancement.

Polysaccharides: Carbohydrates containing a large number of "sugar groups." Starch, glycogen, dextrin and cellulose are examples.

Proline: A non-essential amino acid. Proline improves skin texture and aids collagen formation and helps contain the loss of collagen during aging. Found in meat sources.

Proteins: Highly complex nitrogen-containing compounds found in all animal and vegetable tissues. They are made up of amino acids and are essential for growth and repair in the body. A gram of protein contains four calories. Those from animal sources are high in biological value since they contain the essential amino acids. Those from vegetable sources contain some but not all of the essential amino acids. Proteins are broken up by the body to produce amino acids that are used to build new proteins. Proteins are the building blocks of muscle, enzymes and some hormones.

Protein Efficiency: The measure of the ability to supply complete proteins that are the best absorbed and utilized by the body.

Proteolysis: Specifically, the breakdown of protein.

Polyunsaturated Fatty Acids (PUFAs): Healthy fats containing omega-3. Can help cholesterol reduction.

Pyruvate: The end product of glycolysis.

Recommended Daily Intake (RDI): Daily intake of an essential nutrient and/or energy source that will maintain health in practically all healthy individuals on average. RDI levels and percentage daily intake levels derived from RDI levels are put on food box labels in compliance with U.S. Food and Drug Administration regulations.

Resting Energy Expenditure (REE): This is the number of calories you burn each day just sitting on the couch.

Resting Metabolic Rate (RMR): The number of calories the body burns at rest.

Recommended Daily Allowance (RDA): The RDA is a set of recommendations set by the Food and Nutrition Board of the National Research Council for the intake of substances that the body needs to function normally.

RTDs (ready-to-drinks): Use as a meal-replacement. The ready-to-drink nutrition shake provides high-quality protein and over 50 percent of the RDA for virtually every essential vitamin and mineral.

Saturated Fats: These are bad fats. They are called "saturated" because they contain no open spots on their "carbon skeletons." Saturated fats include myristic acid, palmitic acid, stearic acid, arachidic acid and lignoceric acid. These bad fats have been shown to raise cholesterol levels in the body. Sources of these fats include animal foods and hydrogenated vegetable oils, such as margarine. These fats serve no biological function in the body, other than to supply calories.

Scoville Heat Units (SHU): SHU is a measure of the amount of heat-producing nutrients found in the product.

Serine: A non-essential amino acid. Serine is required for the metabolism of fat, tissue growth and the immune system as it assists in the production of immunoglobulins and antibodies. Found in meats and dairy products, wheat gluten, peanuts and soy products.

Small Frequent Meals (SFMs): Stabilize both food and blood sugar insulin levels throughout the day. Also tend to promote the consistent expression of leptin, which in turn helps decrease feelings of hunger.

Soy Protein: A non-animal source of protein. Helps decrease the amount of muscle breakdown.

Static Training: Involves contracting a muscle against an immovable object.

Sucrose: Most commonly known as table sugar. Industrially, sucrose is derived from sugar cane or sugar beets. When you eat it, the body breaks sucrose into fructose and glucose.

Supercompensation: Short-term recovery that leads to lasting adaptions.

Supersets: Involve the use of two or more exercises performed back to back in a circuit.

Synthesis: The building up of tissue mass.

Threonine: An essential amino acid. Threonine helps prevent fat buildup in the liver; helps the digestive and intestinal tracts function more smoothly; assists metabolism and assimilation.

Training Stimulus: An individual workout that stresses the body by depleting energy supplies, disrupting muscle tissue, changing hormonal patterns and so forth.

Training Volume: The amount of work you perform in a given time period.

Trans Fat: Raises the LDL (bad) cholesterol that increases your risk for coronary heart disease (CHD). It can be found in vegetable shortenings, some margarines, crackers, cookies, snack foods and other foods made with or fried in partially hydrogenated oils.

Transient Hyperinsulinemia: The opportunity to replenish muscle glycogen stores and build new muscle proteins very rapidly.

Tryptophan: An essential amino acid. Tryptophan helps alleviate insomnia by inducing normal sleep; reduces anxiety and depression; helps in the treatment of migraine headaches; helps the immune system; helps reduce the risk of artery and heart spasms; and works with lysine in reducing cholesterol levels.

Tyrosine: A non-essential amino acid. Tyrosine's main purpose is to support the formation of neurotransmitters. Neurotransmitters are important because they carry "messages" from one nerve cell to another and play a vital role in our muscular function. A loss in these neurotransmitters can lead to physical and mental burnout and fatigue. Found in dairy products, meats, fish, wheat and oats.

United States Department of Agriculture (USDA): A government agency responsible for the safety of meat, poultry and eggs. Conducts ongoing nutrition research and supports the production of agriculture.

Valine: An essential amino acid. Valine is an essential protein building block. It promotes muscle recovery after physical exercise and plays a role in wound healing and the growth of new tissue. Found in meat, poultry, fish, eggs and dairy products.

VO_2 Max: The maximum rate of oxygen consumption in an individual.

Whey: A main protein in milk. Found in protein powders, meal-replacement powders and ready-to-drinks. Contains all essential amino acids and high in branch chain amino acids. It's a fast-acting protein (absorbs quickly).

APPENDIX A

Amino Acids and Protein

Protein is a nutrient essential to physical performance and overall health due to its role in structure, repair and maintenance of body tissues. At the molecular level, protein is made up of smaller units called amino acids, which are connected together in different combinations. Your body breaks down dietary protein into amino acids and "reshuffles" them into new protein to build and rebuild/repair tissue, including muscle. Protein also keeps the immune system working well and helps carry nutrients.

Table of Amino Acids: The Building Blocks

The "9" Essential: The following nine amino acids are essential to eat in your daily diet because the body cannot make them.

➤ Histidine	➤ Phenylalanine	➤ Isoleucine
➤ Lysine	➤ Methionine	➤ Threonine
➤ Tryptophan	➤ Valine	➤ Leucine

The "11" Non-essential: The body can make these 11 non-essential amino acids, which are also the building blocks of protein.

➤ Alanine	➤ Cystine	➤ Glycine	➤ Arginine
➤ Asparagine	➤ Glutamic acid	➤ Proline	➤ Serine
➤ Aspartic acid	➤ Glutamine	➤ Tyrosine	

Note:
Although amino acids work together to form body proteins, individual amino acids have specific roles to play in the body. Certain amino acids such as tryptophan and tyrosine are involved in neurotransmitters (chemical messengers) for the brain. A trio of amino acids, leucine, isoleucine and valine, technically known as branched-chain amino acids, are constituents of muscle tissue. Protein is usually not touted as a good "energy fuel source," one exception exists with these branched chain-amino acids. Research shows that these amino acids are used for energy in endurance exercise lasting at least 60 to 90 minutes. In very high-intensity aerobic exercise, leucine is particularly used up.

Good Sources of Dietary Protein

Protein can be obtained from both animal sources and plant sources. Note that you need to eat a larger portion of plant protein to equal the amount in animal foods.

Animal Sources	Grams	Standard Serving
Egg	6 grams	1 large
Egg white	3.5	from 1 large
Milk skim	8	1 cup (8oz)
Cheese, cheddar	7	1 ounce
Yogurt	8-11	1 cup (8oz)
Cottage cheese	12-15	1 cup
Beef, lean	24-32	3-4 ounces cooked
Fish, tuna fish	24-32	3-4 ounces cooked
Chicken breast	24-32	3-4 ounces cooked
Lean pork loin	24-32	3-4 ounces cooked
Hamburger	30	4 ounces broiled
Lunch meat (lean)	10-15	2-3 ounces

Plant Sources	Grams	Standard Serving
Soymilk	8 grams	1 cup
Peas (green)	4-6	½ cup
Peanuts, roasted	18	½ cup
Pumpkin seeds	20	½ cup
Peanut butter	4	1 tablespoon
Soynut butter		1 tablespoon
Kidney beans	6	½ cup
Soybeans, cooked	14	½ cup
Hummus	6	½ cup
Refried beans	7	½ cup
Baked beans	14	1 cup
Tofu, extra firm	11	3.5 ounces
Lentil soup	11	10.5 ounces

Sources: Data from food labels and J. Pennington. *Bowes and Church's Food Values of Portions Commonly Used* (Sixteenth edition) (Lippicott, 1992).

Sources: Rosenbloom, K. *Sports Nutrition: A Guide for professionals working with active people* (Third Edition) (American Dietetic Association, 2000). Coleman, E and Nelson Steen, S. *The Ultimate Sports Nutrition Handbook* (Bull Publishing, 1996).

APPENDIX B

Vitamins and Minerals

U.S. Recommended Dietary Allowances for Vitamins

ADULT U.S. RDA FEMALE/MALE	PHYSIOLOGICAL AND EXERCISE-RELATED FUNCTIONS	BEST FOOD SOURCES	SIDE EFFECTS AND TOXICITY (OVER SUPPLEMENTATION ISSUES)	COMMENTS
Vitamin B Complex				
Thiamin(B_1) 1.1/1.5mg or .5mg per 1000 calories consumed	Carbohydrate metabolism, energy production, maintenance of healthy nervous system	Meat, whole grains, wheat germ, brewer's yeast, bran, milk, beans	None known	
Riboflavin(B_2) 1.2mg/1.2mg	Energy metabolism (fuels), cellular respiration	Milk, eggs, lean meats and broccoli	None known	
Pyridoxine(B_6) 1.6/2.0mg	Protein metabolism, formation of oxygen carrying red blood cells(hemoglobin), energy production, required for production of antibodies	Whole grains and cereals, bananas, spinach, cabbage, lima beans and meats	Liver and nerve damage	
Vitamin(B_{12}) (Cyanocobalamin) 2 micrograms	Energy metabolism (fuels), Red blood cell synthesis and production, central nervous system, may help protect against heart disease	Animal foods: Meat, dairy products, eggs, liver and fish	Liver damage, allergic reactions	
Other Vitamins:				
Niacin 15/19mg	Cellular energy production, Synthesis of fat and amino acids, metabolism of energy (fuels), improves circulation may reduce cholesterol levels and be cancer-protective	Whole grain cereals, wheat germ, peanut butter, greens, meat, poultry, fish	Liver damage, jaundice, skin flushing, and itching, nausea	

ADULT U.S. RDA FEMALE/MALE	PHYSIOLOGICAL AND EXERCISE-RELATED FUNCTIONS	BEST FOOD SOURCES	SIDE EFFECTS AND TOXICITY (OVER SUPPLEMENTATION ISSUES)	COMMENTS
Folic Acid 180/200 mcg	Regulation new cell growth, Red blood cell formation, protection against neural tube defects in newborns	Greens leafy vegetables, liver, mushrooms, fortified foods	Gastric problems; can mask certain anemias	Important nutrient prior to and during pregnancy
Vitamin A 800/1000 mcg/IU	Vision, growth/repair body structures, immunity, antioxidant, may reduce risks of certain cancers and protect heart health	Milk, green leafy and yellow/ orange veggies, egg yolk, liver, yogurt	Digestive system upset, damage to bones and certain organs	
Vitamin D 5mcg or 200IU	Normal bone formation and growth, aids absorption of calcium, may help prevent osteoporosis	Sunlight, fortified dairy products, eggs, fish	Nausea, vomiting, hardening of soft tissues, kidney damage	Needs may increase over 50 per osteoporosis research. Consult health professional
Vitamin K 65/80 mcg	Involved in blood clotting mechanism, glycogen formation and normal liver functioning	Lower GI tract produces source, vegetables, yogurt, liver	Allergic reactions, breakdown of red blood cells	
Biotin 30-100mcg	Component breakdown of dietary fats	Egg yolks and liver	None known	
Pantothenic Acid 4-7mg	Cellular energy production; fatty acid oxidation, required for production of antibodies, may help premature aging	Found widely in foods	None known	

Adapted from *The Ultimate Sports Nutrition Handbook* (Coleman and Steen) and *High Performance Nutrition* (Kleiner).

U.S. Recommended Dietary Allowances for Minerals

ADULT U.S. RDA FEMALE/MALE	PHYSIOLOGICAL AND EXERCISE-RELATED FUNCTIONS	BEST FOOD SOURCES	SIDE EFFECTS AND TOXICITY (OVER SUPPLEMENTATION ISSUES)	COMMENTS
Calcium 800mg(RDA) additional may be needed	Bone formation, enzyme reactions, muscle contraction and nerve transmission, plays a part in muscle growth	Dairy products, fortified food products, green leafy vegetables	Constipation, mineral absorption problems, excessive calcification of some tissues	Used in the prevention and treatment of osteoporosis, new research as an important nutrient for treating hypertension
Iron 15mg/10mg	Hemoglobin formation, oxygen transport to cells for energy, muscle growth and function	Lean meats, beans, dried Fruit, some green leafy vegetables, liver, oysters	Large amounts are toxic	
Magnesium 280/350mg	Energy production by assisting with metabolism of proteins and carbohydrates, muscle relaxation, nerve conduction	Whole grains, legumes, green vegetables, nuts, meats, seafood, beans	Large amounts are toxic	Assists in bone growth, and in absorption of other essential minerals, may protect against heart disease
Sodium Estimated minimum requirement = 500mg	Body fluid balance, muscle contraction and nerve transmission,	Table salt, found in most foods	Water retention, hypertension	
Potassium Estimated minimum requirement = 2000mg	Maintenance of normal fluid balance, muscle action, nerve impulses, assists in conversion of glucose to glycogen, synthesis of muscle protein from amino acids	Bananas, potatoes, orange juice, other fruits and vegetables	Heart disturbances	
Zinc 12/15mg	Tissue growth and healing, immunity, gonadal development, needed for absorption and action of certain vitamins, component of many enzymes involved with metabolism, works with vitamin C in healing	Animal proteins, shellfish, oysters, whole grains and products, brewer's yeast	Doses higher than 20mg/day interfere with copper absorption; reduce HDL cholesterol, and impair functioning of immune system	Known as antioxidant mineral; plays a protective role in free radical damage

APPENDIX

ADULT U.S. RDA FEMALE/MALE	PHYSIOLOGICAL AND EXERCISE-RELATED FUNCTIONS	BEST FOOD SOURCES	SIDE EFFECTS AND TOXICITY (OVER SUPPLEMENTATION ISSUES)	COMMENTS
Copper *ESI = 1.5/3 mg	Hemoglobin formation by assisting with iron absorption, energy production, immunity, involved with (SOD), one of the key antioxidant enzymes.	Whole grains and cereals, beans, nuts, dried fruit, shellfish, eggs, green leafy vegetables	Toxicity is rare.	Known as antioxidant mineral; plays a protective role in free radical damage
Selenium 77/70 mcg	Enhances vitamin E interacting in normal growth and development, antioxidant, provides possible protection against cancer, produces antioxidant enzymes	Meats, seafood, grains, cereal bran, egg yolk, milk, broccoli, garlic and onions.	According to some research, approximately 5mg/day has resulted in hair loss and fingernail changes. Higher daily does associated with nausea, abdominal pain, diarrhea, fatigue and irritability.	Known as an antioxidant mineral; plays a protective role in free radical damage
Manganese *ESI=2/5mg	An enzyme activator involved in many metabolic processes; bone and tissue development, fat synthesis	Nuts, whole grains, beans, tea, egg yolks, vegetables	Large doses cause vomiting and intestinal problems	Involved with superoxidase dismutase, one of the key antioxidant enzymes
Chromium *ESI= 50/200mcg	Plays a role in glucose tolerance factor, helps insulin, normal blood sugar and fat metabolism	Whole grains, corn oil, meats, brewer's yeast, cheese, beer	Liver and kidney damage	Has been touted as a "fat burner" and marketed for weight loss
Iodine 150mg	Regulates metabolism, energy production; growth and development	Iodized salt, seafood, and mushrooms	Thyroid enlargement	
Fluoride 1.5/4mg	Formation of bone and tooth enamel	Tap water (fluoridated)	Large amounts are toxic	
Phosphorus 800mg	Builds bones and teeth, metabolism of fuels; growth, repair, maintenance of cells, energy production; stimulation of muscle contractions	Meats, fish, poultry, dairy products, eggs, whole grains, seeds, nuts, and carbonated drinks	None known	Works with calcium in maintaining healthy bones
Molybdenum 75-250 mcg	Involved in fat metabolism	Milk, beans, breads, and whole grain cereals	Diarrhea, anemia, and depressed growth rate	

Adapted from *The Ultimate Sports Nutrition Handbook* (Coleman and Steen) and *High Performance Nutrition* (Kleiner).

Micronutrients from A to Z
RDAs, DVs & ULs

This chart should only be used as a quick reference for looking up general micronutrient information; not as the end-all answer for vitamin and mineral supplementation. You should always check with your physician to determine if you have any serious vitamin or mineral deficiencies.

Micronutrients	1997-2001 RDA/AI[1]	DV[2] for 4 yrs and older	1997-2001 Tolerable UL[3] (Adults 19-70 yr)
VITAMINS			
Vitamin A (Beta-carotene, Retinol)	Males, 19-50 yr 900 RAE (3,000 IU) Females, 19-50 yr 700 RAE (2,330 IU)	5,000 IU	3,000 RAE (10,000 IU) preformed <u>only</u>; does not apply to beta carotene; Vitamin A toxicity (hypervitaminosis A) can occur with an acute dose of 500,000 IU or chronic intake of 50,000 IU per day. Toxicity symptoms can include nausea, irritability, blurred vision, weakness, hair loss and dry skin.
Vitamin D	Males, 19-50 yr 5 mcg (AI) (200 IU) Females, 19-50 yr 5 mcg (AI) (200 IU)	400 IU (10 mcg)	50 mcg (2000 IU) Vitamin D can be toxic. An intake of 5 times over the RDA over a period of time can be harmful, especially to children. Excess levels of Vitamin D may cause over-absorption of calcium and calcium deposits in kidneys, heart, and blood vessels.
Vitamin E (also called tocopherol)	Males, 19-50 yr 15 mg Females, 19-50 yr 15 mg	30 IU (20 mg)	1,000 mg Consequences of consuming high doses can be diarrhea and cramping.
Vitamin K (phylloquinones from plants and menaquionones from fish oils and meats)	Males, 19-50 yr 120 mcg Females, 19-50 yr 90 mcg	80 mcg	Not established Toxicity is not likely as it is readily excreted from the body.
Vitamin C (Ascorbic acid)	Males, 19-50 yr 90 mg Females, 19-50 yr 75 mg	60 mg	2,000 mg Toxicity is not likely, but excessive intakes of 10,000 mg (10g) or more may cause uncomfortable side effects such as diarrhea, nausea and cramping.
B[1] (Thiamin)	Males, 19-50 yr 1.2 mg Females, 19-50 yr 1.1 mg	1.5 mg	Not established Thiamin is rapidly excreted in the urine via the kidneys. There is no known level of toxicity.
B[2] (Riboflavin	Males, 19-50 yr 1.3 mg Females, 19-50 yr 1.1 mg	1.7 mg	Not established Excess riboflavin is excreted in the urine via the kidneys. There is no known toxicity.
B[3] (Niacin)	Males, 19-50 yr 16 mg Females, 19-50 yr 14 mg	20 mg	35 mg Doses over 75 mg niacin (not niacinamide) can dilate blood vessels which may cause a skin flushing effect. Excess niacin (not niacinamide) can lead to flushing, headaches and diarrhea.

B$_5$ (Pantothenic Acid)	Males, 19-50 yr 5 mg (AI) Females, 19-50 yr 5 mg (AI)	10 mg	Not established No known toxicity; excesses are rapidly excreted.
B$_6$ (Pyroxidine)	Males, 19-50 yr 1.3 mg Females, 19-50 yr 1.3 mg	2 mg	100 mg High doses every day for an extended period of time may cause neurotoxicity and lead to numbness and muscular weakness.
B$_{12}$ (Cyanocobolamin)	Males, 19-50 yr 2.4 mcg Females, 19-50 yr 2.4 mcg	6 mcg	Not established No known toxicity; excesses are rapidly excreted.
B$_9$ Folic Acid (Folate)	Males, 19-50 yr 400 mcg Females, 19-50 yr 400 mcg	400 mcg	1000 mcg May cover up signs of vitamin B$_{12}$ deficiecy (pernicious anemia).
Biotin (Vitamin H)	Males, 19-50 yr 30 mcg (AI) Females, 19-50 yr 30 mcg (AI)	300 mcg	Not established Large doses have been administered over a period of time without harmful side effects.

MINERALS

Calcium	Males, 19-50 yr 1000 mg (AI) Females, 19-50 yr 1000 mg (AI)	1,000 mg	2,500 mg Excessive consumption can lead to decreased absorption of other minerals including zinc and iron as well as constipation.
Chromium	Males, 19-50 yr 35 mcg (AI) Females, 19-50 yr 25 mcg (A)	120 mcg	Not established Toxicity of dietary chromium is unlikely; however, kidney and skin damage can result in extremely high doses.
Copper	Males, 19-50 yr 900 mcg Females, 19-50 yr 900 mcg	2 mg	10 mg Doses of 10 – 15 mg at one sitting may cause vomiting, diarrhea and tremors. Wilson's disease can result from excessive accumulation in the liver and kidneys.
Iodine	Males, 19-50 yr 150 mcg Females, 19-50 yr 150 mcg	150 mcg	1,100 mcg Chronic high doses of iodine may inhibit thyroid hormone synthesis which produces effects as if there were an iodine deficiency.
Iron	Males, 19-50 yr 8 mg Females, 19-50 yr 18 mg	18 mg	45 mg Excess levels can lead to constipation, vomiting, abdominal pain, decreased zinc absorption. Acute excessive intake in children can be fatal.

Magnesium	Males, 19-30 yr 400 mg Male, 31-50 yr 420 mg Females, 19-30 yr 310 mg Female, 31-50 yr 320 mg	400 mg	350 mg Excess consumption can lead to diarrhea, dehydration and impaired nerve activity.
Manganese	Males, 19-50 yr 2.3 mg (AI) Females, 19-50 yr 1.8 mg (AI)	2 mg	11 mg Excess consumption can lead to impairments in the nervous system, muscle spasms and diarrhea.
Molybdenum	Males, 19-50 yr 45 mcg Females, 19-50 yr 45 mcg	75 mcg	2,000 mcg Excess consumption can impair absorption of other minerals.
Phosphorous	Males, 19-50 yr 700 mg Females, 19-50 yr 700 mg	1000 mg	4,000 mg Excess consumption can lead to muscle spasms.
Potassium	No DRI	3,500 mg	Not established Potassium is not toxic unless the kidneys are not functioning properly in which case the buildup of potassium in the blood could lead to irregularity in heartbeat and heart function.
Selenium	Males, 19-50 yr 55 mcg Females, 19-50 yr 55 mcg	70 mcg	400 mcg High daily intakes over a period of months may lead to selenosis. Symptoms include hair and fingernail loss, weakness, nausea, diarrhea and liver damage.
Sodium	No DRI; Less than 2,400 mg	Less than 2,400 mg	Not established Toxicity for sodium is not established. Some experts recommend limiting sodium intake. In susceptible individuals (sodium sensitive), high blood pressure can occur with excessive intake of sodium.
Zinc	Males, 19-50 yr 11 mg Females, 19-50 yr 8 mg	15 mg	40 mg Ingesting a high intake over an extended period of time can inhibit copper absorption; can cause diarrhea, nausea, cramps, vomiting and weakness.

IU = International Units
mcg = micrograms
mg = milligrams
g = grams
RAE = retinol activity equivalents (3.33 IU = 1 RAE)
DFE = dietary folate equivalents

[4] The Recommended Dietary Allowances (RDA) and Adequate Intakes (AI) reflect the average daily amount of a nutrient considered adequate to meet the needs of most healthy people. If there is insufficient evidence to determine an RDA, an AI is set and is like a tentative RDA. Reference: *Dietary Reference Intakes* (2001) by the National Academy of Sciences, National Academy Press, Washington, D.C.
[5] Daily Values (DVs) are established by the Food and Drug Administration (FDA) for use in nutrition labeling of foods.
[6] Upper Limit (UL) represents the maximum amount of a nutrient that appears safe for most healthy people to consume on a regular basis. If you suspect overdose, discuss with your physician or health care physician immediately. This is not a complete list of possible adverse symptoms. Reference: *Dietary Reference Intakes* (2001) by the National Academy of Sciences, National Academy Press, Washington, D.C.

APPENDIX

APPENDIX C

Calculating Your 40/40/20 Balance

40/40/20 is shorthand for "40 percent protein, 40 percent carbohydrates, 20 percent fat." Meaning that 40 percent of your daily caloric intake will come from protein, 40 percent from carbs and 20 percent from fat. That's pretty easy. But calculating the actual calorie and gram level for each of these nutrients can be a bit trickier. Here's how you do it:

First, figure out your overall daily calorie goal. Let's say, for example, that it's 2,000 calories per day. To figure how many calories each nutrient will provide under the 40/40/20 plan, simply multiply your total calories by the percentage of calories for that nutrient. As follows:

➤ **For protein:** 2,000 x .40 = 800 calories from protein
➤ **For carbs:** 2,000 x .40 = 800 calories from carbs
➤ **For fat:** 2,000 x .20 = 400 calories for fat

To calculate how many grams this represents for each nutrient, you have to divide the calories for each separate nutrient by the number of calories that specific nutrient contains per gram. Protein and carbs both contain 4 calories per gram. And fat contains 9 calories per gram. So you can calculate the grams for each nutrient as follows:

➤ **For protein:** 800 protein calories / 4 calories per protein gram = 200 grams of protein
➤ **For carbs:** 800 carb calories / 4 calories per carb gram = 200 grams of carbs
➤ **For fat:** 400 fat calories / 9 calories per fat gram = 44 grams of fat

That's it: A 2,000-calorie diet with a 40/40/20 profile will consist of 200 grams of protein, 200 grams of carbs and 44 grams of fat.

APPENDIX D

Grocery Staples

Standard stock-up/ingredients for quick meal ideas. As you come up with your own quick meal ideas, you can add to this list.

Pantry	Refrigerator	Freezer
Spaghetti	Low-fat skim milk	Multigrain bread
Rice	Low-fat yogurt	Bagels/English muffins
Jar pasta sauce	Low-fat string cheese	Pita bread
Potatoes	Low-fat cottage cheese	Broccoli or other frozen veggies
Wheat crackers	Grated Parmesan cheese	Frozen spinach, peas
Rye krisp/wasa crackers	Eggs	Frozen pastas (ravioli/tortellini)
Pretzels	Oranges, apples, bananas	Frozen mashed potatoes
Tuna, salmon, clams	Carrots, green peppers	Chicken breasts, or tenders
Canned beans	Tortillas	Ground lean turkey
Fat-free refried beans	100 percent fruit juice	Extra-lean ground beef
All-natural peanut butter	V-8 juice-low sodium	Skillet meals, low-fat
Soups (lentil, bean, tomato)	Low-fat cheese (chunk/shredded)	Frozen meals, low-fat
High-fiber cereal	Tofu-light	Frozen orange juice
Oatmeal		Frozen cut green pepper/onion
Granola bars		Frozen low-fat soups
Raisins/dried fruit		Frozen lean veggie burgers
Canned tomatoes/sauce		

** Then you can reinforce your staples weekly with fresh produce and items like roasted chicken, bagged salads, fresh fruits and the like.

Cookbook List

American Heart Association. *American Heart Association Meals in Minutes: Over 200 All-New Quick and Easy Recipes* (Clarkson Potter, 2002).

American Heart Association. *Quick & Easy Cookbook: More Than 200 Healthful Recipes You Can Make in Minutes* (Clarkson Potter, 2001).

Irwin, Dena. *The Weeknight Survival Cookbook: How to Make Healthy Meals in 10 Minutes* (John Wiley & Sons, 1998).

Phillips, Bill. *Eating for Life: Your Guide to Great Health, Fat Loss and Increased Energy* (High Point Media, 2003).

Ponichtera, Brenda. *Quick & Healthy Recipes and Ideas: For People Who Say They Don't Have Time to Cook Healthy Meals* (Scaledown, 1995).

Tribole, Evelyn. *Eating on the Run* (Second Edition). (Human Kinetics, 2001).

Weight Watchers. *Weight Watchers Make It in Minutes: Easy Recipes in 15, 20, and 30 Minutes* (John Wiley & Sons, 2001).

APPENDIX E

Determination of Healthy Body Weight and Body Composition

There are a number of different techniques utilized to determine healthy body weight and body composition. Body weight and composition can change with growth, development and aging. Monitoring these changes assists health and fitness professionals with their assessment of nutritional status, physical fitness and physical performance. Specifically, measurement of body size allows for tracking the changes in the physical dimensions of the body, while measurement of body composition allows for following changes in its gross chemical composition (i.e., fat and fat-free mass).

Excess body weight, especially in the form of body fat, often reflects high calorie intake with lower energy expenditure, and can contribute to poor physical performance in some individuals. Excess body fat is believed to contribute to disease risk, has been linked positively with a higher risk of developing heart disease, diabetes and other chronic diseases.

Extremely low body weight and low body fat are associated with poor physical performance, under-nutrition, muscle wasting, and eating disorders such as anorexia nervosa. The healthy goal is to have a good balance of healthy body weight in proportion with an individual's body composition to maintain good health, minimize risk factors for chronic disease and enhance physical performance. One of the more simple and convenient methods of determining body composition is measuring your body fat percentage.

Body Fat Percentage

Weight alone is not a clear indicator of good health because it does not distinguish between pounds that come from body fat and those that come from lean body mass or muscle. Carrying too much fat is a condition called obesity, and puts a person at risk for developing many serious medical conditions including heart disease and diabetes. It is now recognized that weight alone is also not a suitable indicator of performance capability. Measuring body fat is important for determining fitness more than the scale alone.

For this method, you will need to have a skilled professional to measure your body fat percentage. There are a few methods to do this.
➤ A generalized and time trusted method is by getting skin fold measurements with the caliper method: Appropriate measurements can be done by "3-site" or "7-site" method. Other measurements for calculating body fat percentage are newer technologies such as Bioimpedence and Infra-red (Futron™) are available, usually at health clubs or medical offices.

Healthy Body Fat Standards:

For Men:
- ➤ Desirable for general health is around 15 percent.
- ➤ 3 percent is considered "essential"—meaning a man cannot reduce body fat below this limit without impairing physiological function and capacity for exercise.

For Women
- ➤ Desirable for general health is around 22 percent
- ➤ The percentage of body fat considered "essential" is 12 percent.

OVERALL:
- ➤ Different sports have published ranges most suitable for good performance
- ➤ An active person involved in fitness, sport or athletics ideal percent body fat is really where he/she performs best and is healthy. Attempting to reach an unrealistic percent body fat can set individuals back as much as attempting to achieve an unrealistic weight.

Adapted from: *Nutrition for Health, Fitness, & Sport. 5th Edition,* by M. Williams (McGraw-Hill 1999), Rosenbloom, K. *Sports Nutrition: A Guide for Professionals Working with Active People Third Edition,* by K. Rosenbloom, American Dietetic Association (Jackson-Pollack 2000)

APPENDIX F

Calculating Your Maintenance Calorie Level and Daily Calorie Goal

	Examples
Average daily caloric intake	➤ 2,400 calories*
Weight lost or gained over the last six months	➤ Gained six pounds = 3,500 extra calories each month ➤ Example: Lost six pounds = 3,500 fewer calories each month ➤ No weight lost or gained: 2,400 average daily caloric intake is your maintenance calorie level
Excess or negative calories consumed over the last six months	➤ Gained six pounds = 3,500 extra calories/30 days = 117 extra calories each day ➤ Lost six pounds = 3,500 fewer calories/30 days = 117 too few calories a day if weight loss is not desired
Maintenance caloric level: Average daily caloric intake minus excess calories or plus negative calories	➤ 2,400 average daily caloric intake – 117 excess calories = 2,283 calories = maintenance calorie level ➤ 2,400 average daily caloric intake + 117 negative calories = 2,517 calories = maintenance calorie level

* You can determine your average daily calorie intake by keeping a detailed food journal for seven days.

Calculate your Daily Calorie Goal as follows:

➤ Let's assume your MCL is 2,200 calories.

➤ Multiply your MCL by 85 percent to get your calorie goal: 2,200 x 0.85 = 1,870.

➤ Your daily calorie goal (DCG) is 1,870 calories.

➤ Summary equation: MCL x 0.85 = DCG.

APPENDIX G

Personalized Fat-Loss Nutrition Plan Calculation Worksheet
(** Sample based on a 2,000-calorie MCL)

Your Maintenance Calorie Level (MCL) =	2,000	
Daily Calorie Goal (DCG) = MCL x .85 =	1,700	
Daily Protein Goal (DPG) = (DCG x .40)/4 =	170	grams
Daily Carb Goal (DCrG) = (DCG x .40)/4 =	170	grams
Daily Fat Goal (DFG) = (DCG x .20)/9 =	38	grams

Meal Goals

Breakfast		
Calories = DCG x .30 =	510	
Protein = DPG x .23 =	39	grams
Carbs = DCrG x .33 =	56	grams
Fat = DFG x .30 =	11	grams

Morning Snack		
Calories = DCG x .13 =	221	
Protein = DPG x .13 =	22	grams
Carbs = DCrG x .13 =	22	grams
Fat = DFG x .09 =	3	grams

Lunch		
Calories = DCG x .27 =	459	
Protein = DPG x .23 =	39	grams
Carbs = DCrG x .28 =	48	grams
Fat = DFG x .30 =	11	grams

Afternoon Snack		
Calories = DCG x .13 =	221	
Protein = DPG x .13 =	22	grams
Carbs = DCrG x .13 =	22	grams
Fat = DFG x .09 =	3	grams

Dinner		
Calories = DCG x .17 =	289	
Protein = DPG x .28 =	48	grams
Carbs = DCrG x .13 =	22	grams
Fat = DFG x .22 =	8	grams

APPENDIX H

Personalized Fat-Loss Nutrition Plan Calculation Worksheet

Your Maintenance Calorie Level (MCL) =		
Daily Calorie Goal (DCG) = MCL x .85 =		
Daily Protein Goal (DPG) = (DCG x .40)/4 =		grams
Daily Carb Goal (DCrG) = (DCG x .40)/4 =		grams
Daily Fat Goal (DFG) = (DCG x .20)/9 =		grams

Meal Goals

Breakfast

Calories = DCG x .30 =		
Protein = DPG x .23 =		grams
Carbs = DCrG x .33 =		grams
Fat = DFG x .30 =		grams

Morning Snack

Calories = DCG x .13 =		
Protein = DPG x .13 =		grams
Carbs = DCrG x .13 =		grams
Fat = DFG x .09 =		grams

Lunch

Calories = DCG x .27 =		
Protein = DPG x .23 =		grams
Carbs = DCrG x .28 =		grams
Fat = DFG x .30 =		grams

Afternoon Snack

Calories = DCG x .13 =		
Protein = DPG x .13 =		grams
Carbs = DCrG x .13 =		grams
Fat = DFG x .09 =		grams

Dinner

Calories = DCG x .17 =		
Protein = DPG x .28 =		grams
Carbs = DCrG x .13 =		grams
Fat = DFG x .22 =		grams

APPENDIX I

Fat-Loss Nutrition Plan					
(*Sample based on a 1,700 daily calorie goal)					
Meal	Time	% Total calories	% Total Protein	% Total Carbs	% Total Fat
Breakfast	7:00 a.m.	30%	23%	33%	30%
Snack	10:00 a.m.	13%	13%	13%	9%
Lunch	1:00 p.m.	27%	23%	28%	30%
Snack	4:00 p.m.	13%	13%	13%	9%
Dinner	7:00 p.m.	17%	28%	13%	22%

(*e.g. 1,700 calorie DCG)					
Meal	Time	Total Calories	Protein Grams	Carb Grams	Fat Grams
Breakfast	7:00 a.m.	510	39	56	11
Snack	10:00 a.m.	221	22	22	3
Lunch	1:00 p.m.	459	39	48	11
Snack	4:00 p.m.	221	22	22	3
Dinner	7:00 p.m.	289	48	22	8
	Totals =	1,700	170	170	36

APPENDIX J

Glycemic Index of Various Common Foods

The Glycemic Index (GI) is defined as the response of blood glucose after ingestion to a 50-gram carbohydrate portion of food expressed as a percentage of the response to the same amount of carbohydrate from a standard or comparison food, usually white bread or glucose—in other words, a food's ability to contribute glucose to the blood stream.

In sports nutrition, generally the GI can be used in two ways:
1. The first is the use of foods with a low GI pre-exercise for those athletes or active people who are sensitive or can experience hypoglycemia during exercise.
2. The second is the use of high-GI foods after exercise to help restore muscle glycogen stores.

It is important to note that the GI is only a "tool" for food selection for athletes and active folks. There are limitations to using this tool and athletes should use the information as a guideline, not as an absolute. There is a large variability for a GI for each group of foods. It will vary due to the form of food, how the food is processed, how the food is cooked, amount of fat added, how the food is chewed, the rate of emptying from the stomach, the fiber content and the response of the individual can all affect the GI of a food. In addition, the intensity of the exercise, and if calorie needs are met all factor into the response. The other limitation researchers discuss is that most of the research on GI has been done in diabetes research and on the response of "single foods" and digestion, whereas most of us eat more than one "single food" for a pre- and post-workout snack or meal, which can alter the GI response. Bottom line, GI can be useful but must be used as a guideline and tested to see how you respond and which food or combination of foods offer the best benefit.

HIGH GLYCEMIC INDEX (>85)	HIGH GLYCEMIC INDEX (60-85)	LOW GLYCEMIC INDEX (<60)
Glucose	Rice cakes	brown rice
Sports drinks	Orange juice with pulp	apple
Potato, baked/boiled	Bagel	white rice
Honey	sucrose (sugar)	fructose
Corn flakes	grape nuts	corn
Jelly beans	cherrios	skim milk, chocolate
Milk	Cream of Wheat	most other dairy
Most breads	Oatmeal	yogurt
Most high-sugar breakfast cereals	Raisins	plums
Corn chips	high-fiber cereals	lentils and lentil soup
graham crackers	Saltines	kidney beans
Sweet Potatoes		chick peas
Soft drinks soda		split peas
banana, over-ripe		lima
vanilla wafers		peaches
ice cream		nuts
watermelon		banana, under-ripe
bran muffin		pear
potato chips		apricots dried
angel food cake		barley
		grapefruit

Note: Nutrition bars vary on GI, depending on type of sweetener used, high- or low-carb type and other ingredients. Check with manufacturer.

Adapted from: Data from food companies, Foster-Powell, K and Brand Miller, J. International Tables of Glycemic Index. *Am J Clin Nutr* 62 (1995): 871S-893S and Rosenbloom, K. *Sports Nutrition: A Guide for Professionals Working with Active People* (Third Edition) (American Dietetic Association, 2000).

APPENDIX K

Winning the Mind Game Goal-Setting Chart

Here's your roadmap for making a fitness commitment and sticking with it once and for all. Just follow the steps, fill in the blanks and get going. Don't forget to make some copies of this sheet first as this one page probably won't carry you through to your ultimate vision.

I. DEVELOP YOUR VISION

The first step to a lifetime of health and fitness is to decide what your long-term goal or vision is. Answer this question: *From a fitness perspective, what do I want to achieve or how do I want to change in the next six months to a year?* And don't forget to include your motivation at the end, following the word "because."

_____

_____

_____

II. DETERMINE YOUR STAGE OF CHANGE

The next step is to figure out how far along you are in the process. In other words, which stage of change are you in now? If you aren't sure and haven't taken the self-evaluation quiz already, turn to **Chapter 12**.

Write your stage here:

_____

_____

_____

III. SET YOUR GOALS
This is your last step before you get started on your journey. Remember, goals must be specific, measurable, have a timeline and be designed to move you on to the next stage. Go back to the section entitled "Match Your Goals to Your Stage of Change" for goal-setting tips if you need them.

Mid-term Goal (halfway to your vision):

_____

_____

_____

Short-term Goals (weekly or bi-weekly):

1) _____

_____

2) _____

_____

3) _____

_____

4) _____

_____

5) _____

_____

6) _____

_____

APPENDIX L

Common Weight-Training Exercise Descriptions and Illustrations

SQUATS

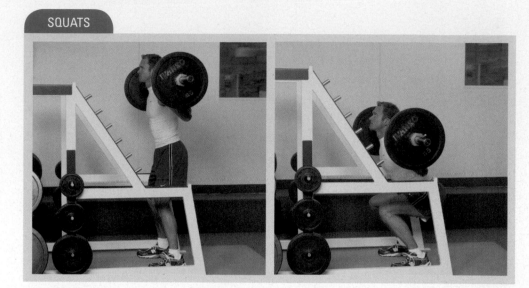

Place your hands evenly on the bar (a close grip with elbows under the bar will allow for a more upright posture), and with your feet squarely under the bar, lift it from the rack by extending your legs. Next, step back just enough to avoid bumping the rack during the exercise, and position feet approximately shoulder-width apart. The weight should remain centered over the back half of the feet, not on the heels or toes. Slowly descend into a near-bottom position, keeping the torso and back erect so the hips remain under the bar at all times. Do not allow the hips to drift backward or the torso to incline forward.

LEG CURLS

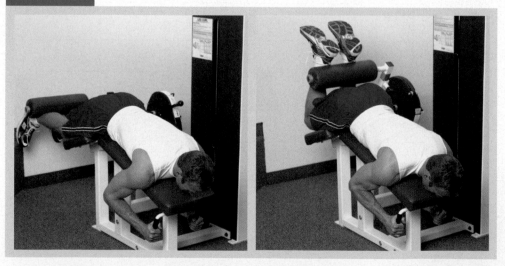

Using a dedicated leg curl machine, simply "curl" the weight by contracting your hamstrings. Pause at the top, and then lower back to the starting position.

SWISS BALL CRUNCHES

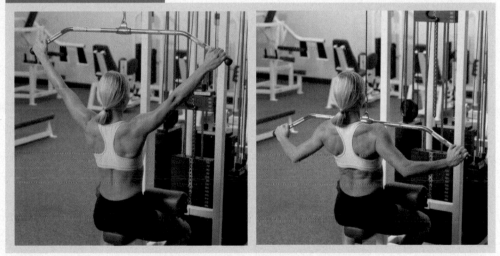

Sit on the ball, and "walk" forward until lying on the ball. Perform crunches in the normal manner, keeping in mind that a greater range of motion is achieved as the back drapes over the ball. The ball's instability and curved surface increase the level of difficulty of the crunch exercise, while simultaneously increasing the comfort of the movement.

LAT PULLDOWNS

Assume a seated position under the bar and pull the bar down to the clavicles (never behind the neck, which lessens the exercise's benefit and increases the possibility of neck injuries). This is done not simply by flexing at the elbows, but also by simultaneously retracting the shoulder blades and arching the back slightly. Think of pushing the chest to the bar rather than pulling the bar to the chest. Do not lean backward during the pull, even slightly. Many lifters unconsciously do this as a matter of habit as fatigue increases.

LOW CABLE ROWS

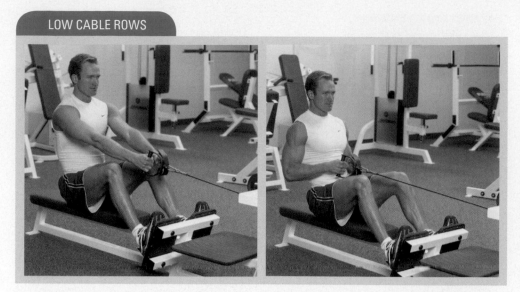

Maintaining normal spinal curvature, pull the handle to the torso at about navel height (not higher). At the finish of the concentric phase, shoulder blades should be retracted. Next, allow the shoulder blades to separate while returning back to the starting position. Keep your torso perpendicular to the floor.

BARBELL CURLS

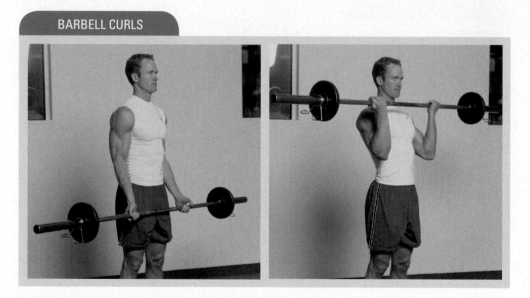

Without moving at the shoulders, and with each elbow locked firmly in place, flex your arms at the elbow, raising the bar in an upward arc until both arms are completely flexed with the bar pressed against the lifter's chest. The bar is then lowered through the same arcing path, and this movement is repeated for the desired number of repetitions.

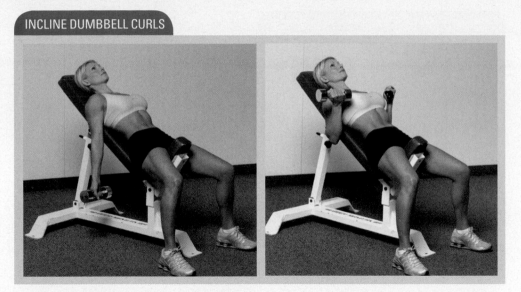

Do not allow the elbows to shift forward during the concentric (lifting) portion of the lift! Allow the arm to completely straighten on the bottom. Squeeze hard at the top.

BENCH PRESSES

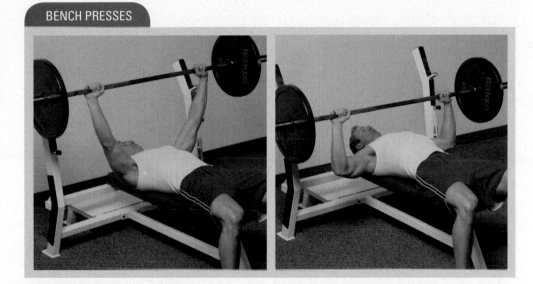

Grasp the bar so both hands are equidistant to the center, and make sure your thumbs are wrapped around the bar, rather than on the same side as your other fingers. At the start, the bar should be directly over your nose. Inhale and un-rack the bar from the supports. As you lower the bar to your chest, keep your elbows directly under the bar, rather than in front of, or ahead of, the bar. At the bottom of the movement, the bar lightly touches your chest at nipple level. Return the bar to the starting position.

LYING DUMBBELL TRICEPS EXTENSIONS

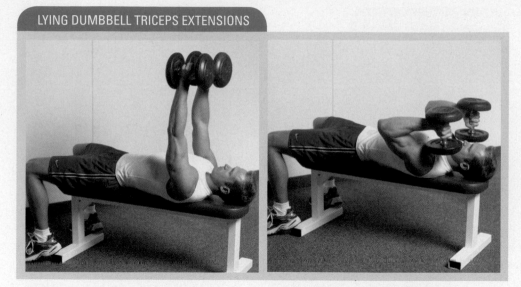

Position yourself face-up on a bench. With a dumbbell in each hand, extend your arms until they are perpendicular to your torso. From this position, relax your triceps to allow your elbows to flex until the dumbbells touch your shoulders. (When using a bar, full flexion is realized when your biceps make contact with your forearms.) Reverse this action to return to the starting position, keeping your elbows stabilized (motionless) throughout the exercise.

TRICEPS PUSHDOWNS

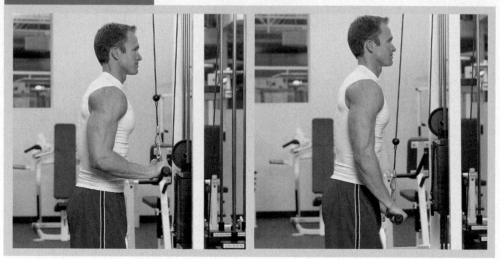

Using either a straight bar or a "triceps rope," grasp the handle and pull yourself into position using your lats to extend your shoulders until your elbows are against your sides. From here, fully flex and extend your elbows while keeping your elbows "pinned" to your sides. Keep the back of the wrists flat.

SEATED DUMBBELL OVERHEAD PRESSES

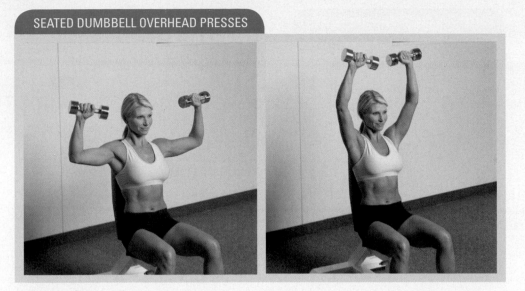

From a seated position with a dumbbell in each hand, simply press the bells directly overhead, and then reverse this motion to return to the starting position.

DUMBBELL LATERAL RAISES

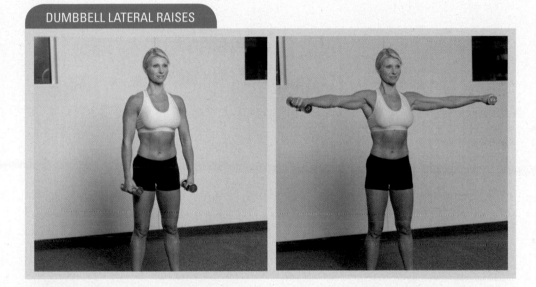

From a standing position with arms at your sides and a dumbbell in each hand, simply raise your arms directly to the sides, keeping your elbows slightly bent. Pause momentarily at the top and then reverse this motion to return to the starting position.

BENT DUMBBELL LATERAL RAISES

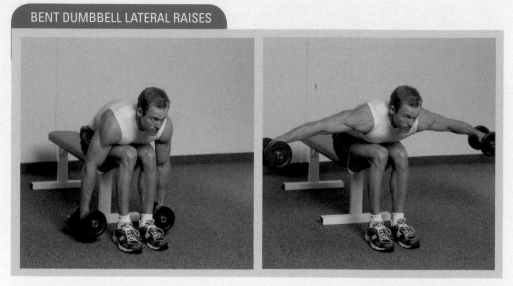

Assume a seated, bent-forward position with arms hanging straight down and with a dumbbell in each hand. Next, simply raise your arms directly to the sides, keeping your elbows slightly bent. Pause momentarily at the top and then reverse this motion to return to the starting position.

LEG EXTENSIONS

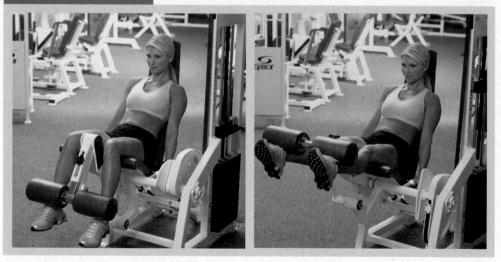

Using a dedicated machine, assume a seated position with your shins under the foot rollers (or pad). From this position, simply lift the weight by extending your knees. Pause momentarily at the top and then reverse this motion to return to the starting position.

APPENDIX M

Performance Nutrition Recipes

1. CHILAQUILLES

Serves 2

1 teaspoon oil
2 each (2 ounces) green onions
1 ounce baked yellow corn tortilla chips, broken
¾ cup egg substitute
¼ teaspoon chili powder
2 slices (2 ounces) non-fat sharp American cheese
2 teaspoons salsa

Combine the egg and chili powder in a small bowl. Sauté the onion with the oil in a medium skillet over medium heat for two minutes. Add the broken up chips and cook another two minutes. Stir in the egg and cheese. Cook, stirring constantly until mixture is scrambled to desired consistency. Serve with a little salsa on top.

Nutritional value per serving:
Calories: 232
Fat: 10 grams
Protein: 20 grams
Carbs: 16 grams

2. MUSCLE TOAST

Serves 3

3 large eggs
2 ½ scoops protein powder
½ cup soy milk
1 teaspoon vanilla
½ teaspoon cinnamon
1 teaspoon vegetable oil
6 slices whole-wheat bread
4 tablespoons maple syrup

Heat a large non-stick skillet or griddle over medium heat. Meanwhile, mix the eggs and protein powder in a medium-size bowl until smooth. Stir in soy milk, vanilla and cinnamon. Lightly coat heated pan with oil. Dip each piece of bread in batter, turning to coat completely and letting the bread soak up a little. Cook on each side until browned. Serve with heated syrup.

Nutritional value per serving:
Calories: 568
Fat: 14 grams
Protein: 57 grams
Carbs: 54 grams

3. POWER PANCAKES
Serves 2

2 large eggs
2 scoops protein powder
¾ cup soy milk
1 cup multi-grain pancake mix

Combine eggs and protein powder in a bowl. Mix until smooth. Stir in the milk and pancake mix. Heat a non-stick pan or griddle over medium heat. Coat with a little oil and spoon onto pan. Cook first side until bubbles appear. Turn over and brown second side. Serve with heated syrup or honey.

Nutritional value per serving:
Calories: 457
Fat: 12 grams
Protein: 36 grams
Carbs: 50 grams

4. SMOKED SALMON AND EGGS ON MUFFINS
Serves 2

½ teaspoon canola oil
¾ cup egg substitute
3 ounces smoked salmon
1 tablespoon onion and chive light cream cheese
1 each (61 grams) English muffin, toasted

Toast muffins and keep warm. Heat oil in a non-stick skillet over medium heat, stir in egg and cream cheese. Cook until almost done, and then stir in salmon. Top each muffin with salmon and egg scramble, serve immediately.

Nutritional value per serving:
Calories: 212
Fat: 7 grams
Protein: 23 grams
Carbs: 14 grams

5. BBQ CHICKEN FAJITAS
Serves 4

¼ cup lemon juice
¼ teaspoon dried oregano
¼ teaspoon ground cumin
¼ teaspoon cayenne
¼ teaspoon garlic powder
¼ teaspoon salt
2 teaspoons olive oil
4 medium, boneless, skinless chicken breasts
1 medium red onion, cut into strips
1 large red or yellow bell pepper, cut into strips
1 medium Anaheim chili, cut into strips
4 medium flour tortillas
1 can (14 ounces) pinto beans, heated
½ cup prepared salsa
¼ cup cilantro (fresh), chopped

Preheat the grill to medium-high heat. Mix the lemon juice, oregano, cumin, cayenne, garlic, salt and oil in a medium-sized bowl. Slice the chicken breasts crossways into thin strips. Add to mixing bowl and toss to coat. Let chicken marinate for 15 minutes. Add onion and peppers to bowl and stir to coat. Place a perforated grill top stir fry pan on grill to preheat. Add the chicken pepper mixture to the pan and cook, stirring often, until vegetables are crisp tender and chicken is cook through. You can also stir fry mixture stove top in a large non-stick skillet over medium-high heat if desired. Transfer to serving dish. Serve with the warm tortillas, cilantro, salsa and beans. Shredded cheddar cheese can be added to increase carbs if desired.

Nutritional value per serving:
Calories: 395
Fat: 4 grams
Protein: 64 grams
Carbs: 22 grams

6. FAST HONEY JERKED SHRIMP
Serves 2

1 teaspoon olive oil
2 tablespoons honey
¼ cup fresh lime juice
2 teaspoons prepared Jamaican jerk seasoning
1 pound large shrimp, peeled, deveined

Mix the oil, honey, juice and seasoning in a medium-sized bowl. Add the shrimp and stir to coat. Marinate the shrimp for 20 minutes while the grill is preheating to medium high. Cook the shrimp for about 3 to 5 minutes each side until firm. Do not overcook. Serve with a portion of steamed brown rice or black beans.

Nutritional value per serving:
Calories: 332
Fat: 6 grams
Protein: 46 grams
Carbs: 22 grams

7. GOURMET MUSHROOM TURKEY BURGERS
Serves 4

¼ cup Worcestershire sauce
¼ cup ketchup
2 tablespoons soy sauce
¼ teaspoon garlic powder
½ cup chopped scallions
¼ cup bread crumbs
1 tablespoon capers
1.5 pounds lean ground turkey
4 slices low-fat cheddar cheese
4 each (2 ounces) onion rolls
1 medium tomato, sliced
4 medium spicy dill pickles
10 sprigs watercress, washed

Preheat grill to medium heat. Combine all ingredients in a large bowl. Form into four to six patties. Season outside with a little salt and pepper. Brush with additional BBQ sauce if desired. Grill for about 6 minutes on each side or until cooked through. Top each burger with cheese at last minute to melt. Build your burger with sliced tomato, pickle slabs and a few sprigs of watercress.

Nutritional value per serving:
Calories: 463
Fat: 8 grams
Protein: 54 grams
Carbs: 41 grams

8. GRILLED ORANGE TERIYAKI PORK TENDERLOIN
Serves 4

1 cup prepared teriyaki glaze
½ cup orange marmalade
1 clove fresh garlic, minced
2 pounds pork tenderloin, trimmed
2 medium tomatoes
6 cups mixed salad greens
½ cup non-fat salad dressing

Mix the teriyaki, marmalade and garlic together in a small bowl. Place the pork in a Ziploc bag or suitable mixing bowl together with the glaze. Let marinate for at least one hour. Preheat grill to medium-high heat. Lightly oil grate and grill, covered, for 15 to 20 minutes turning occasionally and brushing with the glaze. You can check doneness with an instant read thermometer, inserted into the center until temperature reaches 155 degrees F. Let pork rest for 5 minutes before slicing. Serve with mixed greens and tomato salad.

Nutritional value per serving:
Calories: 554
Fat: 13 grams
Protein: 54 grams
Carbs: 53 grams

9. PLANTATION BARBEQUE HALIBUT STEAKS
Serves 2

2 teaspoons olive oil
3 tablespoons brown sugar
3 cloves fresh garlic, minced
2 tablespoons lemon juice
3 teaspoons soy sauce
¼ teaspoon crushed red pepper flakes
14-ounce halibut fillet
4 medium zucchini
1 cup fresh mango chunks

Preheat grill to medium-high heat and wipe the grill with a little oil. Combine the oil, sugar, garlic, lemon juice, soy sauce and pepper in a small saucepan. Cook over medium heat until the sugar dissolves. Slice the zucchini diagonally into ¼-inch thick pieces. Brush the zucchini and the fish with the sauce. Grill the fish for about 5 minutes each side, basting frequently, or until the fish flakes easily with a fork. Put the zucchini on the grill about halfway into cooking the fish and cook until just tender (about 3 minutes per side). Top each piece of halibut with the chopped mango and serve.

Nutritional value per serving:
Calories: 452
Fat: 10 grams
Protein: 46 grams
Carbs: 48 grams

10. FREEDOM BEANS
Serves 4

6 slices turkey bacon; chopped
3 clove garlic; minced
1 medium onion; chopped
8 ounces low-fat ham; chopped
2 cans great northern white beans
1 can black beans; drained
1 large bay leaf
1 teaspoon hot pepper sauce

In a medium-sized soup pot, cook the bacon and garlic together, over medium heat, until the bacon has browned. Add the onion and ham, cook another 5 minutes until onion has softened. Stir in remaining ingredients, cover and reduce heat to low. Simmer for a half hour or so until flavors have blended. Serve with a small portion of low-fat protein.

Nutritional value per serving:
Calories: 176
Fat: 5 grams
Protein: 13.5 grams
Carbs: 27 grams

11. MINUTE MAN STEAKS
Serves 4

24 ounces of eye of round beef steaks; sliced (¼-inch)
½ cup fresh lime juice
2 tablespoons olive oil
4 cloves fresh garlic; chopped
1 tablespoon paprika
½ teaspoon ground cumin
½ teaspoon black pepper
1 teaspoon salt

In a medium-sized mixing bowl, combine all ingredients except the steak. Mix well. Place the steak in a Ziploc bag and add the mixture. Marinate the steak in the mixture for at least one hour. Preheat the grill to medium high heat. Cook the steaks for about one to three minutes per side or to desired doneness. Serve immediately.

Nutritional value per serving:
Calories: 283
Fat: 6 grams
Protein: 41 grams
Carbs: 5 grams

12. OLD GLORY CHICKEN
Serves 4

4 large boneless, skinless chicken breasts
½ cup dry white wine
½ cup fresh lemon juice
3 tablespoon olive oil
½ teaspoon onion powder
½ teaspoon garlic powder
½ teaspoon salt
½ teaspoon black pepper

On a solid work surface or cutting board, pound the chicken breasts with a meat hammer, heavy pot or fry pan until breast is about ¼-inch thick and even (it may help to cover the breast with a piece of plastic wrap before pounding.) Lay them flat on several large plates. Mix remaining ingredients together in a small bowl and pour evenly over each of the breasts. Let rest for about an hour in refrigerator. Preheat grill to medium high heat. Cook chicken about two to three minutes per side, basting with some of the marinade. Do not overcook. Serve with additional fresh lemon wedges and olive oil.

Nutritional value per serving:
Calories: 200
Fat: 8 grams
Protein: 21 grams
Carbs: 3 grams

13. PATRIOT HAM AND TUNA
Serves 4

3 (6-ounce) cans tuna; drained, flaked
3 ounces low-fat ham; diced

¼ medium red onion; minced

1 medium stalk celery; diced

1 teaspoon capers; drained

3 tablespoons fat-free sour cream

1 tablespoon fat-free mayonnaise

3 teaspoons Dijon mustard

½ teaspoon liquid smoke seasoning

¼ cup fresh parsley; chopped

1 tablespoon fresh tarragon; chopped

½ teaspoon salt

½ teaspoon black pepper

1 medium cucumber; sliced thinly

1 medium baguette (about 16 inches long)

In a medium-sized mixing bowl, combine all ingredients except the cucumber and bread (this can be done a day ahead of time). To make the open-faced sandwiches, split the baguette in half lengthwise (you can substitute with another bread, like, hoagie rolls if desired). Remove about half of the soft bread inside hollow it out and make a channel. Layer the sliced cucumber in the channels of each half. Top with the tuna mixture, pressing it into the channel slightly. Cut each bread half into two pieces to serve.

Try adding hot peppers, chopped tomato or dill pickle to this sandwich.

Nutritional value per serving:
Calories: 156
Fat: 6 grams
Protein: 20 grams
Carbs: 12 grams

14. STAR-SPANGLED GRILLED PIZZA
Serves 4

2 pizza crusts, Boboli, personal size, about 8 to 10 inches

12 ounces (2 cups) grilled chicken breast; diced

6 ounces non-fat shredded mozzarella cheese

½ cup marinated artichoke hearts; drained, chopped

½ cup prepared marinara or pizza sauce

½ teaspoon dried oregano

1 pinch salt

1 pinch black pepper

Preheat grill to medium heat. Top each shell with ¼ cup sauce. Divide the remaining ingredients equally between the two pizzas, finishing with the cheese. Place the pizzas on the upper rack, or away from direct flame on a double piece of greased aluminum foil. Cover grill and cook for about eight to 10 minutes until cheese is melted and hot. Check the bottom of crust half way through cooking to be sure it is not overcooking. (Aluminum foil under the pizza will help slow the crust browning if needed.)

Nutritional value per serving:
Calories: 178
Fat: 6 grams
Protein: 36 grams
Carbs: 17 grams

15. BAJA FISH TACOS
Serves 4

1 pound orange roughy
1 ounce lime juice (fresh), 1 lime
1 teaspoon blackened fish seasoning blend
1 tablespoon olive oil
1 medium Anaheim chili, seeded, cut into thin strips
½ medium red onion, cut into thin strips
½ medium tomato, chopped
3 cups cabbage, shredded
1 cup non-fat Monterey Jack or cheddar cheese, shredded
¼ cup pickled banana peppers
8 medium (6-inch) soft corn or flour tortillas
3 limes, cut into wedges

Place the fish on a plate and season with the lime juice, then the spice blend. Set aside while preparing vegetables. Wrap tortillas in foil and place in 300 degrees F oven to warm. Heat a large non-stick skillet over medium-high heat. Add the oil, chili strips and onion. Sauté for about 5 minutes until vegetables are crisp and tender. Stir in tomato at the very end just to warm. Remove to a serving bowl and cover to keep warm. In the same skillet (don't bother to clean it) cook the fish over medium-high heat until the fish flakes easily (about 6 to 8 minutes). Remove to another serving bowl, flake fish apart into bite-sized chunks. Cover to keep warm. Assemble your tacos by placing a portion of fish on the center of the tortilla first, followed with portions of chili/onion mixture, cheese, cabbage and banana peppers (optional). Have some hot sauce, salsa and fresh lime wedges on hand to season tacos as desired. Wrap up and eat immediately.

Nutritional value per serving:
Calories: 382
Fat: 7 grams
Protein: 45 grams
Carbs: 39 grams

16. CHICKEN QUESADILLAS
Serves 4

1 pound boneless, skinless chicken breast, sliced crossways into thin strips
1 large bell pepper (red, green, yellow), chopped
½ medium red onion, chopped
1 jalapeno pepper, minced
1 ounce fresh lime juice
2 teaspoons chili powder
1 teaspoon garlic powder
1 teaspoon dried oregano
1 tablespoon olive oil
½ cup fresh cilantro, chopped
2 cups non fat jack cheese, shredded
4 large (10-inch) flour tortillas

Combine the chicken, peppers, onion, lime juice, chili powder, garlic and oregano in a medium sized mixing bowl. In a large non-stick skillet, over medium-high heat, cook the mixture in the oil for about 6 minutes, stirring often, until chicken is cooked and vegetables are crisp and tender. Remove from heat and cover to keep warm. Meanwhile, preheat oven to 400 degrees F. Line a large baking sheet with foil and spray with a little vegetable release (like Pam). Place tortillas on the baking sheet. Using a slotted spoon, portion the chicken mixture on the tortillas keeping mixture off to one side so you can fold. Top mixture with cheese and cilantro and fold. Press down so top stays put. Bake for about 15 minutes, turning over with spatula half way through cooking. Tortilla should be crisp and beginning to brown. Cut into four pieces and serve.

Nutritional value per serving:
Calories: 146
Fat: 3 grams
Protein: 17 grams
Carbs: 14 grams

17. GROUND TURKEY TOSTADAS
Serves 4

1 tablespoon vegetable oil
½ medium red onion, diced
1 medium poblano chili, seeded, chopped
¼ cup sun-dried tomatoes, chopped
1 pound lean ground turkey
1¼ ounces (1 package) prepared taco seasoning mix
¾ cup water
¼ cup fresh cilantro, chopped

½ cup non-fat jack cheese, shredded

2 cups lettuce, shredded

1 medium tomato, diced

4 large tostada shells

In a large non-stick skillet, over medium heat, cook the onion, chilis and sun-dried tomatoes in the oil for 5 minutes. Add turkey and continue cooking, breaking up ground turkey with a spatula, until turkey is no longer pink. Add seasoning packet and water. Continue to cook another 5 to 7 minutes, stirring occasionally. Remove from heat. Place tostada shells on plates. Top each with a portion of the turkey mixture (about 1 cup), followed by the cheese, cilantro, lettuce and tomato. Serve with salsa on the side if desired.

Nutritional value per serving:

Calories: 236

Fat: 6 grams

Protein: 37 grams

Carbs: 10 grams

18. OLD MEXICO PORK GREEN CHILI STEW

Serves 8

1 teaspoon canola oil

1 medium onion, chopped

2 small ($^1/_8$ cup) jalapeno peppers, seeded, minced

4 medium carrots, peeled, chopped

2 pounds lean pork, cut into ½-inch pieces

3 tablespoons red chili powder

1 teaspoon garlic powder

½ teaspoon dried oregano

1 cup water

1 can (15 ounces) southwestern style tomatoes

1 can (15 ounces) golden hominy, drained

1 can (15 ounces) chili beans

2 cans (14 ounces) diced green chilis

In a large heavy-bottomed stew pot, heat the oil over medium heat. Add the onion, peppers and carrots. Sauté for 5 minutes. Stir in the pork and cook another 5 minutes to brown the meat. Add remaining ingredients. Cover, reduce heat to low, and simmer 1 ½ hours or until flavors have blended and pork is tender, stirring occasionally. Serve in bowls with heated tortillas for dipping.

Nutritional value per serving:
Calories: 308
Fat: 7 grams
Protein: 30 grams
Carbs: 30 grams

19. POWER BERRY MARGARITA
Serves 4

8 ounces margarita mix
2 cups frozen mixed berries
1 cup orange juice
1 ounce fresh lime juice
3 scoops protein powder
6 ice cubes
4 ounces tequila (optional!)

Put all ingredients into the blender. Process until smooth. Serve with a fresh lime wedge. (Tequila is optional, but included in the nutritional information.)

Nutritional value per serving:
Calories: 257
Fat: less than 1 gram
Protein: 20 grams
Carbs: 27 grams

20. ASIAN CHICKEN AND NOODLES
Serves 4

1 teaspoon olive oil
1 clove garlic, minced
3 each (1 cup) scallions, chopped
2 cups broccoli floret, cut into 1-inch pieces
1 cup (4 ounces) mushrooms, sliced
1½ pounds chicken breast (boneless), sliced crossways into thin slices
1 package (3 ounces) top ramen noodles, chicken flavored
2 cups chicken broth

In a large non-stick skillet, over medium-high heat, cook the garlic in oil 2 minutes to release flavors. Add the onion, broccoli and mushrooms. Continue to stir fry for 2 minutes until mushrooms begin to soften. Stir in sliced chicken. Cook another 3 minutes, stirring constantly. Add the chicken broth. Break the noodles up into 4 pieces, add to pan and push them down into the liquid. Sprinkle on contents of the seasoning packet. Cover, bring to a simmer and cook about 5 minutes until noodles are tender, stirring once to push noodles into the broth. Top with some fresh chopped scallions and toasted sesame seeds if desired.

Nutritional value per serving:
Calories: 315
Fat: 9 grams
Protein: 27 grams
Carbs: 15 grams

21. ESCAROLE AND SAUSAGE SKILLET

Serves 4

1 pound low-fat turkey Italian sausage, hot
3 cloves garlic, minced
2 tablespoons shallots, minced
2 medium red bell peppers, chopped
1 teaspoon olive oil
10 cups escarole, washed, chopped into 1-inch pieces
1 pinch salt
1 pinch black pepper
3 cups navy beans, cooked

Cut sausages crossways into 1-inch pieces. Set aside. In a large, deep skillet, cook the garlic in the oil over medium-high heat for 2 minutes until just barely golden brown. Add peppers, shallot and sausage. Cover and cook about 10 minutes, stirring often, until sausage is cooked thoroughly.
Stir in the escarole and cook another 5 to 7 minutes, turning the mixture over often, until the escarole is wilted and hot. Add the salt and pepper.
Serve immediately with the heated navy beans along side.

Nutritional value per serving:
Calories: 208
Fat: 6 grams
Protein: 16 grams
Carbs: 24 grams

22. RANCHERO EGGS
Serves 4

2 cups egg substitute, liquid, southwestern style or plain
½ medium yellow onion, chopped
½ medium red bell pepper, seeded, chopped
1 teaspoon olive oil
1 package taco seasoning mix
¼ cup water
¾ pound extra lean ground turkey

In a large non-stick skillet, over medium-high heat, cook the onions and peppers in the oil for 2 minutes until the onion begins to brown. Add the ground turkey and brown thoroughly, breaking up meat into smaller chunks with a flat spatula. Add seasoning packet and water. Simmer 2 to 3 minutes until mixture thickens. Stir in southwestern liquid egg substitute (like Egg Beaters) and scramble until eggs is firm. Serve with warm tortillas and salsa.

Nutritional value per serving:
Calories: 203
Fat: 6 grams
Protein: 32 grams
Carbs: 4 grams

23. SEAFOOD PAELLA
Serves 4

2 teaspoons olive oil
½ medium yellow onion, chopped
1 medium tomato, chopped
12 ounces shrimp (raw, medium-size), peeled, deveined
8 ounces scallops
1 cup hot water
1 box (6.8 ounces) Spanish rice mix
4 ounces imitation crab meat, cut into 1-inch pieces

In a large non-stick skillet, over medium-high heat, cook the onion in the oil for 2 to 3 minutes until softened. Stir in the tomato, shrimp and scallops. Cook another 5 minutes until the shrimp begin to turn pink. Stir in rice mix, seasoning packet and water. Cover, reduce heat to medium low, and simmer 20 minutes until the rice is tender. Add the imitation crab meat to heat during the last 5 minutes of cooking time. Garnish with fresh chopped parsley and chopped black or green olives.

Nutritional value per serving:
Calories: 350
Fat: 5 grams
Protein: 37 grams
Carbs: 38 grams

24. SKILLET PORK WITH APPLES AND BEANS
Serves 4

1 teaspoon canola oil
1½ pounds boneless pork loin chops, ¾-inch, trimmed of all fat
1 large onion, chopped
2 large red apples, cored, cut into ½-inch pieces
1 can (20 ounces) fat-free baked beans
1 tablespoon BBQ sauce

In a large non-stick skillet over medium-high heat, cook the pork in a little oil about 4 minutes per side until lightly browned. Remove to a plate and set aside. Without cleaning the pan, add the onion and sauté about 2 minutes until softened and beginning to brown. Stir in the apples, beans and BBQ sauce. Lay the pork over the beans and press into the mixture. Reduce heat to low, partially cover and simmer for about 30 minutes, or until the pork is no longer pink inside, turning chops over once during cooking time. Place each serving of pork on a deep plate and top with the bean/apple mixture. Serve with a tossed salad or other greens on a separate salad plate.

Nutritional value per serving:
Calories: 230
Fat: 11 grams
Protein: 23 grams
Carbs: 25 grams

25. CHILLED WRAPPED ASPARAGUS
Serves 4

1 pound fresh asparagus (about 16 stalks), stems trimmed
1 pound sliced low-fat ham (about 8 slices)
1 pound low-fat turkey (about 8 slices)
6 ounces light cream cheese with garden vegetables
½ cup roasted red peppers, drained, minced
1 teaspoon fresh chopped parsley
¼ teaspoon crushed red pepper flakes

Bring salted water to a boil in a medium-sized stock pot big enough for the asparagus. Cook the asparagus in the water for about 2 minutes until it is crisp tender. Drain and immediately plunge asparagus into ice water to stop the cooking process. Drain well. Lay the slices of meat out on a cutting board and spread each with a teaspoon or so of the flavored cream cheese. Sprinkle with about ½ teaspoon of the minced red pepper. Lay a stalk of asparagus on one edge of the sliced meat and roll up. Put on a serving plate and sprinkle with the parsley and crushed red pepper. These may be prepared well in advance.

Nutritional value per serving:
Calories: 161
Fat: 3 grams
Protein: 25 grams
Carbs: 12 grams

26. COOL TROPICAL FRUIT AND TURKEY SALAD
Serves 6

1½ pound cooked white meat turkey, cut into ¼-inch pieces
2 small stalks celery, diced
1 fresh mango, skin removed, diced
1 small fresh papaya, peeled, seeded, diced
1½ cups fresh pineapple, peeled, diced
2 small green onions, minced
¾ cup non-fat plain yogurt
2 tablespoons honey
2 tablespoons fat-free sour cream
2 tablespoons fresh mint, chopped
½ teaspoon salt
½ cup almonds or peanuts, toasted, chopped

Combine the turkey, celery, mango, papaya, pineapple and onion in a large mixing bowl. Stir together remaining ingredients (except nuts) in a small mixing bowl to combine. Pour dressing over turkey/fruit mixture and stir gently to combine. Cover and chill for 15 minutes. Serve on lettuce leaves topped with the toasted chopped nuts.

Nutritional value per serving:
Calories: 271
Fat: 6 grams
Protein: 24 grams
Carbs: 33 grams

27. SLICED CHICKEN WITH GAZPACHO SAUCE
Serves 4

4 large boneless, skinless chicken breasts
2 large tomatoes, seeded, cut into ½-inch chunks
½ large cucumber; seeded, chopped into ½-inch chunks
1 tablespoon jalapeno peppers, minced
1 cup V-8 vegetable juice
1 clove garlic, chopped
½ medium red bell pepper, seeded, chopped into ½-inch chunks
1 tablespoon fresh lemon juice
1 medium green onion, minced
¼ cup fresh cilantro, chopped

In a blender, place the tomato, cucumber, jalapeno, V-8 juice, garlic and bell pepper. Pulse-chop mixture until pieces are about $\frac{1}{8}$-inch in size. Transfer to a mixing bowl and stir in remaining ingredients and chill for at least one hour, covered. Meanwhile, cook chicken as desired, on the grill or in a pan. Cover and set aside to cool. To serve, slice each breast crossways into thin slices. Place on smaller serving plates. Use plates that will hold some liquid without spilling over the sides. Top each breast with a cup of the gazpacho, and serve with fresh cracked pepper. Crusty bread is good to serve with this dish for dipping.

Nutritional value per serving:
Calories: 243
Fat: 2 grams
Protein: 24 grams
Carbs: 10 grams

28. SUMMER CEVICHE
Serves 4

8 ounces medium-sized shrimp, peeled, de veined
8 ounces sea scallops, cut into ¼-inch pieces
8 ounces sea bass, cut into ¼-inch pieces
½ cup fresh lime juice
¼ cup fresh orange juice
¼ cup fresh lemon juice
1 tablespoon fresh garlic, minced
1 cup cherry tomatoes, quartered
¼ cup red onion, diced
1 medium jalapeno peppers, minced
1 tablespoon extra virgin olive oil
1 medium avocado, sliced
¼ cup fresh cilantro, chopped
3 cups Bibb lettuce leaves

Bring a medium-sized stock pot of salted water to a boil. Add the shrimp and scallops and cook for 1 minute until the shrimp turn pink. Immediately plunge the shrimp and scallops in a bowl of very cold water to stop the cooking process. Drain well. Cut the shrimp lengthwise into halves. Combine the scallops, shrimp and sea bass (or, another meaty mild white fish) in a large shallow bowl. Sprinkle with a little salt and pepper. Combine the juices and garlic in a bowl, pour over the seafood mixture. Toss to coat. Marinate, cover and refrigerate, for 2 hours, stirring occasionally. Add the tomato, onion, jalapeno and olive oil; mix gently. Marinate for at least another hour until the fishes are opaque. Stir in the cilantro.

Prepare serving dishes with Bibb lettuce leaves. Using a slotted spoon, place a portion of the Ceviche on each along with avocado slices. Spoon a little of the marinade over each.

Nutritional value per serving:
Calories: 234
Fat: 6 grams
Protein: 33 grams
Carbs: 12 grams